Fuel Cells, Solar Panels and Storage Devices

Scrivener Publishing
100 Cummings Center, Suite 541J
Beverly, MA 01915-6106

Publishers at Scrivener
Martin Scrivener (martin@scrivenerpublishing.com)
Phillip Carmical (pcarmical@scrivenerpublishing.com)

Fuel Cells, Solar Panels and Storage Devices

Materials and Methods

Johannes Karl Fink

Scrivener Publishing

WILEY

This edition first published 2018 by John Wiley & Sons, Inc., 111 River Street, Hoboken, NJ 07030, USA and Scrivener Publishing LLC, 100 Cummings Center, Suite 541J, Beverly, MA 01915, USA

For more information about Scrivener publications please visit www.scrivenerpublishing.com.

Wiley Global Headquarters
111 River Street, Hoboken, NJ 07030, USA

For details of our global editorial offices, customer services, and more information about Wiley products visit us at www.wiley.com.

Library of Congress Cataloging-in-Publication Data
ISBN 978-1-119-48010-5

Cover images: Pixabay.Com
Cover design by: Russell Richardson

Set in size of 11pt and Minion Pro by Exeter Premedia Services Private Ltd., Chennai, India

10 9 8 7 6 5 4 3 2 1

Contents

Preface

This book focuses on the materials used for fuel cells, solar panels, and storage devices such as rechargeable batteries.

Fuel cell devices, such as direct methanol fuel cells, direct ethanol fuel cells, direct urea fuel cells, as well as biological fuel cells and the electrolytes, membranes, and catalysts used therein are detailed. Separate chapters are devoted to polymer electrode materials and membranes.

With regard to solar cells, the types of solar cells are detailed, such as, inorganic-organic hybrid solar cells, solar powered biological fuel cells, heterojunction cells, multijunction cells, and others. Also, the fabrication methods are described. In addition, the electrolytes, membranes, and catalysts used therein are detailed.

The chapter dealing with rechargeable batteries explains the types of rechargeable devices, such as aluminium-based batteries, zinc batteries, magnesium batteries, and most importantly lithium batteries. Materials that are used for cathodes, anodes and electrolytes are detailed.

The text focuses on the basic issues and also the literature of the past decade. Beyond education, this book may serve the needs of polymer specialists as well as other specialists, e.g., materials scientists, electrochemical engineers, etc., who have only a passing knowledge of these issues, but need to know more.

How to Use This Book

Utmost care has been taken to present reliable data. Because of the vast variety of material presented here, however, the text cannot be complete in all aspects, and it is recommended that the reader study the original literature for more complete information.

Index

There are three indices: an index of acronyms, an index of chemicals, and a general index. In the index of chemicals, compounds that occur extensively are not included at every occurrence, but rather when they appear in an important context. When a compound is found in a figure, the entry is marked in boldface letters in the chemical index.

Acknowledgements

I am indebted to our university librarians, Dr. Christian Hasen-hüttl, Dr. Johann Delanoy, Franz Jurek, Margit Keshmiri, Dolores Knabl Steinhäufl, Friedrich Scheer, Christian Slamenik, Renate Tschabuschnig, and Elisabeth Groß for their support in literature acquisition. In addition, many thanks to the head of my department, ProfessorWolfgang Kern, for his interest and permission to prepare this text.

I also want to express my gratitude to all the scientists who have carefully published their results concerning the topics dealt with herein. This book could not have been otherwise compiled.

Last, but not least, I want to thank the publisher, Martin Scrivener, for his abiding interest and help in the preparation of the text. In addition, my thanks go to Jean Markovic, who made the final copyedit with utmost care.

Johannes Fink
Leoben, 9th October 2017

1

Fuel Cells

Fuel cells produce more electricity than batteries or combustion engines, with far fewer emissions. An introduction to the principles and practicalities behind fuel cell technology has been presented (1). Beginning with the underlying concepts, the discussion explores the thermodynamics of fuel cells, kinetics, transport, and modeling before moving onto the application side with guidance on system types and design, performance, costs, and environmental impact.

The latest technological advances and relevant calculations have been presented, along with enhanced chapters on advanced fuel cell design and electrochemical and hydrogen energy systems (1).

Fuel cells are commonly classified on the basis of their electrolyte according to which they can be divided into five main groups (2,3):

1. Alkaline fuel cells (AFC),
2. Phosphoric acid fuel cells (PAFC),
3. Polymer electrolyte fuel cells (PEFC),
4. Molten carbonate fuel cell (MAFC), and
5. Solid oxide fuel cells (SOFC).

Polymer electrolyte fuel cells can be further subdivided into three general groups: The polymer electrolyte fuel cells feed on hydrogen, direct methanol fuel cells and direct ethanol fuel cells.

The basic issues of fuel cells have been collected in a way also suitable for beginners (2,4).

Also, the issues of direct liquid fuel cells have been reviewed (5). Direct liquid fuel cells are one of the most promising types of fuel cells due to their high energy density, simple structure, small fuel cartridge, instant recharging, and ease of storage and transport. Alcohols such as methanol and ethanol are the most common types of fuel.

1.1 Conventional Fuel Cells

A schematic view of a polymer electrolyte membrane fuel cell is shown in Figure 1.1.

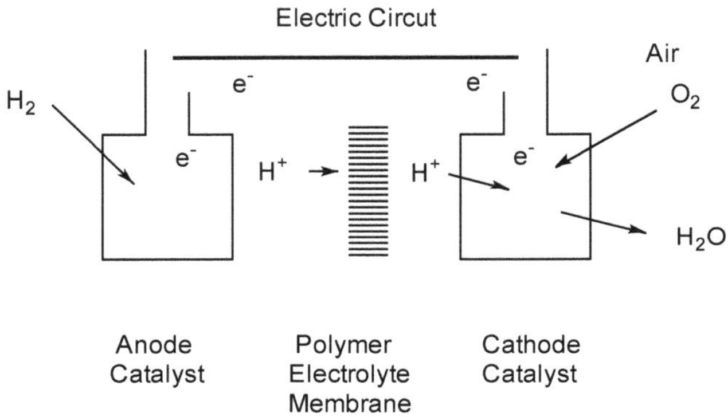

Figure 1.1 Polymer Electrolyte Membrane Fuel Cell (6).

1.1.1 *Sealing Material for Solid Polymer Fuel Cell Separator*

A sealing material for solid polymer fuel cells includes a silicone rubber composition and, compounded therewith, a layered double hydroxide has an excellent resistance to hydrofluoric acid (7).

The molecular structure of the organohydrogen poly(siloxane) may be a linear, cyclic, branched or three-dimensional network structure. Illustrative examples of the organohydrogen poly(siloxane) component are summarized in Table 1.1. Some of the components are shown in Figure 1.2.

1.1.2 *Water Management in a Polymer Electrolyte Fuel Cell*

Water management of polymer electrolyte fuel cell has been extensively studied because of its effect on the performance of a polymer

Table 1.1 Organohydrogen poly(siloxane) (7).

Compound
1,1,3,3-Tetramethyldisiloxane
1,3,5,7-Tetramethylcyclotetrasiloxane
Tris(hydrogendimethylsiloxy)methylsilane
Tris(hydrogendimethylsiloxy)phenylsilane
Methylhydrogencyclo poly(siloxane)
Methylhydrogensiloxane-dimethylsiloxane cyclic copolymers
Methylhydrogen poly(siloxane) capped at both ends with trimethylsiloxy groups
Dimethylsiloxane-methylhydrogensiloxane copolymers capped at both ends with trimethylsiloxy groups
Dimethyl poly(siloxane) capped at both ends with dimethylhydrogensiloxy groups
Dimethylsiloxane-methylhydrogensiloxane copolymers capped at both ends with dimethylhydrogensiloxy groups
Methylhydrogensiloxane-diphenylsiloxane copolymers capped at both ends with trimethylsiloxy groups
Methylhydrogensiloxane-diphenylsiloxane-dimethylsiloxane copolymers capped at both ends with trimethylsiloxy groups
Methylhydrogensiloxane-methylphenylsiloxane-dimethylsiloxane copolymers capped at both ends with trimethylsiloxy groups
Methylhydrogensiloxane-dimethylsiloxane-diphenylsiloxane copolymers capped at both ends with dimethylhydrogensiloxy groups
Methylhydrogensiloxane-dimethylsiloxane-methylphenylsiloxane copolymers capped at both ends with dimethylhydrogensiloxy groups
Copolymers consisting of $(CH_3)_2HSiO_{\frac{1}{2}}$ units and $SiO_{\frac{4}{2}}$ units

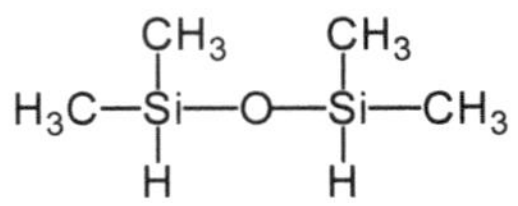

1,1,3,3-Tetramethyldisiloxane

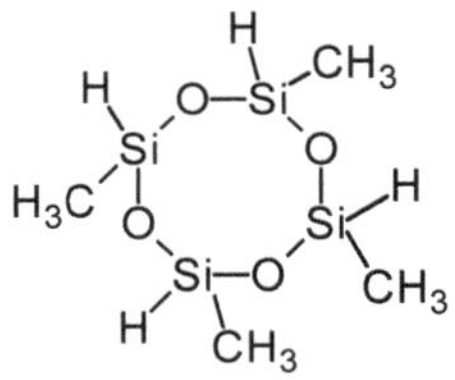

1,3,5,7-Tetramethylcyclotetrasiloxane

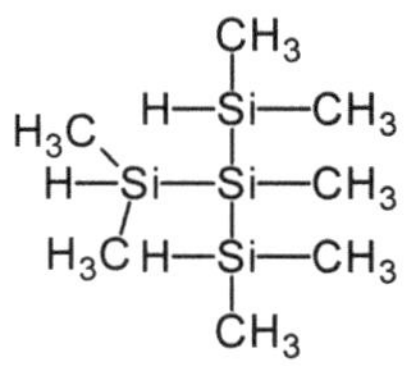

Tris(hydrogendimethylsiloxy)methylsilane

Figure 1.2 Siloxanes (7).

electrolyte fuel cell system (8). The transport and congelation of water significantly affect the efficiency and durability of a polymer electrolyte fuel cell.

The electrochemical reaction in a polymer electrolyte fuel cell produces water, thereby dampening the electrolyte membrane. The electrochemical reaction at the anode is

$$H_2 \rightarrow 2H^+ 2e^- \tag{1.1}$$

and the reaction at the cathode is

$$\frac{1}{2}O_2 + 2H^+ + 2e^- \rightarrow H_2O \quad . \tag{1.2}$$

Nafion®, c.f. Figure 1.3, is typically used as the electrolyte membrane. However, Nafion exhibits a proton conductivity only in the presence of water.

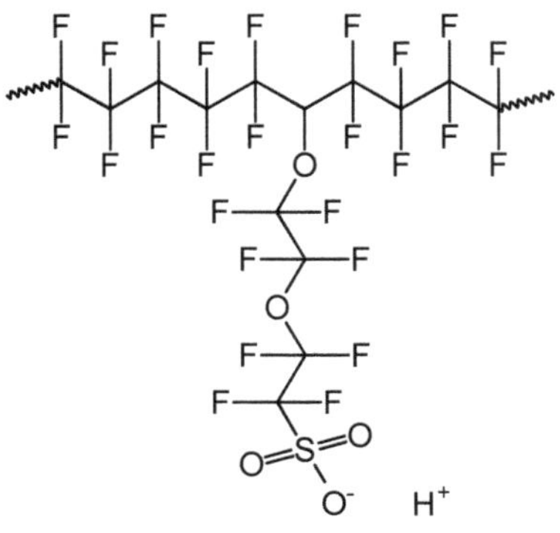

Figure 1.3 Nafion®.

Therefore, the reactive gases supplied to the fuel cell should be humidified in order to ensure an efficient transport of protons. Unfortunately, an excessive amount of accumulated water in the gas diffusion layer reduces the performance and the durability of a cell (9).

In contrast, operating with a high current density and back diffusion dehydrates the gas diffusion layer of the anode and the membrane (10).

An efficient water management is essential to maintain the performance of a polymer electrolyte fuel cell. Therefore, water in a polymer electrolyte fuel cell system should be accurately analyzed for understanding the water balance. Therefore, the water balance and the removal of water from a polymer electrolyte fuel cell system are the key parameters that govern its efficiency and durability (8).

Several empirical methods have been used to visualize the distribution of water in a polymer electrolyte fuel cell. These methods include (8):

1. Optical imaging (11–13),
2. Magnetic resonance imaging (MRI) (14),
3. Neutron radiography (15–18), and
4. X-ray imaging techniques.

Experimental studies using high-resolution imaging techniques have been conducted to reveal the unknown morphological aspects that reduce the performance of a polymer electrolyte fuel cell system.

The X-ray imaging technique is the preferred method over other imaging techniques because of its high spatial and temporal resolution. Recently, X-ray micro computed tomography has been introduced to better characterize the anisotropic structure of a gas diffusion layer by reconstructing its three-dimensional structure. Due to the development of advanced software and hardware, the X-ray imaging technique has become essential in the visualization of the water management in polymer electrolyte fuel cells (8).

In particular, X-ray imaging experiments have been detailed in order to visualize the water contents and water management in a polymer electrolyte fuel cell system (8).

A highly focused X-ray beam, a high-density scintillator, highly magnified optics, and a digital detector with small pixel size are used here.

The light intensity of the X-ray beam that passes through a test sample can be described by the Beer-Lambert law.

The complementarity properties of the neutron imaging method and synchrotron X-ray radiography have been shown (19). The synchrotron X-ray they employed had a spatial resolution of 3 μm and a temporal resolution of 5 s, whereas those of the neutron imaging system were 150 μm and 10 s, respectively. The field of view for the synchrotron X-ray radiography was only 7×7 mm^2, whereas that of the neutron imaging was more than 100 mm^2, which is sufficiently large to cover the entire active area of the cells.

The formation of liquid water was investigated as a function of the current density in the in-plane direction of polymer electrolyte fuel cells (20). The synchrotron X-ray imaging setup used in the study is similar to that in the study described in reference (19), with a spatial resolution of 3 μm and a temporal resolution of 5 s. The amount of water in the gas channels exhibited a cyclic eruption of water. The liquid water formation was mostly located beneath the rib, caused by the reduced porosity as a result of compression and the increase of electrical conductivity (8).

Also, the results of several other techniques have been detailed (8). In summary, X-ray radiography is a suitable method for studying the water management in a polymer electrolyte fuel cell, because it has a higher spatial and temporal resolution compared to other imaging techniques. X-ray μCT provides details of the water transport in a gas diffusion layer by adopting a tomograph.

1.1.3 Alkaline Fuel Cells

An alkaline fuel cell is also known as a Bacon fuel cell, named after its inventor, Francis Thomas Bacon (21,22).

Alkaline fuel cells are among the most efficient fuel cells, with the potential to reach 70% (23).

This type of fuel cell produces electrical power by the following reactions. At the anode hydrogen is oxidized in the presence of alkali according to the following reaction:

$$2H_2 + 4OH^- \rightarrow 4H_2O + 4e^- \tag{1.3}$$

Here water is produced and electrons are released. On the cathode, oxygen is reduced according to the following reaction:

$$O_2 + 2H_2O + 4e^- \rightarrow 4OH^-. \tag{1.4}$$

Here, the hydroxide ions are given back and the electrons are consumed (23).

The anode and cathode are separated by a porous matrix saturated with an aqueous alkaline electrolyte solution. The hydroxyl ions flow from the cathode back to the anode through the electrolyte.

1.1.4 Alkaline Direct Alcohol Fuel Cells

The faster kinetics of the alcohol oxidation and oxygen reduction reactions in alkaline direct alcohol fuel cells opens the possibility of using less expensive metal catalysts, such as silver, nickel and palladium (24). This makes the alkaline direct alcohol fuel cell to a potentially low-cost technology in comparison to the acid direct alcohol fuel cell technology, which employs platinum catalysts.

A boost in the research regarding alkaline fuel cells, fueled with hydrogen or alcohols, has resulted in the development of alkaline anion exchange membranes, which allows the problem of the progressive carbonation of the alkaline electrolyte to be overcome.

An overview of catalysts and membranes for alkaline direct alcohol fuel cells has been presented.

Also, methods of testing of alkaline direct alcohol fuel cells, fueled with methanol, ethanol and ethylene glycol, formed by these materials have been described (24).

1.1.5 Vanadium Redox Flow Battery

The concept of the vanadium redox flow battery has received wide attention due to its attractive features for large-scale energy storage (25). The key material of a vanadium redox flow battery is an ion exchange membrane that prevents cross mixing of the positive and negative electrolyte components, while still allowing the transport of ions to complete the circuit during the passage of current.

The aspects related to ion exchange membranes have been detailed that are relevant to an understanding of ion exchange membranes. An overview of the general issues of vanadium redox flow batteries has been given.

The role of an ion exchange membrane has been outlined together with the material requirements for advanced alternative ion exchange membranes. Also, the recent progress of ion exchange membranes in vanadium redox flow batteries has been reviewed (25).

1.1.6 *Miniaturization of a Polymer-Type Fuel Cell*

A solid polymer-type fuel cell may be miniaturized to reduce its weight because of generation of high power density and low-temperature operability. Such a device is expected to be put to practical use as a power source for automobiles, a power source for stationary electric power generation, or power generation equipment for mobile devices (26).

A solid polymer-type fuel cell has been provided with a pair of electrodes disposed on both sides of a proton conductive solid polymer electrolyte membrane, and generates electric power by supplying pure hydrogen or reformed hydrogen as a fuel gas to one electrode, the fuel electrode, and an oxygen gas or air as an oxidant to the other electrode, the air electrode.

An electrode for such a fuel cell is composed of an electrode electrolyte on which a catalyst component is dispersed. The electrode catalyst layer on the fuel electrode side generates protons and electrons from the fuel gas, while the electrode catalyst layer on the air electrode side generates water from oxygen, protons and electrons, enabling the solid polymer electrolyte membrane to ionically conduct protons. Thus, electric power is generated from such electrode catalyst layers.

A conventional solid polymer-type fuel cell has used a perfluoroalkylsulfonic acid-type polymer represented by Nafion™ as an electrode electrolyte. Although this material is excellent in proton conductivity, it is very expensive and its low combustibility resulting from many fluorine atoms within its molecule makes it very difficult to recover and recycle expensive noble metals such as platinum used as an electrode catalyst.

On the other hand, various non-perfluoroalkylsulfonic acid-type polymers have been investigated as alternative materials. In order to use those polymers at a high-temperature condition where the efficiency of power generation is high an attempt has been made to use high heat-resistant aromatic sulfonic acid-type polymers as an electrode electrolyte.

However, such materials, conventionally known as an electrolyte, in some cases developed a reversible elimination reaction of the sulfonic acid group or a crosslinking reaction involving the sulfonic acid under a high temperature. This causes some problems, such as lowering of power generation output of a fuel cell due to the lowered proton conductivity or the embrittlement of a membrane, and failure to generate power due to the rupture of the membrane.

These problems can be solved by the introduction of nitrogen-containing heterocyclic aromatic groups into a polymer containing sulfonic acid groups. This gives an improved stability of the sulfonic acid groups under high temperature conditions and suppresses the elimination of the sulfonic acid groups and crosslinking of the sulfonic acid groups.

Furthermore, such compositions contain no fluorine atom or only in a substantially reduced amount. This may be a solution for the problem of recovering and recycling the catalyst metals. A lot of monomers that can be used in this case have been detailed (26).

A method to synthesize such compounds is the nucleophilic substitution reaction between the compound represented by halogen-containing aromatic compound and nitrogen-containing heterocyclic compound. Examples of such compounds are listed in Table 1.2 and in Table 1.3.

Table 1.2 Halogen-containing aromatic monomers (26).

Aromatic Monomer
2,4-Dichloro-4′-fluorobenzophenone
2,5-Dichloro-4′-fluorobenzophenone
2,6-Dichloro-4′-fluorobenzophenone
2,4-Dichloro-2′-fluorobenzophenone
2,5-Dichloro-2′-fluorobenzophenone
2,6-dichloro-2′-fluorobenzophenone
2,4-Dichlorophenyl-4′-fluorophenyl sulfone
2,5-Dichlorophenyl-4′-fluorophenyl sulfone
2,6-Dichlorophenyl-4′-fluorophenyl sulfone
2,4-Dichlorophenyl-2′-fluorophenyl sulfone

Some of the monomers are shown in Figures 1.4 and 1.5.

The monomers are at first copolymerized to yield a precursor in order to obtain the final polymer.

The copolymerization is carried out in the presence of a catalyst. The catalyst used is a catalyst system containing a transition metal compound. The catalyst system contains as essential components

Table 1.3 Nitrogen-containing heterocyclic monomers (26).

Heterocyclic Monomer	
Pyrrole	Thiazole
Isothiazole	Oxazole
Isoxazole	Pyridine
Imidazole	Imidazoline
Pyrazole	1,3,5-Triazine
Pyrimidine	Pyridazine
Pyrazine	Indole
Quinoline	Isoquinoline
Purine	Benzimidazole
Benzoxazole	Benzothiazole
Tetrazole	Tetrazine
Triazole	Carbazole
Acridine	Quinoxaline
Quinazoline	2-Hydroxypyridine
3-Hydroxypyridine	4-Hydroxypyridine
3-Hydroxyquinoline	8-Hydroxyquinoline
2-Hydroxypyrimidine	2-Mercaptopyridine
3-Mercaptopyridine	4-Mercaptopyridine
2-Mercaptopyrimidine	2-Mercaptobenzothiazole

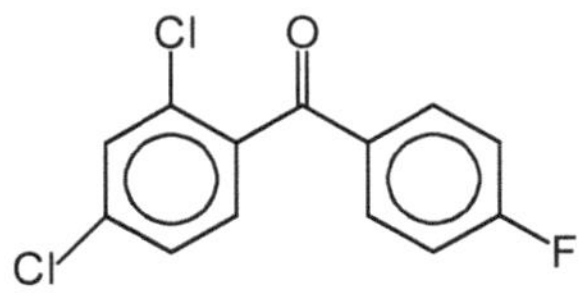

2,4-Dichloro-4´-fluorobenzophenone

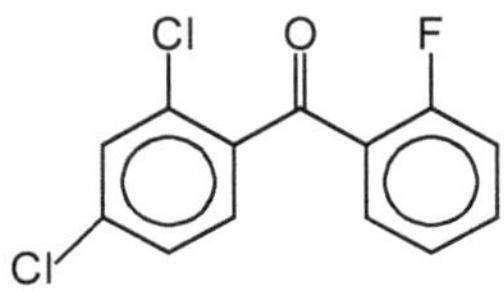

2,4-Dichloro-2´-fluorobenzophenone

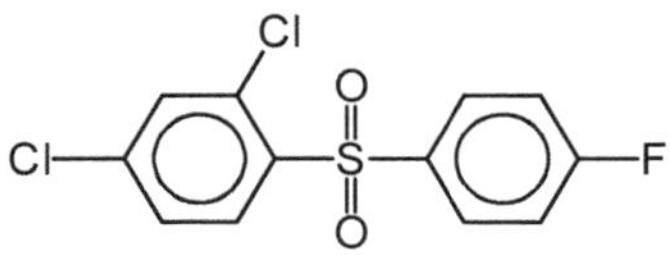

2,4-Dichlorophenyl-4´-fluorophenyl sulfone

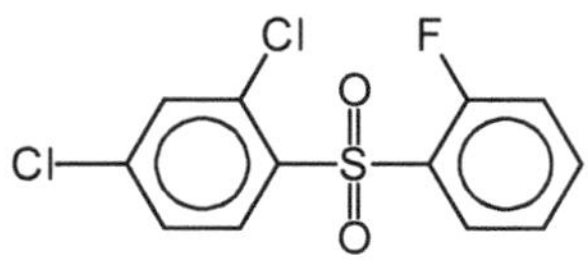

2,4-Dichlorophenyl-2´-fluorophenyl sulfone

Figure 1.4 Monomers.

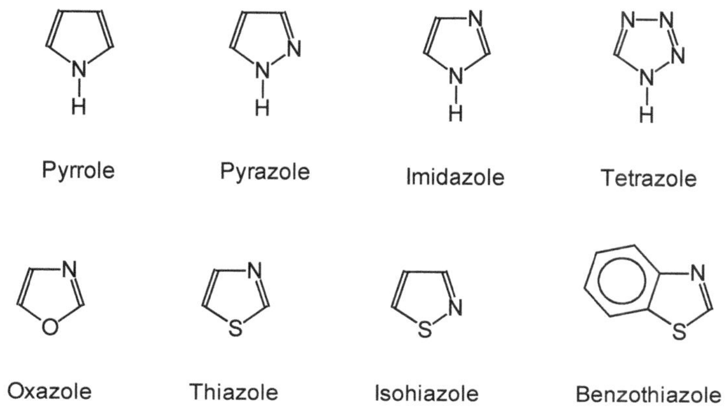

Figure 1.5 Monomers.

a transition metal salt and a compound to serve as a ligand or a transition metal complex coordinated with a ligand (including a copper salt). A reducing agent and a salt may be further added in order to increase the polymerization rate (26).

For example, nickel chloride, nickel bromide can be preferably used as a transition metal salt and triphenylphosphine, tri-*o*-tolylphosphine, cf. Figure 1.6, tri-*m*-tolylphosphine, tri-*p*-tolylphosphine, tributylphosphine, tri-*tert*-butylphosphine, trioctylphosphine, 2,2-bipyridine and similar compounds are preferably used as the compound to serve as the ligand. Bis(triphenylphosphine) nickel chloride and 2,2′-bipyridine)nickel chloride can be suitably used as a transition metal salt (26).

1.1.7 Polymer Fuel Cell Structure

A polymer electrolyte fuel cell structure contains a proton exchange membrane (27). An anode catalyst layer is located on one side of the proton exchange membrane. A cathode catalyst layer is located on the opposite side of the proton exchange membrane, and a gas distribution layer is arranged on each side of the proton exchange membrane. The anode side gas distribution layer is a flat, porous structure having water channels formed in the surface facing the membrane.

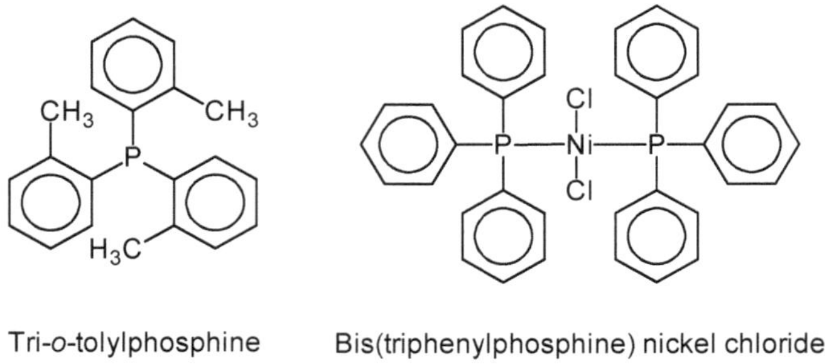

Figure 1.6 Tri-*o*-tolylphosphine and Bis(triphenylphosphine) nickel chloride.

The anode side gas distribution layer is enclosed by a coplanar, sealing plate with water inlet channels coupled to the water channels in the gas distribution layer (27).

A fuel cell that directly supplies the liquid fuel to the anode is called a direct-type fuel cell, in which the supplied liquid fuel is decomposed on a catalyst carried by the anode, so that positive ion, electron and an intermediate product are given (28). In a fuel cell of this type, the positive ion thus generated further migrates to the cathode through the solid polymer electrolytic membrane, while the generated electron migrates to the cathode through an external load, to be reacted with oxygen in the atmosphere on the cathode, thereby generating electricity.

In a direct methanol fuel cell that employs, a methanol aqueous solution as the liquid fuel, the reaction is represented by the following chemical formulas (28):

$$CH_3OH + H_2O \rightarrow CO_2 + 6H^+ + 6e^- \tag{1.5}$$

$$6H^+ + 6e^- \rightarrow \frac{3}{2}O_2 \rightarrow 3H_2O \tag{1.6}$$

The reaction in Eq. 1.5 takes place on the anode, and the reaction represented by the formula 1.6 takes place on the cathode.

As is apparent from these formulae, theoretically 1 *mol* of methanol and 1 *mol* of water are reacted on the anode, thereby giving

1 *mol* of the reaction product, i.e., carbon dioxide. Since hydrogen ions and electrons are also generated simultaneously, the theoretical concentration of methanol in the methanol aqueous solution, serving as the fuel, is approx. 70 vol% (28).

However, it is known that in the case where the fuel concentration becomes higher and hence a relatively larger amount of alcohol fuel is supplied to the anode than water, what is known as *crossover effect* takes place, in which the alcohol fuel is transmitted through the solid polymer electrolytic membrane without being involved in the reaction represented by Eq. 1.5, to be reacted with the catalyst on the cathode, which results in decreased generation capacity and generation efficiency (28).

Examples of techniques that can suppress the crossover effect include providing a fuel vaporization layer consisting of a porous material or the like that vaporizes the liquid fuel on the upstream side of the anode of the membrane and electrode assembly, to thereby supplying the given vaporized liquid fuel.

1.1.8 Fuel Cell System and Method for Humidifying

Reactant gas supply streams for solid polymer fuel cells may be heated and humidified using the heat generated by the fuel cell and water vapor from the fuel cell exhaust (29). The heat and water vapor in the oxidant exhaust stream are sufficient to heat and humidify a reactant gas supply stream, preferably the oxidant supply stream. The heating and humidifying can be accomplished by flowing a reactant gas supply stream and a fuel cell exhaust gas stream on opposite sides of a water-permeable membrane in a combined heat and humidity exchange apparatus.

The method and apparatus are particularly suitable for use with air-cooled fuel cell systems and systems which employ near ambient pressure air as the oxidant gas supply (29).

1.2 Direct Methanol Fuel Cells

The overall reaction in a direct methanol fuel cell is

$$CH_3OH + \frac{3}{2}O_2 \rightarrow 2H_2O + CO_2 \quad . \qquad (1.7)$$

The anode reaction is

$$CH_3OH + 6OH^- \rightarrow 5H_2O + CO_2 + 6e^- \tag{1.8}$$

and the reaction at the cathode is

$$2OH^- + CO_2 \rightarrow H_2O + CO_3^- \quad . \tag{1.9}$$

The direct methanol fuel cell has the potential to replace lithium-ion rechargeable batteries in portable electronic devices (30). However, significant power density and efficiency losses have been observed due to high methanol crossover through polymer electrolyte membranes (30).

A comprehensive overview of the passive direct methanol fuel cell barriers has been presented (31). These issues are methanol crossover, slow kinetics, water management, heat management, species management, durability and stability and the costs for commercialization. Different approaches to overcome the discussed barriers of passive direct methanol fuel cells have been detailed.

The critical challenge regarding minimization of methanol crossover through the membrane is to the use of various hybrid membranes and methanol transport barrier so that the cell performance can be maximized.

In order to reduce the catalyst cost with better kinetics, the development of non-noble catalysts for passive direct methanol fuel cells is expected. The challenges related to the operating temperature of a passive direct methanol fuel cell are the selection of the methanol concentration, current density, ambient temperature, air humidity, cell orientation, membrane thickness, and cell design. Several methods related to the water management layer are the transport of the water produced on the cathode to the anode through the membrane and the cathode with minimum water flooding (31). The thermodynamic data of some alcohols are summarized in Table 1.4.

Alcohols have a very good energy density W_e, close to that of hydrocarbons, and gasoline of around 10–11 $kWh\,kg^{-1}$, so they appear to be a reasonable alternative energy carrier for an electric vehicle.

Table 1.4 Thermodynamic data of some alcohols (32).

Alcohol	ΔG^0 $kJ\,mol^{-1}$	E_{cell} V	W_e $kWh\,kg^{-1}$
CH_3OH	-702	1.213	6.09
C_2H_2OH	-1325	1.145	8.00
C_3H_3OH	-1853	1.067	8.58
C_4H_9OH	-2381	1.029	8.93
Gasoline			10.5

However, in contrast to these promising thermodynamic data, the kinetics of alcohol oxidation is more difficult, leading to high anodic overvoltages, in particular for the high molecular alcohols. For example, the overvoltage of the methanol electrooxidation reaches 0.5 V at 200 $mA\,cm^{-2}$ on pure platinum. But the development of better electrocatalysts allows this to be greatly decreased (32).

1.2.1 *Modeling Liquid Feed Direct Methanol Fuel Cells*

A multiphysics model for liquid-feed direct methanol fuel cells has been presented (33). The model accounts for two-dimensional across-the-channel anisotropic mass and charge transport in the anode and cathode gas diffusion layers, including the effect of gas diffusion layer assembly compression and electrical contact resistances at the bipolar plate and membrane interfaces.

A one-dimensional across-the-membrane model has been used to describe the diffusion of local species through the microporous layers, methanol/water crossover, proton transport, and electrochemical reactions, thereby coupling both gas diffusion layer submodels.

The two-dimensional/one-dimensional model has been extended to the third dimension and supplemented with one-dimensional descriptions of the flow channels to yield a three-dimensional/one-dimensional + one-dimensional model that could be successfully validated.

A parametric study has been conducted on the two-dimensional/one-dimensional model to examine the effect of the operating conditions on the cell performance. The results show that an optimum methanol concentration exists that maximizes power output due to the trade-off between anode polarization and cathode mixed overpotential. For a fixed methanol concentration, the cell performance is largely affected by the oxygen supply rate, cell temperature, and liquid/gas saturation levels. There is also an optimal gas diffusion layer compression due to the trade-off between ohmic and concentration losses, which strongly depends on bipolar plate material and, more weakly, on the actual operating conditions (33).

1.2.2 *Vapor Feed Direct Methanol Fuel Cells*

In a vapor feed direct methanol fuel cell, the liquid methanol transports from a reservoir tank to the vaporizer to generate vaporized methanol (34). The vaporizer can be an external heater, i.e., an electric vaporizer, or a pervaporation membrane.

Vapor feed direct methanol fuel cells can be classified as active or passive direct methanol fuel cells

In an active feed direct methanol fuel cell, the methanol solution is delivered due to a peristaltic pump to the anode side, while the oxygen from the surrounding air is supplied by a blower or fan to the cathode side.

In the passive direct methanol fuel cell, the reactants, methanol and oxygen are delivered to the catalyst layer and the products, carbon dioxide and water are removed from the cell by passive processes, e.g., diffusion, natural convection and capillary forces (35,36).

A passive direct methanol fuel cell is advantageous over an active direct methanol fuel cell because of its simpler and more compact design and low costs. On the other hand, an active direct methanol fuel cell may be more suitable for a bulky high power system.

Various critical challenges limit the widespread commercial application of direct methanol fuel cells. A review of the experimental and numerical studies on the vapor feed direct methanol fuel cells has been presented (34). The critical challenges of a vapor feed direct methanol fuel cell are methanol crossover, water management layer, carbon dioxide release and the operation at high temperature.

It has been shown that the critical challenge regarding the methanol crossover is how to feed vapor methanol with minimum methanol crossover through the membrane so that the cell performance can be maximized. Several methods related to the water management layer deal with the transport of the water produced on the cathode to the anode through the membrane and help to operate the anode with vapor methanol and the cathode with minimum water flooding. The critical challenge related to the high temperature vapor feed direct methanol fuel cell is the selection of the membrane electrode assembly materials so that it can be operated at high temperature which critically affects the cell performance. The various vaporization methods of supplying liquid methanol to direct methanol fuel cell have been discussed in detail.

The recent developments in the stacking of vapor feed direct methanol fuel cell to increase the power density have also been discussed. A statistical flow chart has been proposed to optimize a passive vapor feed direct methanol fuel cell with concentrated methanol (34).

1.2.3 *Mixed Feed Direct Methanol Fuel Cells*

Experiments were conducted to establish the effect of the vapor fraction on the performance of a direct methanol fuel cell by varying the vapor fraction in the feed from 0% (liquid) to 100% (vapor) of the methanol solution (37). The methanol concentrations were varied between 1 *M* and 3 *M* to find the optimal concentration for performance.

Also, the effects of neat methanol were studied. It was found that both the increase in the vapor fraction of feed, and the increase in the concentration of the feed increase the performance of the fuel cell (37).

1.2.4 *Metalized Polymer Film*

A concept for a flexible direct methanol micro-fuel cell based on the microstructuring of a Cr/Au metalized, thin polymer film of photosensitive SU-8 has been evaluated (38). SU-8 is a photosensitive and very firm epoxy resin and is shown in Figure 1.7.

The inscribed microchannels in the electrodes are 200 $\mu m \times 200$ μm in cross section and span an active fuel cell area of 10 $mm \times 10$ mm with a Pt black catalyst on the cathode side of the membrane electrode assembly and a Pt-Ru alloy catalyst on the anode side.

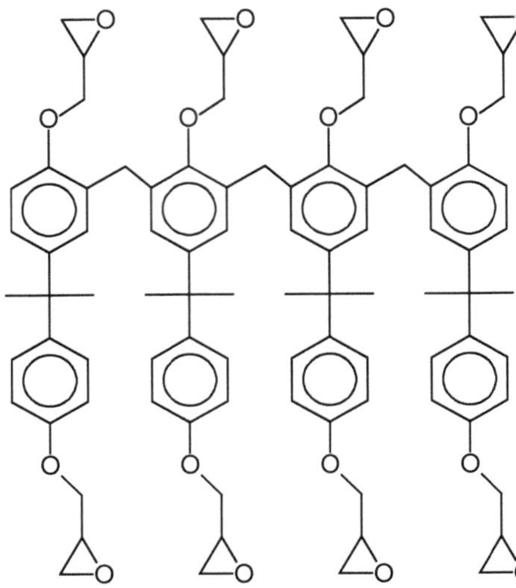

Figure 1.7 SU-8.

An optimal operating condition with long-term stability has been found for the fuel cell which employs a serpentine flow field for both electrodes and has a volume flow rate of 0.14 $ml\,min^{-1}$ of a 1 *M* methanol solution at the anode side with a gas volume flow rate of 8 $ml\,min^{-1}$ of humidified oxygen at the cathode side, yielding a power density of 19.0 $mW\,cm^{-2}$ at 75 $mA\,cm^{-2}$ at a temperature of 60°C (38).

1.2.5 *Catalysts*

1.2.5.1 Poly(oxometalate) Functionalized Graphene

Catalysts for direct methanol fuel cells have been developed based on poly(oxometalate) functionalized graphene quantum dots with several monometallic and bimetallic nanoparticles, such as platinum nanoparticles, palladium nanoparticles and platinum-palladium nanoparticles (39).

According to transmission electron microscope images, the average particle sizes of the platinum nanoparticles and palladium nanoparticles were found to be approximately 20–30 *nm*. The platinum-palladium nanoparticle-based catalysts exhibited a higher peak current for methanol oxidation than those of the other catalysts, thus providing evidence for their higher electrocatalytic activity (39).

1.2.5.2 *Core-Shell Nanoparticles*

Core-shell structured $PtRuNi_x$ nanoparticles with Ni-rich core and PtRu-rich shell are successfully synthesized on poly(ethylene imine) functionalized carbon nanotubes through successively dealloying and annealing of PtRuNi alloy nanoparticles (40).

The best results could be obtained after annealing the dealloyed PtRuNi nanoparticles at 450°C. Here a PtRu-rich shell is formed and Ni-rich core structure with a surface composition of Pt:Ru:Ni = 1.0:1.13:0.24.

$PtRuNi_x$ shows significantly low onset potential and a high activity for the methanol oxidation reaction. This is significantly higher than the values measured on PtRuNi before dealloying and an annealing treatment, and 155 $A\,g_{Pt}^{-1}$ on the conversional Johnson Matthey PtRu/C electrocatalysts. At 0.4 V vs. Ag/AgCl, the stable current for the MOR on $PtRuNi_x$ electrocatalysts is 34.3 $A\,g_{Pt}^{-1}$ after polarization for 5000 s, which is significantly higher than 10.2 $A\,g_{Pt}^{-1}$ of PtRuNi and 9 $A\,g_{Pt}^{-1}$ of the conversional PtRu/C.

Also, the $PtRuNi_x$ exhibits significantly improved microstructural stability under an accelerated degradation test. The enhanced activity and stability is most likely related to the formation of an intermetallic PtRu skinned shell and Ni-rich core structures (40).

1.2.5.3 *Hierarchical Branched Platinum Copper Nanoparticles*

Hierarchical branched nanoparticles are a promising nanostructure with a three-dimensional open porous structure composed of integrated branches for superior catalysis (41).

Pt-Cu hierarchical branched nanoparticles have been synthesized with a small size of about 30 *nm*. Integrated ultrathin branches are obtained by using a modified polyol process with introduction of poly(vinylpyrrolidone) and HCl.

This strategy is expected to be a general strategy to prepare metallic nanostructures for catalysis. Because of the special open porous structure, the so-prepared hierarchical branched nanoparticles show a highly enhanced specific activity toward the methanol oxidation reaction of as much as 2.5 and 1.7 times in comparison to commercially available Pt-Cu and Pt-Cu/C catalysts (41).

1.2.5.4 *Platinum Ruthenium Nafion Catalysts*

The influence of catalyst layer thicknesses at the anode of a direct methanol fuel cell has been investigated (42). The catalysts were applied with the drawdown method with varied thicknesses ranging from 25.4 μm to 205 μm with a Pt/Ru anode loading of 0.25 $mg\,cm^{-2}$ to 2.0 $mg\,cm^{-2}$. The membrane electrode assemblies with thicker individual layers performed better compared to those with thinner layers.

The peak power densities for the different loading levels followed an exponential decrease of Pt/Ru utilization at higher loading levels.

The highest power density achieved was 49 $mW\,cm^{-2}$ with the 100 μm layers at 2.0 $mg\,cm^{-2}$ catalyst loading, whereas the highest normalized power density was 116 $mW\,mg^{-1}$ with the 205 μm layers at 0.25 $mg\,cm^{-2}$ loading (42).

The effect of the organic solvent polarity on the properties of unsupported Pt-Ru catalyst inks and on the performance of the catalyst layers that are prepared with these materials for the methanol electrooxidation, has been studied (43).

Results of light scattering indicate that the Pt-Ru-Nafion aggregates in the inks prepared with *n*-butyl acetate (NBA) are larger than those prepared with 2-propanol. The lower polarity of the former favors the aggregation of Nafion and the nanoparticles. The electron microscopy images and porosimetry measurements of the catalyst layers show that the secondary pore volume between the agglomerates is larger for *n*-butyl acetate (43).

The linear sweep voltammetry and EIS results for the methanol electrooxidation in the three-electrode cell denote the higher active surface area for *n*-butyl acetate and comparable specific oxidation rates of the intermediates in both catalyst layers. The current densities for Pt-Ru anode catalyst layers in single direct methanol fuel cells are higher when the solvent is *n*-butyl acetate, the mass transport limitations being much more apparent with 2-propanol. The adapted transmission line equivalent circuit to interpret the impedance results in a single direct methanol fuel cell indicates that the proton resistance for *n*-butyl acetate is significantly lower than for

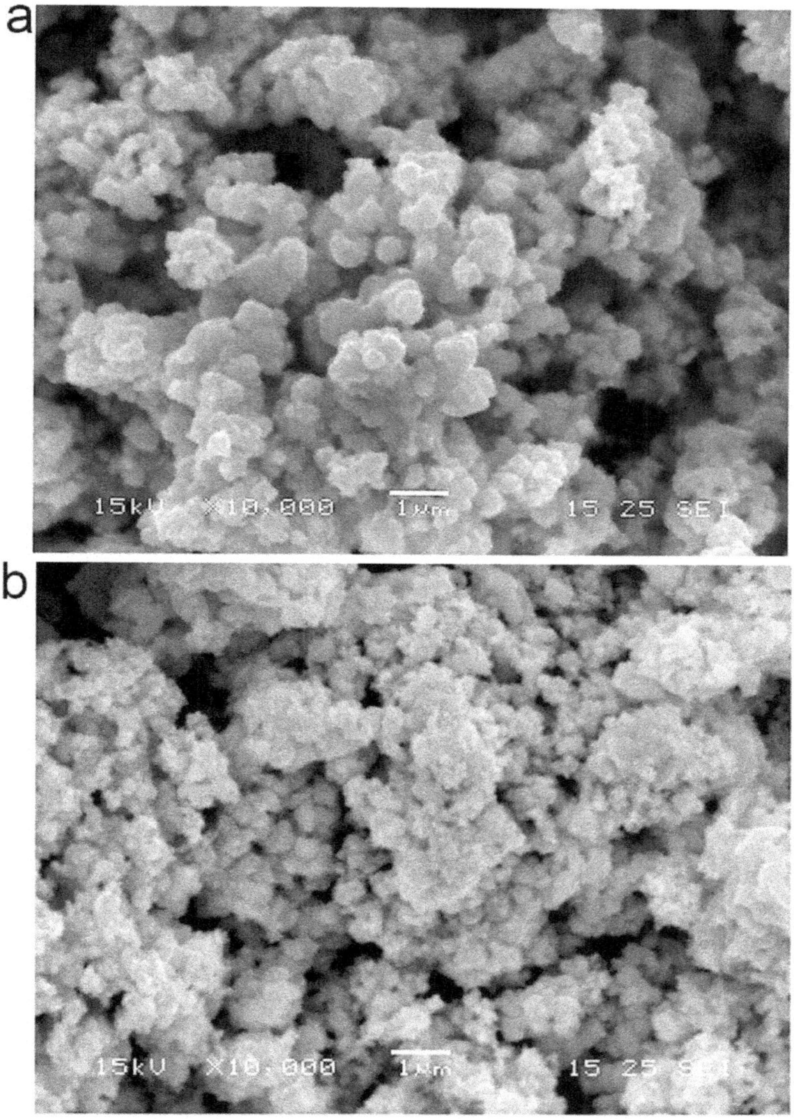

Figure 1.8 Electron microscopy images of selected Pt Ru catalyst layers prepared using (a) NBA and (b) IPA as organic solvents, reprinted from (43) with permission from Elsevier.

2-propanol, thus suggesting that the greater number of accessible active sites for methanol oxidation in the former are well connected to the Nafion ionomers and more easily transported to the membrane (43).

It has been stated that state-of-the-art Pt-based cathode catalysts suffer from low efficiency which is severely affected by poisoning of methanol fuel crossing the membrane that separates the electrodes and high cost (44).

1.2.5.5 Platinum-Based Cathodes

The Pt-based cathodes in direct methanol fuel cells suffer significantly from performance loss due to a severe methanol crossover from anode to cathode (45). The migrated methanol in the cathodes tends to contaminate Pt active sites through yielding a mixed potential region resulting from oxygen reduction reaction and methanol oxidation reaction.

1.2.5.6 Non-Platinum-Containing Catalyst

A highly active non-platinum group metals catalyst for oxygen reduction reaction has been synthesized (46).

The electrochemical activity towards oxygen reduction reaction and tolerance to methanol poisoning of the catalyst were studied by the rotating disk electrode method. A performance analysis was carried out at the cathode of a direct methanol fuel cell comprising the variation of fuel concentration and temperature. A peak power density of about 50 $W g^{-1}$ was recorded at 90°C in a wide range of methanol concentration of 1–10 *M*.

It was found that the non-platinum group metals catalyst has an extraordinarily high tolerance to methanol crossover, with no significant decay of performance up to 10 *M* of alcohol concentration, making this material state-of-the-art in direct methanol fuel cell application. Chronoamperometric tests in direct methanol fuel cell at 90°C and 5 *M* methanol concentration for 100 *h* also showed a suitable stability (46).

Also, a non-platinum group metals catalyst based on iron-nitrogen-carbon for the oxygen reduction reaction derived from pyrolyzed Fe-aminobenzimidazole was synthesized by sacrificial support method, and characterized by several physical-chemical techniques (47).

1.2.5.7 *Bimetallic Oxides of Cobalt and Nickel*

Two $NiCo_2O_4$ bimetallic oxides have been synthesized via a hydrothermal method (48).

Preparation 1–1: In a typical synthesis procedure, 0.002 *mol* $Ni(NO_3)_2 \times 6H_2O$ and 0.004 mol $Co(NO_3)_2 \times 6H_2O$ were dissolved in 40 *ml* distilled water. Next, 0.03 *mol* $(NH_2)_2CO$ were added to the mixture, which was then magnetically stirred for 2 *h* at room temperature to obtain a transparent pink solution. This mixture was transferred to a 50 *mL* Teflon-lined stainless steel autoclave, which was then sealed and heated to 120°C for 6 *h*. After the mixture was cooled to room temperature, a brown precipitate was obtained and washed with distilled water several times until the pH was 7. The resulting product was dried at 60°C in an oven for 24 *h* and then calcined at 350°C in air in a muffle furnace for 3 *h* to obtain $NiCo_2O_4$ with a dandelion-like structure.

The flower-like compound was synthesized, using basically the same procedure as described above, except the hydrothermal reaction was performed in the autoclave at 170°C for 8 *h*.

Scanning electron microscope (SEM) and transfer electron microscopic observations showed that these materials have three-dimensional dandelion-like and flower-like morphologies. The images are shown in Figure 1.9.

Their large specific surface areas of 90.68 $m^2\ g^{-1}$ and 19.8 $m^2\ g^{-1}$ and porous structures provide many active sites and effective transport pathways for the oxygen reduction reaction.

Electrochemical measurements using a rotating ring-disc electrode indicated that the electron transfer numbers for the oxygen reduction reaction of the dandelion-like compound is 3.97 and for the flower-like compound 3.91 is found. These compounds have been used in fuel cells.

A high catalytic activity of $NiCo_2O_4$ was found which is mainly attributed to the presence of many Co^{3+} cations that directly donate electrons to oxygen to reduce it via a more efficient and effective route. The catalytic performance of the dandelion-like material is superior to that of the flower-like material, because it has a higher specific surface area and is less crystalline (48).

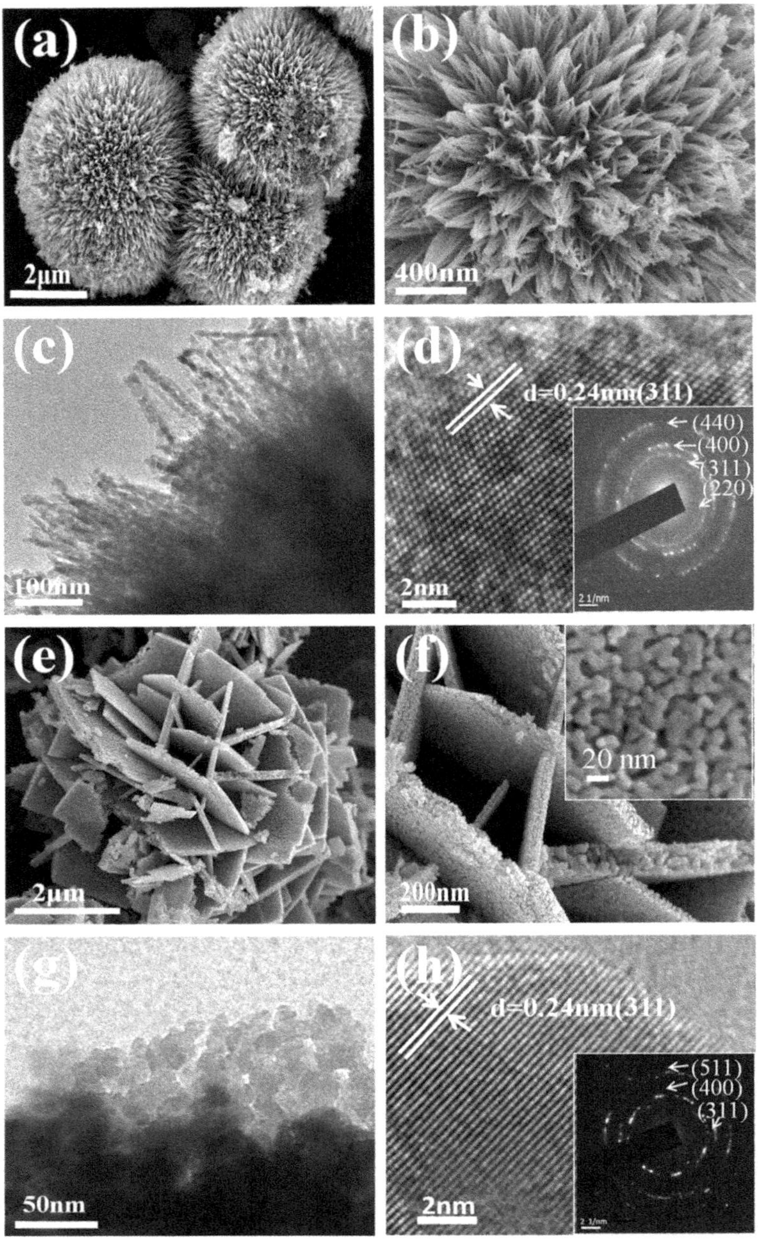

Figure 1.9 (a) Low- and (b) high-magnification SEM, (c) TEM and (d) HRTEM images of NiCo2O4-DL (inset in [d]: SAED pattern); (e) low- and (f and inset) high-magnification SEM, (g) TEM and (h) HRTEM images of NiCo2O4-FL (inset in [h]: SAED pattern), reprinted from (48) with permission from Elsevier.

1.2.5.8 *Iron Aminobenzimidazole Catalyst*

In a half-cell electrochemical configuration, the iron aminobenzimidazole catalyst presented a significant improvement of the oxygen reduction reaction activity with respect to a recently reported non-non-platinum group metals formulation based on Fe-aminoantipyrine (46), with an enhancement of the half-wave potential of about 85 mV in an oxygen saturated sulfuric acid solution. The structures of 2-aminobenzimidazole and 4-aminoantipyrine are shown in Figure 1.10.

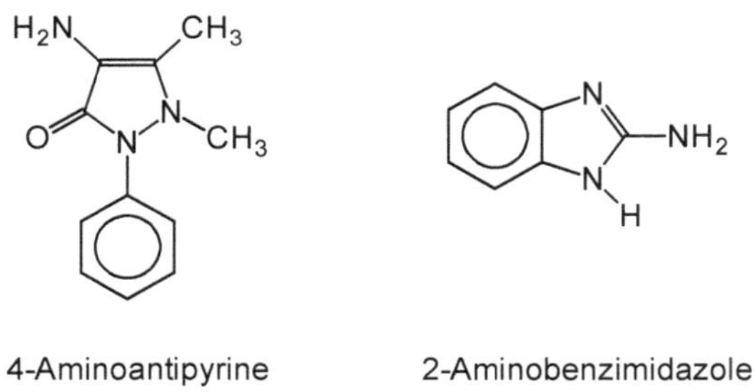

Figure 1.10 Iron-based catalyst precursors.

The Fe-aminobenzimidazole catalyst showed a remarkably high tolerance to methanol, resulting in a superior oxygen reduction reaction performance compared to Pt/C at methanol concentrations higher than 0.02 M. In a direct methanol fuel cell good performances could also be obtained.

A durability test of 100 h at 90°C, feeding 5 M methanol, was carried out. A certain decrease of performance was recorded, amounting to -0.20 $mW\,cm^{-2}h^{-1}$ at the very beginning of the test and -0.05 $mW\,cm^{-2}h^{-1}$ at the end. However, the Fe-aminobenzimidazole is more adequate than previously reported formulations in terms of both oxygen reduction reaction activity and stability (47).

1.2.5.9 *Fe-N-C Catalysts*

Other platinum group metal-free catalysts based on Fe-N-C have also been investigated in an acidic medium (49). The posttreatment of the catalyst improves the oxygen reduction reaction activity in comparison with other previously published platinum group metal-free formulations and shows an excellent tolerance to the presence of methanol.

A reduced graphene oxide-based Fe-N-C cathode exhibits a high methanol tolerance (45). In the compositions, the morphology of two-dimensional reduced graphene oxide is largely preserved, but the resulting Fe-N-reduced graphene oxide catalyst provides a more unique porous structure.

Non-precious metal catalysts for electrochemical oxygen reduction have been synthesized by the pyrolysis of multiwalled carbon nanotubes in the presence of nitrogen and iron precursors (50).

The catalyst synthesis was carried out by a simple pyrolysis using cheap precursors, dicyandiamide and $FeCl_3$, followed by an acid treatment and a second pyrolysis step.

The Fe-containing nitrogen-doped carbon nanotubes exhibit an enhanced electrocatalytic performance in comparison to their metal-free counterparts and their electrocatalytic activity is comparable to that of a commercial Pt/C catalyst. Thus, these materials can be considered as promising cathode catalysts for application in alkaline fuel cells (50).

1.2.5.10 *Ruthenium Selenium Catalysts*

Non-platinum RuSe catalysts with a size of 3–15 *nm* have been synthesized using microwave irradiation technique. Here, nanomaterials are produced with a high efficiency and short time spans (44).

Several atomic ratios of Ru to Se were used for the preparation using both elemental Se powder and H_2SeO_3 as precursors. The use of H_2SeO_3 as Se source provides catalysts with a controlled composition.

An electrochemical study of the oxygen reduction reaction on these catalysts was done with the rotating disk electrode technique. All the investigated materials showed a good electrocatalytic activity towards oxygen reduction and maintained high activity in the presence of high methanol contamination.

It has been found that a Ru to Se ratio of 2 to 1 yields the highest kinetic currents. Stability tests at 0.4 *V* in strong acidic conditions and at elevated temperatures, for over 600 *h*, did not indicate any degradation (44).

1.2.6 *Electrolytes*

Protonic and superprotonic electrolytes that can be used for the application in direct methanol and direct urea/urine fuel cells have been reviewed (51).

Solid acids are a good choice as the electrolyte for direct methanol fuel cells because they show high proton conductivity and do not require humid conditions, which can simplify the fuel cell system.

The typical formulas of solid acids are $MHXO_4$, $M_3H(XO_4)_2$, and MH(PO3H), where M= Li^+, Cs^+, Rb^+, K^+, Na^+, NH_4^+, and X=S or Se.

Also, a solid oxide electrolyte has received attention because it can be easily prepared and is practicable for a variety of fuels including methanol (52). The conventional solid oxide-based materials require a high temperature.

Solid acids exhibit an anhydrous proton transport and a high-temperature stability. A continuous, stable power generation for both H_2/O_2 and direct methanol fuel cells operated at around 250°C using a humidity-stabilized solid acid CsH_2PO_4 electrolyte (52).

Solid acids that exhibit a phase transition and high ion transport are addressed as superprotonic (51).

1.3 Direct Ethanol Fuel Cells

Direct ethanol fuel cells are attractive as a power source because ethanol is nontoxic and therefore easy to handle and it is a high energy density fuel, leading to a high system energy density.

Two types of direct ethanol fuel cells have been recognized (53):

1. Direct ethanol-proton exchange membrane fuel cells, and
2. Alkaline anion exchange membrane direct ethanol fuel cells.

Basically, there are several issues regarding direct ethanol fuel cells that must be taken into account (53):

1. Low power density,
2. Effect of ethanol crossover on efficiency of fuel utilization,
3. Electrical, mechanical and thermal stability, and
4. Water uptake of the direct ethanol fuel cells electrolyte membrane.

On the other hand, the direct anodic oxidation of an alcohol fuel other than methanol allows the formation of compact power sources with no heavy and bulky fuel reformer (32). They can be fed with a convenient electrochemically reactive and relatively nontoxic and cheap liquid fuel. The schematic principle of a direct ethanol fuel cell is shown in Figure 1.11.

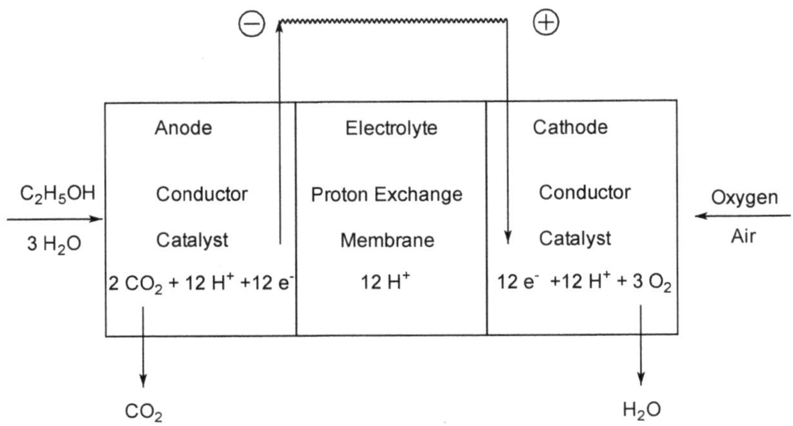

Figure 1.11 Basic principle of a direct ethanol fuel cell (32).

In the usage of ethanol, an anode mixture of ethanol dissolved in water, a few percent by weight to make a 1–2 *M* ethanol solution, is circulated through the anodic compartment, and oxygen or air, respectively, flows through the cathodic compartment.

The anode/water mixture allows the hydration of the proton exchange membrane, particularly when working at higher temperatures of 100–130°C. In this case, some increase in pressure of 2–5 *bars* of the anode compartment is needed to keep the alcohol solution in liquid form (32).

The direct electrochemical oxidation of ethanol occurs at the anode, according to the following reaction:

$$C_2H_5OH + 3H_2O \rightarrow 2CO_2 + 12H^+ + 12e^- \quad (1.10)$$

In contrast, direct methanol fuel cells produce only 6 electrons for the complete oxidation of methanol to carbon dioxide.

Such a direct ethanol fuel cell system, which does not follow Carnot's theorem, can produce electricity with a high energy efficiency ε of 97% under reversible conditions (32).

It has been stated that the performance of ethanol in direct oxidation fuel cells is better than that of methanol due to the lower crossover rate of the fuel, which decreases the effect on cathode performance (54).

Ethanol is a sustainable compound due to its natural availability (55, 56). Ethanol has also been classified as a renewable energetic compound because it can be produced in bulk from agricultural bioprocesses via a fermentation process of biomass from agriculture, forestry and urban residues (56–59).

1.3.1 *Transport Phenomena in Alkaline Direct Ethanol Fuel Cells*

The transport phenomena of various species in alkaline direct ethanol fuel cells have been reviewed (60). The design and structural parameters of membrane electrode assemblies and the operating parameters affect the fuel cell performance.

The conventional architecture design of alkaline direct ethanol fuel cells that purely relies on an hydroxide exchange membrane and hydroxide exchange ionomers to conduct ions exhibited extremely low performance, which is primarily attributed to the low conductivity of the state-of-the-art hydroxide exchange membranes and corresponding hydroxide exchange ionomers (61).

Ethanol can be completely oxidized into carbon dioxide on some electrocatalysts in alkaline media (62). However, the main product of the ethanol oxidation reaction on Pd-based electrocatalysts is acetate. Therefore, the anodic reaction becomes (63):

$$CH_3CH_2OH + 5OH^- \rightarrow CH_3COO^- + 4e^- + 4H_2O \qquad (1.11)$$

Then, the water in the anode is transported through the membrane and arrives at the cathode, and the produced electrons are transported through the external circuit to the cathode.

On the cathode, the oxygen is transported through the cathode DL to the cathode catalyst layer, where oxygen reacts with the electrons and water to produce hydroxide ions:

$$O_2 + H_2O + 4e^- \rightarrow 4OH^- \tag{1.12}$$

The hydroxide ions in the cathode migrate through the hydroxide exchange membrane to the anode for the ethanol oxidation reaction. The combination of the ethanol oxidation reaction given by Eq. 1.11 and the oxygen reduction reaction given by Eq. 1.12 results in the following overall reaction:

$$CH_3CH_2OH + OH^- + O_2 \rightarrow CH_3COO^- + 2H_2O \tag{1.13}$$

An anion-conducting ionomer, referred to as A3, has been developed by Tokuyama as a binder for alkaline membrane fuel cells (61). Alkaline membrane fuel cells have been detailed (64).

The A3 binder was evaluated and the influence of its content in the anode and cathode catalyst layers for alkaline direct methanol fuel cells was investigated. An optimum A3 content was found to be 45.4% for both anode and cathode electrodes (65).

This anion-conducting ionomer was also investigated for direct ethanol fuel cells. The experimental results for the case of feeding C_2H_5OH solution without added KOH indicate that the cell performance varies with A3 ionomer content in the anode CL, and the best performance is obtained from a membrane electrode assembly with 10% A3 impregnated into the anode catalyst layer (61).

Future perspectives and challenges with regard to transport phenomena in this fuel cell system have also been highlighted. The critical transport issues that need to be further addressed in the near future include (60):

- Ethanol transport: Maintaining an appropriate ethanol concentration level in the anode catalyst layer is the direction to maximize the cell performance.
- Water transport: The direction of water management is to transport water through the membrane to the cathode at an appropriate rate.
- Alkali transport: The direction of alkali management is to alleviate or eliminate the alkali crossover.

- Carbon dioxide: When the air is used as oxidant, CO_2 from the air can react with hydroxide ions generated by the oxygen reduction reaction and penetrated from the anode to form carbonate, limiting the fuel cell performance and durability.
- Oxygen transport: The direction of oxygen transport is how to enhance the oxygen supply to the cathode catalyst layer and the water removal from the cathode diffusion layer by utilizing passive forces or regulating the gas flow rates.
- Hydrogen peroxide transport: Maintaining an appropriate hydrogen peroxide concentration level in the cathode catalyst layer is the direction to maximize the cell performance. On the other hand, the issue associated with hydrogen peroxide decomposition has to be addressed before the fuel cell technology using hydrogen peroxide as oxidant becomes possible; the rate of hydrogen peroxide decomposition can be reduced by optimizing the pH value, the hydrogen peroxide concentration, the temperature of the aqueous solution, and the electrochemical properties of electrode materials.

1.3.2 *Nanoporous Palladium Anode*

The operation of micro-solid oxide fuel cells has been demonstrated using a nanoscale proton-conducting Y–$BaZrO_3$ electrolyte, in order to avoid the fuel crossover problem for direct ethanol fuel cells (66). The micro-solid oxide fuel cells were operated with the direct utilization of ethanol vapor as a fuel and Pd as anode in a temperature range of 300–400°C. The nanoporous Pd anode is achieved by direct current sputtering at high Ar pressure of 80 *m torr*. The Pd-anode/Y–$BaZrO_3$-electrolyte/Pt-cathode cell shows peak power densities of 72.4 $mW\,cm^{-2}$ using hydrogen and 15.3 $mW\,cm^{-2}$ using ethanol at 400°C. No obvious carbon deposition is seen from X-ray photoelectron spectroscopy analysis after a fuel cell test using ethanol as fuel (66).

1.3.3 *Catalysts for Ethanol Fuel Cells*

In the past, two types of ethanol fuel cells have been developed: the acid- and alkaline-type direct ethanol fuel cell. For both types of fuel cells, platinum was found to be an excellent catalyst for the electrochemical reaction (67).

The catalyst in a direct ethanol fuel cell system is a site, which provides a surface for the ethanol electrooxidation to occur at lower activation energy and at a higher rate. The lower activation energy significantly affects the energy consumed during the breaking and forming of the reactant and product bonds. A higher rate of reaction reduces the time required for the reaction to proceed.

Palladium is the least reactive catalyst in acidic media, however, palladium displayed a superior performance in alkaline media compared to platinum.

It has been demonstrated that palladium is a potential substitute for the costly platinum as the primary catalyst. Several studies have indicated that palladium is superior over platinum, in particular in an alkaline environment.

It has been shown that palladium performed approximately four times better than platinum as a catalyst under alkaline conditions, especially for ethanol oxidations (68).

The addition of a co-catalyst is to improve the monometallic palladium catalyst performance. It has been found that the Ni addition works consistently with the performance in ethanol fuel cells with acidic media. Also, it has been found that Ni provides a synergetic effect by weakening the bond formed between the surface intermediates active during adsorption/desorption phase, thus reducing the probability of the poison formation (69).

1.3.3.1 *Carbon-Supported Platinum-Based Nanocatalysts*

Bifunctional electrocatalysts have been proposed to decrease the precious noble metal content in the catalyst composition and to promote the conversion of this fuel, leading to the preparation of Pt-based materials containing oxophilic co-catalysts such as tin, osmium, iridium and ruthenium (70).

These materials allow the oxidation of ethanol at low potentials, and also remove CO-like adsorbed species from the surface of the electrode. The performance of a single direct ethanol fuel cell using various Pt-based anode nanomaterials for oxidizing ethanol in an acidic environment have been discussed. The activity of electrocatalysts has been reported by examining their capability of converting ethanol to different reaction products.

Also, the intermediate species in the course of the reaction have been described. The performance in a direct ethanol fuel cell can be obtained by a direct measurement of the anodic and cathodic potentials. This depends on the ethanol oxidation occurring at low overpotentials and also on the oxygen reduction reaction (70).

1.3.3.2 *Platinum-Free Catalysts*

Palladium-Based Catalysts. Metal-based catalyst materials, non-containing platinum, for preferred application to form both alcohol-tolerant cathodes for oxygen reduction and anodes for oxidation of various fuel molecules, and methods of making these catalysts have been provided (71). Also, methods for preparing anodes and cathodes for these fuel cells have been shown.

Nitrogen-oxygen-carbon polymers can be obtained by the condensation of a 4-1-[(2,4-di(substituted)-phenyl)-hydrazono]-alkyl-benzene-1,3-diol, cf. Figure 1.12, with a phenol or a 3-substituted phenol or a 3,5-disubstituted phenol and formaldehyde or paraformaldehyde in the presence of either a basic (e.g., NaOH) or acid (e.g., HCl) catalyst (71).

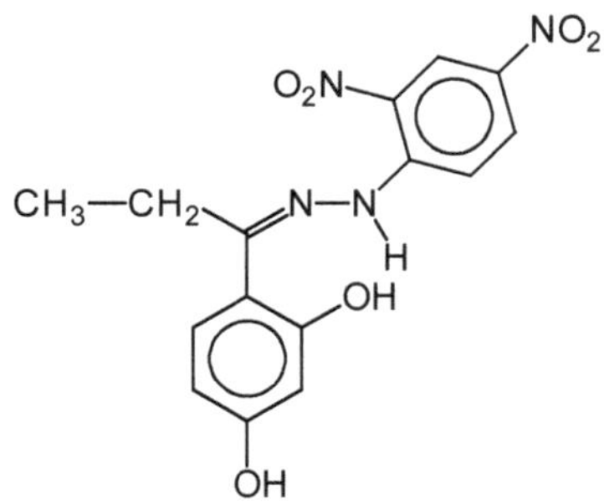

Figure 1.12 4-1-[(2,4-Dinitrophenyl)-hydrazono]-ethylbenzene-1,3-diol.

An enhancement in the performance of alkaline direct ethanol fuel cells has been found by using non-functionalized (Vulcan) and functionalized (Vulcan-F) carbon-supported Pd, PdSn, PdNi and PdNiSn anodic electrocatalysts (72). The compounds were produced by an impregnation-reduction method.

Thermogravimetric analysis (TGA) measurements of Vulcan showed characteristic weight losses which were attributed to the presence of surface functional groups due to the acid treatment. X-Ray diffraction (XRD) measurements showed that a higher degree of alloying is reached between Pd and Sn, whereas the Ni in PdNi and PdNiSn exists mostly segregated in the oxide form. TEM analysis indicates an agglomeration of Pd and PdSn particles, whereas a more uniform particle distribution is observed for PdNi and PdNiSn samples.

Cyclic voltammetry experiments showed that the onset potential is shifted towards negative values for binary and ternary samples supported on functionalized Vulcan (Vulcan-F), indicating that the ethanol oxidation is facilitated on the functionalized surface. Alkaline direct ethanol fuel cell tests revealed that the highest open-circuit voltage (VOC) and maximum power density can be achieved for the PdNiSn supported on Vulcan-F in which improved textural properties were found (72).

The structure and the electrochemical activity of Ag/C, Mn_3O_4/C and $AgMnO_2$/C electrocatalysts were investigated by transmission electron microscopy, energy dispersive X-ray spectroscopy, XRD, and cyclic voltammetry. The nanocatalysts displayed an ethanol-tolerance for the oxygen reduction reaction in 0.1 *M* KOH containing ethanol electrolytes at various temperatures (73).

All the electrocatalysts prevented the oxidation from ethanol crossover through the membrane from the anode to cathode compartments in alkaline direct ethanol fuel cells. $AgMnO_2$/C catalysts exhibited the best results toward the oxygen reduction reaction in the presence of alkaline ethanol electrolytes (73).

Gold Nanoparticles. Electrocatalysts for the ethanol oxidation reaction in direct ethanol fuel cells have been fabricated (74). A Pd coupled Au nanostructure was obtained, as a non-Pt group for catalysts for direct ethanol fuel cells.

The catalytic proficiency of the bimetallic nanoparticles with a size of 2–10 *nm* has been found to be strongly dependent on the ratio of palladium to gold.

The overvoltage is considerably reduced by around 260 mV with a content of 33% gold in the composition in comparison to palladium alone (74).

1.4 Direct Formate Fuel Cells

Direct formate fuel cells, which convert the chemical energy stored in formate directly into electricity, have attracted more attention, primarily because of the use of the carbon-neutral fuel and the low-cost electrocatalytic and membrane materials (75).

Also, the issues of formic acid-based fuel cells have been reviewed (76). Formic acid has emerged as a highly promising candidate for a commercially viable fuel cell feedstock owing to its favorable oxidation kinetics, thus enabling low operating temperatures, high theoretical cell potential and relatively mild fuel crossover problems (77,78). Catalysts for direct formic acid fuel cells, mainly Pt/Ru and Pt/Pd, have been described (79).

A hybrid structure of $Pd/WO_{2.72}$ with 5 nm Pd nanoparticles anchored on 50×5 nm $WO_{2.72}$ nanorods has been synthesized (80).

The strong $Pd/WO_{2.72}$ coupling results in the lattice expansion of Pd from 0.23 to 0.27 nm and to the decrease of Pd surface electron density. Thus, the $Pd/WO_{2.72}$ shows a much enhanced catalysis toward the electrochemical oxidation of formic acid in 0.1 M $HClO_4$. It shows no obvious activity loss after a 12 h chronoamperometry test at 0.4 V. In this way, the catalyst efficiency of Pd nanoparticles for energy conversion reactions can be enhanced (80).

As an emerging energy technology, direct formate fuel cells have been increasingly investigated. Currently, the state-of-the-art power density is 591 $mW\,cm^{-2}$ at 60°C (75).

The research on the development of this type of fuel cell has been reviewed, including the working principle, mechanisms and materials of the electrocatalytic oxidation of formate, singe-cell designs and performance, as well as innovative system designs (75).

Among various liquid fuels, formate has received increasing attention, primarily because of several advantageous characteristics in comparison to other fuels (75):

1. Formate is a carbon-neutral fuel that can be easily derived from the reduction of carbon dioxide via artificial photosynthesis (81,82),
2. The oxidation of formate is facile in alkaline media, particularly on the palladium (83),
3. The fuel cell running on formate has a theoretical potential of as high as 1.45 *V* with air or oxygen as oxidant, which is 0.24 *V* and 0.31 *V* higher than the fuel cells running on methanol and ethanol, respectively (84),
4. Unlike in acid media, there is no poisoning effect for the formate oxidation in alkaline media (85), and
5. Formate salts can be readily stored, transported, and handled in their solid state and can be easily dissolved in water to form a liquid fuel (86).

On the anode, the fuel solution, typically, formate salts and alkali dissolved in water and formate ions will be oxidized to generate electrons, water, and carbonate ions according to the following reaction:

$$HCOO^- + 3OH^- \rightarrow CO_3^- + 2H_2O + 2e^- \qquad (1.14)$$

On the cathode, the oxygen provided by the cathode flow field is reduced to produce hydroxide ions according to the following reaction:

$$\frac{1}{2}O_2 + H_2O + 2e^- \rightarrow 2OH^- \qquad (1.15)$$

This results in an overall reaction for this fuel cell system:

$$HCOO^- + \frac{1}{2}O_2 + OH^- \rightarrow CO_3^- + 2H_2O \qquad (1.16)$$

The electrocatalytic oxidation of formate on Pd has been studied using potential-sweep and galvanostatic methods (87).

It has been suggested that formate adsorbed on the Pd surface was decomposed into two fragments, such as an adsorbed hydrogen and a carboxyl ion:

$$HCOO^- \rightarrow COO^-_{adsorbed} + H_{adsorbed} \quad (1.17)$$

Also, it has been shown that the electrocatalytic oxidation of formate did not involve a strongly bound poisoning intermediate on the Pd surface.

The electrocatalytic activity of the formate oxidation on platinum is much lower than that on palladium. Therefore, only a few studies have been done using platinum and platinum-based catalysts as electrocatalytic materials for the formate oxidation in alkaline media.

The formate oxidation on platinum black modified electrodes under microbial fuel cell conditions at neutral pH, room temperature and in microbial culture solutions has been investigated (88). The electrode deactivation could be successfully prevented using an oxidative potential reactivation procedure. However, polymer coating fully stopped the formate oxidation.

A fuel cell has been developed using ammonium formate as fuel (89, 90). The electrocatalytic activity of ammonium formate on Pt and Pt–Ir was investigated using cyclic voltammetry. The Pt–Ir catalysts could effectively oxidize ammonium formate. An aqueous solution of ammonium formate showed a very high oxidation current. In particular, the oxidation peak values of ammonium formate were about 2 and 12 times those of formic acid and methanol, respectively. This means that ammonium formate has a very high oxidative activity. This can be explained by the fact that an aqueous solution of ammonium formate is almost neutral, which promotes dissociation, thus producing formate ions that contribute to the oxidation reaction. It was also found that the Pt–Pd catalysts can effectively oxidize ammonium formate (91).

A liquid-electrolyte-free direct formate fuel cell has been fabricated and tested using hydrogen peroxide as oxidant (92). On the anode, as a result of no addition of an alkali to the fuel solution, formate reacts with hydroxide ions to possibly generate electrons, water and bicarbonate ions according to:

$$HCOO^- + 2OH^- \rightarrow HCOO_3^- + H_2O + 2e^- \quad (1.18)$$

On the cathode, the hydrogen peroxide reduction reaction will take place in alkaline media as:

$$H_2O_2 + 2e^- \rightarrow 2OH^- \tag{1.19}$$

Membraneless direct formate fuel cells have been investigated that use highly selective electrocatalysts (85). This technique is simpler than that of conventional membraneless fuel cells achieved by non-mixing laminar flows. Here, Pd/C and Pd/C were used as anode and cathode catalysts, respectively.

The fuel solution containing HCOOK and KOH was fed through a chamber between the anode and cathode anode catalyst layers. The fuel solution flowing through the chamber not only sustains the migration of hydroxide ions, but also delivers reactants to the anode anode catalyst layer (85). The use of a flow chamber in fuel cells indeed avoids the need for inefficient and costly anion exchange membranes, simplifies the cell configuration, as well as lowers the system cost, but the flow chamber limits the power output due to the large gap between two electrodes.

1.5 Direct Urea Fuel Cells

Methanol has a high energy density, which is essential for portable direct methanol fuel cells, and is simpler to store and transport than conventional hydrogen as the fuel (51). However, methanol is not readily available, which makes waste an attractive option for a fuel source, resulting in the development of direct urea fuel cells. Fuel cells that use waste that contains hydrogen, like wastewater or urine, are attractive because of their potential to generate energy from low-cost, abundant sources (51).

Therefore, direct urea fuel cells have received a lot of attention in recent years because of the simple availability of urea as fuel and high hydrogen storage in this compound (93).

A direct urea fuel cell usually uses oxygen as the oxidant and the platinum catalysts as the cathode catalyst. It has been found that O_2 or even air can produce H_2O_2 *in-situ* under the action of a Pd catalyst.

A unique direct urea fuel cell was developed which uses H_2O_2 as the oxidant and Pd/C as the cathode catalyst. The results demonstrate that when H_2O_2 serves as the oxidant, the VOC and maximum power density of direct urea fuel cell are much higher than those of direct urea fuel cell with O_2 as the oxidant. Therefore, if O_2 or air can be *in-situ* converted to H_2O_2, the performance of the fuel cell can be greatly improved (93).

Three-dimensional $Ni(OH)_2$/Ni foam electrodes with low costs could be easily fabricated via a template-free growth method and employed as efficient anodes for a direct urea-hydrogen peroxide fuel cell (94). The surface morphologies of $Ni(OH)_2$ catalysts on the electrodes can be easily controlled by altering the reaction temperatures.

The reaction at the anode runs as (95):

$$\begin{array}{rcl} Ni(OH)_2 + OH^- & \rightarrow & NiOOH + H_2O + e^- \\ CO(HN_2)_2 + 6OH^- & \rightarrow & N_2 + 5H_2O + CO_2 + 6e^- \end{array} \tag{1.20}$$

and the reaction at the cathode runs as:

$$6H_2O + 6e^- \rightarrow 3H_2 + 6OH^- \tag{1.21}$$

The nanosheet $Ni(OH)_2$/Ni foam electrode exhibits the highest catalytic activity towards urea electrooxidation among the four electrodes. The oxidation current density of the nanosheet $Ni(OH)_2$/Ni foam electrode reaches 337 $mA\,cm^{-2}$ at 0.45 V (vs. Ag/AgCl) with a low onset oxidation potential in $0.6V$ urea and 5 $mol\,l^{-1}$ KOH solutions (94).

The direct urea-hydrogen peroxide fuel cell using nanosheet $Ni(OH)_2$/Ni foam anode shows a VOC of 0.86 V and high peak power density of 19.7 $mW\,cm^{-2}$ and 28.8 $mW\,cm^{-2}$ at 20°C and 50°C, respectively, which is much higher than the performance of direct urea fuel cells previously reported. The outstanding cell performance using a cheap nanosheet $Ni(OH)_2$/Ni foam anode indicates direct urea-hydrogen peroxide fuel cell is a promising new type of fuel cell (94).

Similarly, a three-dimensional porous nickel-cobalt (Ni–Co) film on nickel foam could be successfully prepared and further used as an efficient anode for direct urea-hydrogen peroxide fuel cell (96). By varying the cobalt/nickel mole ratios an optimized Ni–Co/Ni foam anode with a ratio of 80% could be obtained.

When human urine is directly fed as fuel, the direct urine-hydrogen peroxide fuel cell reaches a maximum power density of 7.5 $mW\,cm^{-2}$ with a VOC of 0.80 V at 20°C, showing a good application prospect in wastewater treatment (96).

Multilayer graphene-nickel nanocomposites were prepared for use as an anode in a direct urea fuel cell (97). Commercially available sugar was mixed with nickel(II) acetate tetrahydrate in distilled water and then calcined at 800°C for 1 h. The formation of multilayer graphene sheets decorated with nickel nanoparticles could be confirmed by a variety of spectroscopy methods.

In a passive direct urea fuel cell, the observed maximum power density was 4.06 × 10−3 $mW\,cm^{-2}$ with an open-circuit voltage of 0.197 V at room temperature (97).

1.6 Solid Oxide Fuel Cell Systems

The state-of-the-art in the field of solid oxide fuel cells has been described in a monograph. Specific subjects, such as protonic conductors, interconnects, electrocatalytic and catalytic processes and modeling have been detailed (98).

Solid oxide fuel cells have been considered as one of the most promising technologies for very high-efficiency electric energy generation from natural gas, both with simple fuel cell plants and with integrated gas turbine/steam turbine-fuel cell systems (99). The high temperature exhaust gas from these cells can be utilized in other cycles, i.e. Rankine and Brayton, for additional power generation or for heating and cooling purposes. The analysis showed that the resulting maximum efficiency of such combined systems can be up to 90%, depending upon the operating condition and configuration used (99).

Solid oxide fuel cells have emerged as energy conversion devices in achieving a high efficiency of more than 70% with regeneration. The critical components of solid oxide fuel cells include anode, electrolyte, and cathode. However, for a stack of individual solid oxide fuel cells, the evaluation of sealants and interconnects are also essential.

The material selection, fundamentals of operation and underlying mechanisms, processing, microstructural and phase characterization, and the functionality and performance of individual solid oxide fuel cell components have been presented in detail (100).

The major challenges and complexity in functional section of solid oxide fuel cell include (100):

1. Poisoning via sulfur and coke deposition, surface diffusion of adsorbate, and charge transfer at triple-phase boundary in anode,
2. Hindered O^{2-} migration that converts chemical energy into electrical energy in the solid electrolyte; thus, the creation of ion transfer channels, ease of O^{2-} migration, dissociation of vacancy around dopants, straining of lattice, and other factors, such as control of phase and its distribution, grain and grain boundary conductivity, become critical in designing the electrolytes for solid oxide fuel cells,
3. Multiple rate determining factors, such as geometry of active surfaces, and existence of overpotential, in cathode; therefore, comprehensive electrochemical impedance spectroscopy is required for the analysis of solid cathodes in solid oxide fuel cells,
4. Chemical incompatibility and instability in both oxidizing and reducing environments while matching the coefficient of thermal expansion in the interconnects in order to sustain the large number of thermal cycling during the operation of solid oxide fuel cells, and
5. Isolation of the fuel and oxidizing gases while matching the coefficient of thermal expansion of the anode, cathode and interconnects using sealant.

In addition, the glass transition of sealant dictates the maximum allowable working temperature of solid oxide fuel cells. Thus, the necessitated temporal progress in material selection along with a detailed insight into the conceptual role of thermodynamics and kinetics of surface/cell reactions, effect of phases and microstructure on conductivity, fuel flexibility and deterioration in performance of individual fuel cell components, and evolution of new materials have been coherently presented (100).

A solid oxide fuel cell system comprises a solid oxide fuel cell stack and a gas turbine engine (101, 102). The solid oxide fuel cell stack comprises a plurality of solid oxide fuel cells. The gas turbine engine consists of a compressor and a turbine. The compressor supplies oxidant to the cathodes of the fuel cells via an oxidant ejector and the oxidant ejector supplies a portion of the unused oxidant from the cathodes of the fuel cells back to the cathodes of the fuel cells with the oxidant from the compressor.

The fuel cell system further comprises an additional compressor, an electric motor arranged to drive the additional compressor, a cooler and a recuperator. The compressor supplies oxidant via the cooler to the additional compressor and the additional compressor supplies oxidant to the oxidant ejector via the recuperator. The solid oxide fuel cell stack supplies exhaust gases to the turbine and the turbine supplies the exhaust gases through the recuperator to heat the oxidant flowing through the recuperator (102).

1.6.1 Perovskite Oxides

Perovskite oxides play a substantial role in the delivery of sustainable energy among others as electrode or electrolyte components in solid oxide fuel cells (103).

The attractiveness of perovskite oxides arises from the possibility of incorporating different A-site and B-site metal elements into their $ABO_{3-\delta}$ lattice to form special compounds which allow the tailoring of the oxygen non-stoichiometry; and thus the oxygen ionic conductivity, the oxygen reduction reaction activity, and the electronic conductivity to fit a particular application.

The basic aspects and progress concerning these issues have been reviewed. Also, the advantages and limitations of perovskites in such applications have been discussed (103).

Quantum mechanics studies of electrode materials for solid oxide fuel cells have been presented (104).

Theoretically obtained insights into the oxygen ion conductivity in two classes of perovskite-type materials for solid oxide fuel cells applications have been detailed (104): The conventional

$La_{1-x}Sr_xMO_3$ family, with M = Cr, Mn, Fe, Co, along with a promising class of $Sr_2Fe_2-xMo_xO_6$ materials. The electronic structures for the two processes that govern ionic diffusion in these materials have been characterized:

1. Oxygen vacancy formation, and
2. Vacancy-mediated oxygen migration.

It could be shown, how the corresponding macroscopic oxygen diffusion coefficient can be accurately obtained in terms of microscopic quantities calculated with first-principles quantum mechanics. The oxygen vacancy formation energy is a robust descriptor for evaluating the properties of the oxide ion transport. There is a direct relationship with the transition metal-oxygen bond strength and the extent to which electrons left behind by the departing oxygen delocalize onto the oxygen sublattice (104).

1.6.2 Yttria-Stabilized Zirconia

Yttria-stabilized zirconia is a common material used as an electrolyte for high-temperature solid oxide fuel cells (105). Due to the high operating temperature, various design issues are arising.

Therefore, low- to intermediate-temperature solid oxide fuel cells have been developed. Ceria-based materials are among the best options for intermediate-temperature solid oxide fuel cells of 500–800°C.

The synthesis of a gadolinium-doped ceria electrolyte material has been reported. Two different techniques have been used, i.e., sol-gel and co-precipitation. Both techniques have the advantages of high phase purity, homogeneity and low processing temperatures along with strong control on crystallite size. The synthesized materials were characterized by XRD, SEM and other techniques. A cubic fluorite structure has been found for both synthesized compounds.

The co-precipitation synthesis resulted in better control of the crystallite size in comparison to the sol-gel method. The average particle size was found to be in the range of 40–70 *nm*. The electrical conductivity of the pellet was measured in the temperature range of 220–660°C in air and for the pellet synthesized by sol-gel method the highest conductivity value of 2.17 10^{-4} $S\,cm^{-1}$ at 600°C was found with an activation energy of 0.31 *keV* (105).

The anode of NiO and yttria-stabilized zirconia with straight open pores could be prepared by a phase-inversion tape casting method (106). In the so-prepared green tape, its top and middle layers are derived from a slurry of NiO and yttria-stabilized zirconia, while the bottom layer from a slurry of graphite.

The graphite layer can be eliminated by calcination at elevated temperatures, leaving the finger-like porous layer exposed to the gas phase. A cell supported on the as-prepared anode substrate exhibits satisfactory electrochemical performances with a maximum power density of 780 $mW\,cm^{-2}$ at 800°C. The cell does not show a convex-up curvature in I-V plots at high current density is often observed for most anode-supported cells. This indicates the absence of concentration polarization which is in turn attributed to the open pore structure of the phase-inversion derived anode.

The phase-inversion tape casting technique explored in the present study involves almost the same equipment and similar procedures as to conventional tape casting, and after further optimization it may become a simple and effective technique for mass production of anodes for solid oxide fuel cells (106).

1.6.3 *Anodized Aluminum Oxide*

An ultrathin film, low-temperature, high performing solid oxide fuel cell could be successfully fabricated on an anodized aluminum oxide supporting structure using atomic layer deposition (107). A dense and pinhole-free layer of hybrid platinum was applied to reduce the size of the substrate pores in order to facilitate the development of a dense electrolyte on the Pt electrode while maintaining the gaseous fuel access.

As a result, an about 180 nm thick yttria-stabilized zirconia electrolyte could be successfully deposited without pinholes. This ultrathin film, anodized aluminum oxide-supported fuel cell demonstrates the highest performance with a maximum power density of 380 $mW\,cm^{-2}$ at an operating temperature of 450°C (107).

1.6.4 *Copper-Modified Ceria Zirconia*

The activity of copper-modified ceria-zirconia-based anodes was investigated (108). The anodes were prepared through subsequent impregnation steps into a porous yttria-stabilized zirconia matrix. The ceria-zirconia oxide was reduced at increasing temperatures.

The effect of structural changes on anode performance was investigated at 973 K under humidified H_2. The performance of all the cells increased after one redox cycle due to a decrease of both the anode polarization and the ohmic resistance of the cell.

It was observed that subsequent redox cycles lead to an activation and stabilization of the electrodes. This is mainly attributable to a rearrangement of the morphology and microstructure of the CZ oxide at the electrode/electrolyte interface and to an improvement of copper distribution in the porous electrode matrix (108).

1.6.5 *Nanostructured Bilayer Solid Oxide Fuel Cell*

Obtaining high power density at low operating temperatures has been a continuous challenge in the field of solid oxide fuel cells, which are efficient engines to generate electrical energy from fuels (109).

A thin-film three-dimensional (3D) solid oxide fuel cell architecture has been described that can achieve a peak power density of 1.3 W cm^{-2} at 450°C. This is made possible by nanostructuring of the ultrathin (60 *nm*) electrolyte interposed with a nanogranular catalytic interlayer at the cathode/electrolyte interface.

The superior cell performance has been attributed to a significant reduction in both the ohmic and the polarization losses due to the combined effects of employing an ultrathin film electrolyte, enhancement of effective area by 3D architecture, and superior catalytic activity by the ceria-based interlayer at the cathode (109).

1.6.6 *Organic Waste Power Plant*

An organic waste power plant was designed that utilizes both anaerobic digestion and solid oxide fuel cell technologies (110).

Food waste and sewage sludge from a mid-sized Canadian municipality were modeled as a feedstock for anaerobic digestion. The biogas quality and quantity produced from the digestion process were determined by modeling the municipal waste's chemical composition and chemical oxygen demand content. Overall, between

480 *kW* and 1410 *kW* of electrical power can be produced from the solid oxide fuel cell system that is fueled by the biogas.

The compatibility of these two technologies has been demonstrated. The major challenges and benefits associated with implementing this concept have been discussed in detail. In summary, it has been demonstrated that an organic waste power plant is a sustainable solution for both the management of waste and the production of power (110).

1.6.7 Oriented Nanostructures

The role of nanostructured materials for the challenges in energy and natural resources has attracted wide attention (111). In particular, oriented nanostructures demonstrate promising properties for energy harvesting, conversion, and storage.

The synthesis and application of oriented nanostructures have been detailed for energy technologies, namely photovoltaics, batteries, supercapacitors, and thermoelectrics.

Although the applications differ from field to field, a common fundamental challenge is to improve the generation and transport of electrons and ions. The role of high surface area to maximize the surface activity has been highlighted and the importance of optimum dimension and architecture, controlled pore channels, and alignment of the nanocrystalline phase to optimize the transport of electrons and ions was discussed. Finally, the challenges in attaining integrated architectures to achieve the desired performance have been detailed. Brief background information is provided for the relevant technologies, but the emphasis is focused mainly on the nanoscale effects of mostly inorganic-based materials and devices (111).

1.6.8 Silicon-Based Nanothin Film Solid Oxide Fuel Cell

A silicon-based micro-solid oxide fuel cell with an electrolyte membrane array embedded in a thin silicon supporting membrane has been developed (112). The membrane features a unique edge reinforcement structure.

The device was fabricated with simple silicon micromachining processes. The square silicon supporting membrane, fabricated by combining deep reactive ion etching and through-wafer wet etching processes, has thicker edges and corners than the center portion of the membrane, which effectively improves the mechanical stability of the entire fuel cell array during cell fabrication and cell operation.

The 20 μm thick single crystalline silicon membrane supports a large number of 80 nm thick freestanding yttria-stabilized zirconia (YSZ) electrolytes. The fuel cell array was stably maintained at the VOC of 1.04 V for more than 30 h of operation at 350°C. A high peak power density of 317 $mW\,cm^{-2}$ was obtained at 400°C.

During a rigorous can be *in-situ* thermal cycling between 150°C and 400°C at a fast cooling and heating rate of 25 °C min^{-1} the VOC of the micro-solid oxide fuel cell recovered to its high value of 1.07 V without any drop caused by membrane failure, which justifies the superior thermal stability of this cell architecture (112).

1.6.9 *Nanoparticles-Loaded Cathode*

Reluctant oxygen-reduction-reaction (ORR) activity has been a long-standing challenge limiting cell performance for solid oxide fuel cells (SOFCs) in both centralized and distributed power applications. This challenge has been tackled with coloading of (La,Sr)MnO3 (LSM) and Y2O3 stabilized zirconia (YSZ) nanoparticles within a porous YSZ framework. This design dramatically improves the ORR activity, enhances fuel cell output (200–300% power improvement), and enables superior stability (no observed degradation within 500 h of operation) from 600 to 800 °C. The improved performance is attributed to the intimate contacts between nanoparticulate YSZ and LSM particles in the three-phase boundaries in the cathode (113).

1.6.10 *Direct Oxidation of Hydrocarbons in a Solid Oxide Fuel Cell*

The direct electrochemical oxidation of dry hydrocarbon fuels to generate electrical power has the potential to substantially accelerate the use of fuel cells in transportation and distributed power applications (114). Most fuel cell research has involved the use of hydrogen as the fuel, although the practical generation and storage of hydrogen remains an important technological hurdle.

Methane has been successfully oxidized electrochemically, but the susceptibility to carbon formation from other hydrocarbons that may be present or poor power densities have prevented the application of this simple fuel in practical applications. The direct, electrochemical oxidation of various hydrocarbons (methane, ethane, 1-butene, *n*-butane and toluene) have been reported, using a solid oxide fuel cell at 973 and 1,073 K with a composite anode of copper and ceria (or samaria-doped ceria).

It has been demonstrated that the final products of the oxidation are CO_2 and water, and that reasonable power densities can be achieved. The observation that a solid oxide fuel cell can be operated on dry hydrocarbons, including liquid fuels, without reforming, suggests that this type of fuel cell could provide an alternative to hydrogen-based fuel cell technologies (114).

1.7 Biological Fuel Cells

Biological fuel cells offer a clean, renewable and potentially autonomous source of energy in the same vein as other environmental power sources such as solar, geothermal, and wind (115). Biological fuel cells can be separated into two classes.

One class is termed enzymatic because they utilize isolated immobilized enzymes to deliver reducing equivalents to the electrode surface but usually require redox mediators to facilitate electron transfer.

The second class of biological fuel cells is addressed as microbial fuel cells. Microbial fuel cells rely upon the metabolic cycle of living bacteria to generate electrons that are then harvested by the anode and transferred to the cathode where a complementing reduction reaction occurs (115).

The technology involved in biological fuel cells is scalable, e.g., anode, cathode, fluidic chambers, microbe attachment to anode, and could potentially be used in both real-time aquatic and terrestrial applications.

However, the isolation and identification of thousands of bacterial species and their mutants or the activity of millions of enzymes with a wide variety of substrates is a difficult and time-consuming process with little to no standardization between one species and the next.

If the bacteria or enzymes are to be compared in an assay, it is important that a single electrode behaves like a reference electrode in the system, i.e., that the performance of the cathode from one test to another does not vary. It is important that this electrode is invariant so that changes in performance can be determined based entirely on the array performance, and therefore the performance of the biological species being tested.

The rapid identification of mutants or enzymes engineered for power production will ultimately have substantial applications, primarily as a method to enhance the power production capabilities of biological fuel cells.

In 1975 there was already an implantable fuel cell described in the patent literature (116). This cell was developed particularly for operating heartbeat actuators, or artificial hearts. The device utilized an oxidizable body substance, preferably glucose as fuel, and oxygen from the body fluids.

1.7.1 Miniature Biological Fuel Cell

Microbial electrochemical systems use microorganisms to covert the chemical energy stored in biodegradable materials to direct electric current and chemicals (117). Compared to the traditional treatment focused, energy-intensive environmental technologies, this technology offers a solution for integrated waste treatment and energy and resource recovery, because it offers a flexible platform for both oxidation and reduction reaction oriented processes.

Comprehensive reviews of all the different functions of microbial electrochemical cells and system constructions are available (117–119).

All the microbial electrochemical systems share one common principle in the anode chamber, in which biodegradable substrates, such as waste materials, are oxidized and generate electrical current. A great variety of applications have been developed by utilizing this *in-situ* current, such as direct power generation, microbial fuel cells, chemical production by microbial electrolysis cells, microbial electrosynthesis, microbial electrochemical system, or water microbial desalination cell systems (117).

Packages comprising autonomous electronic and electromechanical systems that are implanted in the body of animals, such as sensors and their associated electronic circuits that function to amplify the sensor signals and transmit them to a nearby receiver, require a power source.

These packages have been powered externally by batteries. The smallest batteries are, however, much larger than the implantable sensors and their associated signal amplifier circuits. For this reason, the size of autonomous packages that include a sensor, an amplifier-transmitter, and a power source are generally defined by the battery. Batteries cannot be made as small as the sensors or amplifiers because the batteries require cases and seals, the miniaturization of which is difficult and prohibitively expensive.

Biological fuel cells, also known as biofuel cells, have received much attention in past years. Herein, the term *biological fuel cell* or *biofuel cell* refers to an electrochemical cell having performance attributes that permit its use as a power source for an implanted device in a biological system, such as an animal, including a human or a plant.

Biological fuel cells generate electrical energy using the components found in biological systems such as sugars, alcohols, carboxylic acids, carbohydrates, starches, cellulose, and oxygen.

Such devices have been disclosed and discussed (120, 121).

Numerous biofuel cells have been described in the past. However, only a few of these biofuel cells can operate under physiological conditions, which are the conditions relevant to operation in the body of an animal. Physiological conditions include, for instance, a pH of about 7.2–7.4, a temperature of near 37°C, and a chloride concentration of about 0.14 *M*.

Miniature biofuel cells having oxygen electroreducing cathodes and glucose electrooxidizing anodes are of current interest because such cells may power future autonomous electronic and electromechanical systems implanted in a biological system, and particularly, the human body.

A fuel cell has been provided with an anode and a cathode (122). A membrane is not necessary in these fuel cells by the virtue of two special electrocatalysts. One electrocatalyst is immobilized on the surface of the anode and the other is immobilized on the surface of the cathode.

The anode electrocatalyst is a poor catalyst for oxygen reduction and the cathode electrocatalyst is a poor catalyst for oxidation of the fuel of the cell, such as glucose. In other words, the anode electrocatalyst is so selective for the fuel of the cell, that oxygen is not rapidly electroreduced at the anode, even though the anode is poised at a potential that is much more reducing than the potential of the cathode, where oxygen is reduced. Furthermore, the cathode electrocatalyst is so selective for oxygen, that the fuel of the cell is not rapidly electrooxidized at the cathode, even though the cathode is poised at a potential that is much more oxidizing than the potential of the anode, where the cell fuel is electrooxidized. As a result, the current loss associated with the oxidation of the cell fuel at the cathode, and the current loss associated with the reduction of oxygen at the anode, are both small.

The anode enzyme is preferably an oxidase or a dehydrogenase. The cathode enzyme is a copper-containing enzyme, such as a laccase, an ascorbate oxidase, a ceruloplasmine, or a bilirubin oxidase. One category of suitable enzymes includes thermostable enzymes.

Examples of thermostable enzymes are listed in Table 1.5.

The enzymes can be immobilized in silica polymeric matrices made by sol-gel processes, such as the hydrolysis of tetramethoxysilane or another poly(alkoxysilane) that contains one or more silicon atoms. The condensation of the resulting silanol in the presence of the enzyme results in an entrapment of the enzyme.

This process has been referred to as sol-gel immobilization. Binding of enzymes in silica or other inorganic polymeric matrices formed from sol-gels can stabilize the enzyme. Entrapment of glucose oxidase, a glycoprotein, in a silica sol-gel matrix greatly improves the stability of the enzyme, which retains activity when heated in water to 98°C for 10 *min*.

In general, the addition of a polycation, such as, poly(1-vinyl imidazole) or poly(ethylene imine), prior to the sol-gel immobilization process stabilizes the enzyme. Preferably, the added polycation is a more basic polyelectrolyte than the enzyme. Enzymes with high isoelectric points often need more basic polyelectrolytes for stabilization. Poly(ethylene imine) is more basic than poly(1-vinyl imidazole) (123).

Typically, the polymers used for the redox polymers have nitrogen-containing heterocyclic units, such as pyridine, imidazole, or derivatives thereof, for binding, as ligands to the redox species (123). Suitable polymers for the complexation with redox species, such as

Table 1.5 Thermostable enzymes (123).

Compound	Origin
Laccase	*Myceliophthora thermophila*
Cytochrome C peroxidase	Thermophilic bacterium PS3 and *Thermus thermophilus*
Peroxidase	Soybean
Pyranose oxidase	White rot fungus *Phlebiopsis gigantea*
L-Lactate dehydrogenase	Bacillus
Malate dehydrogenase	Thermus species (expressed in E. coli)
Glucose oxidase	*Aspergillus*
Microbial pyruvate oxidase	
Urate oxidase	Bacillus
α-Amylase	*Bacillus stearothermophilus*
β-Amylase	*Aspergillus*
Glucan-1,4-α-glucosidase	*Rhizopus niveus*
Cellulase	*Aspergillus niger*
endo-1-3(4)-β-Glucanase	*Aspergillus niger*
Dextranase	*Leuconostoc mesenteroides*
α-Glucosidase	*Bacillus stearothermophilus*
β-Glucosidase	*Caldocellum saccharolyticum*
β-Galactosidase	*Aspergillus*
β-Fructofuranosilidase	Yeast
Lactase	*Aspergillus oryzae*

the transition metal complexes, include polymers and copolymers of poly(1-vinyl imidazole) and poly(4-vinyl pyridine), as well as polymers and copolymer of poly(acrylic acid) (PAA) or poly(acrylamide) that have been modified by the addition of pendant nitrogen-containing heterocyclic units, such as pyridine and imidazole.

The modification of PAA may be performed by reaction of at least a portion of the carboxylic acid functionalities with an aminoalkylpyridine or aminoalkylimidazole, such as 4-ethylaminopyridine, to form amides. Suitable copolymer substituents include acrylonitrile, acrylamide, acrylhydrazide, cf. Figure 1.13, and substituted or quaternized *N*-vinyl imidazole. The copolymers can be random or block copolymers (123).

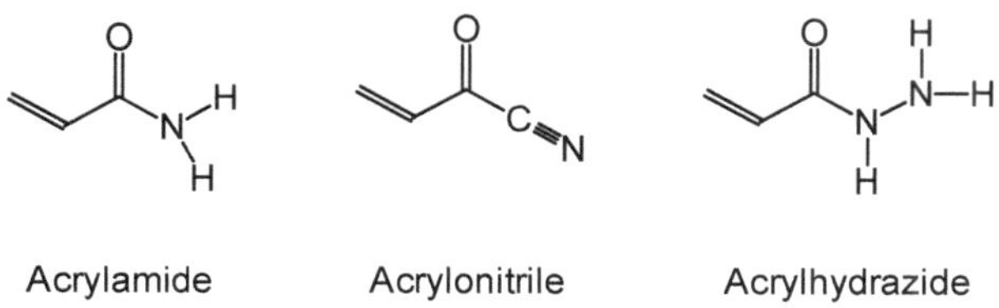

Figure 1.13 Acrylonitrile, Acrylamide, Acrylhydrazide.

A variety of methods can be used to immobilize the redox polymer on an electrode surface. One method is adsorptive immobilization. This method is particularly useful for redox polymers with relatively high molecular weights. The molecular weight of a polymer may be increased, for example, by crosslinking.

The polymer of the redox polymer may contain functional groups, such as, for example, hydrazide, amine, alcohol, heterocyclic nitrogen, vinyl, allyl, and carboxylic acid groups, that can be crosslinked with a crosslinking agent. These functional groups may be provided on the polymer or one or more of the copolymers. Alternatively or additionally, the functional groups may be added by a reaction, such as, for example, quaternization. One example is the quaternization of poly(4-vinyl pyridine) with bromoethylamine groups.

The miniaturization of the biological fuel cell is possible, because the cell does not have corroding or corrosive components (124). Also, the cell reactants react much faster at their respective electrodes than at their respective counter electrodes.

The fuel cell can be used in connection with a biological system, such as a human, as it may operate at physiological conditions. By virtue of its size and operability at physiological conditions, the fuel cell is of particular interest for applications calling for a power source implanted in a human body, such as a variety of medical applications (122).

Several examples have been reported to demonstrate the function of biological fuel cells (125,126)

1.7.2 Cellulose Pellicles

Electrically conducting composite membranes were prepared by incorporating carboxylic multiwalled carbon nanotubes into bacterial cellulose pellicles (127). The biocathode and bioanode were prepared by a simple method of adsorption. An enzymatic biological fuel cell composed of a biocathode and an enzymatic bioanode was developed.

The materials were characterized by field emission scanning electron microscope (FESEM), Fourier transform infrared spectroscopy and TGA. The presence of multiwalled carbon nanotubes on biocathode was certified. Here, the loading of multiwalled carbon nanotubes was calculated as 30.02/100 g.

The enzyme biological fuel cell showed an excellent performance with the largest open-circuit voltage of 0.76 V and a maximum power density value of 55 $\mu W\,cm^{-3}$. In addition, the cell exhibited acceptable stability over the recording period of 30 d (127).

1.7.3 Nanoporous Filters

The use of proton exchange membranes in biological fuel cells limits the diversity of novel designs for increasing output power or enabling autonomous function in unique environments (128).

Some selected nanoporous polymer filters (nylon, cellulose, or poly(carbonate)) can be used effectively in place of proton exchange membranes in a miniature microbial fuel cell, a device with a cross section 2 cm^2, a generating power density of 16 Wm^{-3} with an uncoated graphite felt oxygen reduction reaction cathode.

The incorporation of poly(carbonate) or nylon membranes into biological fuel cell designs produce comparable power and durability to Nafion-117 membranes. Also, high power densities for novel larger (5 cm^3 anode volume, 0.6 Wm^{-3}) and smaller (0.025 cm^3 projected geometric volume, average power density 10 Wm^{-3}) chamberless and pumpless microbial fuel cells were observed.

It turned out that there was an additional benefit, as the nanoporous membranes isolate the anode from invading natural bacteria, thus increasing the potential applications for a miniature microbial fuel cell beyond aquatic sediment environments (128).

1.7.4 *Paper-Based Fuel Cell*

Biological fuel cells have been developed that use a paper-based fuel delivery layer which delivers fuel to the biological anode and cathode via capillary action or evaporation (129).

The paper-based fuel cell is formed by stacking a series of flexible and mechanically robust thin-film layers to form a single self-supporting multi-lamellar stack.

The order of stacking and the composition of the thin-film layers depends on the intended function of the device. Accordingly, the various thin films may be formed from cellulose, regenerated cellulose membranes, polyester, vinyl, poly(styrene), poly(carbonate), poly(tetrafluoroethylene), nitrocellulose, poly(dimethylsiloxane) (silicone rubber) Nafion, Tegaderm, Toray paper, Buckeye paper, and chemically functionalized variants of these thin films, including functionalization with carbon nanotubes, carbon black, graphite, and enzymes (129).

1.7.5 *Fuel Cell Utilizing Mitochondria*

Mitochondria are the power plants of most eucaryotic cells because of their ability to generate energy used by the cell (130). The biology of mitochondria is well known and understood. Mitochondria feature an outer membrane, a highly folded inner membrane, an intermembrane space and a matrix space enclosed by the inner membrane.

Furthermore the techniques for harvesting mitochondria are understood and defined. Importantly, mitochondria can provide a source of hydrogen ion or electrons that may participate in the oxidation-reduction reaction with other materials to provide an electric flow.

While mitochondria offer a potential near limitless source of power, their actual capacity to produce power, and in particular direct current electricity, is not well known or understood.

Pyruvate or succinate or other derivatives of pyruvate may be used as the mitochondrial fuel. Gold, carbon, polymeric or other inert, electronically conductive electrode substrates are used to collect the electrons from mitochondria.

The devices have been found ideal for implantable, renewable power sources because mitochondria are already present in eucaryotic cells, and the larger biological systems that they populate. Harnessing electric energy from mitochondria could save considerable costs associated with isolation and implantation of enzymes.

A bio-hybrid cell incorporates an organic/biological electrode composition for at least one of the anode or cathode.

The power cell includes a cathode, an anode separated by a separator within a container. The container is filled with an electrolyte. The cell produces a direct current that is coupled to a load via leads.

One or both of the cathode and the anode include a biological component. For example, the cathode or the anode may include a layer or formation of mitochondria on a substrate such as glass, metal-plated glass or metal (130).

1.7.6 Grafting of Biomolecules onto Microbial Fuel Cells

A method for enhancing a microbial environment for a fuel cell has been presented (131). The method includes the initial step of oxidizing the outer surface of the fuel cell anode to establish reactive chemical functional groups. The anode surface can be oxidized by washing the anode with a solution of 4-carboxybenzene diazonium tetrafluoroborate, followed by washing with acetone, methanol and water. Once the anode surface has been oxidized, it follows the step of binding a surface graft matrix to the reactive chemical functional groups, i.e., the activated carboxyl groups on the anode surface.

1-Ethyl-3-(3-dimethylaminopropyl) carbodiimide and *N*-hydroxysuccinimide or sulfo-*N*-hydroxysuccinimide can be used to establish a surface graft matrix in order to bind to the activated carboxyl groups. These compounds are shown in Figure 1.14

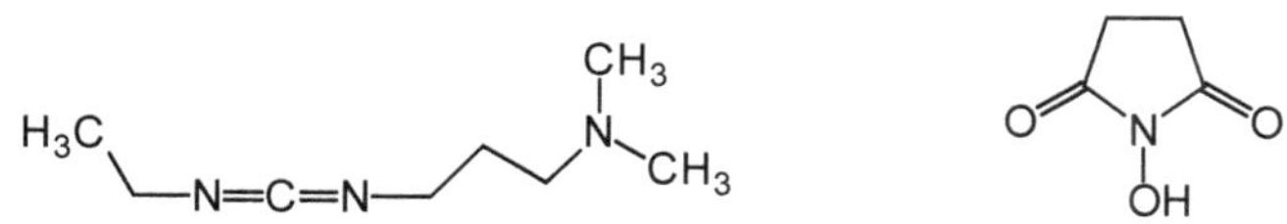

1-Ethyl-3-(3-dimethylaminopropyl) carbodiimide   *N*-Hydroxysuccinimide

Figure 1.14 Compounds for surface grafting.

A biological substance, such as a biological agent or biomolecule, can be chemically attached to the outer terminal reactive groups of the surface graft matrix. The result is a microbial fuel cell with increased power generation and durability properties. The biological agent can be selected from the group consisting of bacteria, toxins, fungi, antigens and antibodies. Also, the biological substance can be a biomolecule selected from the group of polysaccharides, proteins, lipids, nucleic acids and enzymes. One such molecule is chitosan, which can be used in applications where the microbial fuel cell is to be positioned within a body of water for an extended period of time (131).

1.7.7 Biosupercapacitor

A biological supercapacitor comprises a biocathode, a bioanode, a barrier which may comprise a separator positioned between the biocathode and the bioanode, and an electrolytic fuel fluid (132). Both of the electrodes may comprise a carbon element, for example, metallic, glassy carbon or other conventional electrode surfaces onto which one or more enzymes may be immobilized.

The bioelectrodes may comprise buckypaper of various thicknesses (15–250 μm), with a purity of 100% MWNTs.

The carbon nanotube layer can be well dispersed in a redox-polymer-enzyme matrix for mediated charge transfer. Enzymes of a bioelectrode catalyze the redox reactions. The bioelectrode may also be fabricated with the enzymes covalently bonded to the matrix, or attached with an immobilizer, like a linker protein, in which case they may require mediators in the electrolyte fuel fluid to transfer the charge.

The multilayers can also be made from a modified Nafion, bonded redox enzymes, and mediators like poly(methylene green). The bioelectrode material may also be fastened to a metal disk or plate, such as steel, aluminum, copper, or another metal. A separator is positioned between the biocathode and the bioanode. In separating the bioanode from the biocathode, two chambers are defined.

The biological supercapacitor may further comprise an electrically conductive current collector element immobilized with a biological electron donor or acceptor. In some embodiments, the electrically conductive current collector element may consist of nickel, copper, aluminum, titanium, or combinations thereof.

The current collector element may be connected to elements in a circuit, such as: A comparator with hysteresis, microgenerator, active balance circuit, boost converter, single or paired (p-channel) metal-oxide-semiconductor field-effect transistors.

The fabrication of the bioanode may be achieved by immobilizing lactate oxidase on a laser-cut buckypaper anode by mixing the enzymes with a linear poly(ethylenimine) hydrogel and a crosslinking agent.

A variety of biomolecules may be used as fuel. Examples include sugars, such as sucrose, glucose, and fructose; alcohols, such as methanol, ethanol, and glycerol, further acids, such as pyruvate and lactate, and fatty acids (132).

1.7.8 Biological Clean Fuel Processing Systems

Methods for biological carbon capture and conversion systems have been developed and also methods to remove carbon dioxide from emissions (133). A carbon capture process can be integrated into existing fossil fuel combustion sources, including combustion power plants and natural gas-fueled fuel cell plants as a biological carbon capture and conversion system to remove carbon dioxide from emissions.

The resulting biomass produced may be reprocessed as fertilizer, feedstock, biofuel, or the like or may even be directly injected into the combustion facility (such as perhaps in co-fired applications). It is a goal of the present invention to utilize carbon dioxide as a value-added product of fossil-fuel power plants rather than a production-limiting waste product. In this way the carbon originally released from coal combustion can be captured and recycled in perhaps a closed-loop system, thus significantly lowering overall carbon emissions and even improving plant efficiency (133).

1.7.9 Filtration-Active Fuel Cell

Membrane filtration is among the most important methods used for the separation of materials, and various membrane processes are available (134). These basically are distinguished according to their retention capability and the driving force to be applied.

Depending on the respective field of use, microfiltration, ultrafiltration (UF), nanofiltration (NF) and reverse osmosis (RO) are employed in the field of water and wastewater treatment, with these membrane processes being classified according to their retention capability based on the respective pore size or the cut-off value. The cut-off value or molecular weight cut-off (MWCO) is used in membrane technology to characterize ultrafiltration and nanofiltration membranes and also reverse osmosis in respect to their retention capability.

Membrane filtration is a key technology in the field of water and wastewater treatment, in particular for applications in which the purified wastewater has to be reused, for example in a production process. The process is based on the combination of a biological purification stage in which the biological water contamination is degraded microbially aerobically or else anaerobically, with a subsequent membrane separation in which the bacterial biomass is separated from the purified wastewater and retained in the bioreactor.

Such systems are also referred to as membrane bioreactors or membrane activation reactors (MAR). The great retention capability of membrane filtration results in a high sludge maturity and thus a water which has been purified to a high degree and is largely free of particles and germs. Thus, for example, a completely closed water circuit can be realized in an industrial production process. The MAR technology is accordingly a widely used alternative to conventional purification processes in industrial wastewater purification.

In particular, a fuel cell for the filtration of fluids, in particular of liquids, also referred to as filtration-active fuel cell, comprising a filtration-active, electrically conductive membrane layer which simultaneously represents the anode of the fuel cell, a cathode which is preferably an air-breathing cathode, a fluid-permeable separator which separates the cathode spatially and electrically from the anode and an active species which is capable of oxidizing materials which are present in the feed and serve as energy carriers and transfer the electrons liberated to the anode, has been provided (134).

1.7.10 *Sustainable Wastewater Treatment*

The increasing concerns of water resource are becoming an important issue as a severe shortage of water has been seen throughout the world (135). The integrated processes for wastewater treatment based on the principle of microbial fuel cells have been reviewed (135, 136).

Microbial fuel cells have been studied as a promising technology to achieve a sustainable wastewater treatment (137, 138).

Various review papers have been published on microbial fuel cell configuration, substrates, electrode materials, separators and microbiology.

Microbial fuel cells can be rationally incorporated into the treatment process. The integration of microbial fuel cells into other treatment technologies has been proposed (138).

A 120 *l* microbial electrolysis cell was operated on site in Northern England, using raw domestic wastewater to produce virtually pure hydrogen gas for a period of more than 3 months (139). It could be demonstrated that this technology is capable of energy capture as hydrogen gas from low-strength domestic wastewater at ambient temperature.

Also, an electrochemical membrane bioreactor has been developed for the recovery of energy from wastewater and meantime harvest clean water for reuse (140). The bioreactor is shown in Figure 1.15.

With the help of the microorganisms in the biocatalysis and biodegradation process, net electricity could be recovered from a low-strength synthetic wastewater after estimating total energy consumption of this system. In addition, high-quality clean water could be obtained for reuse.

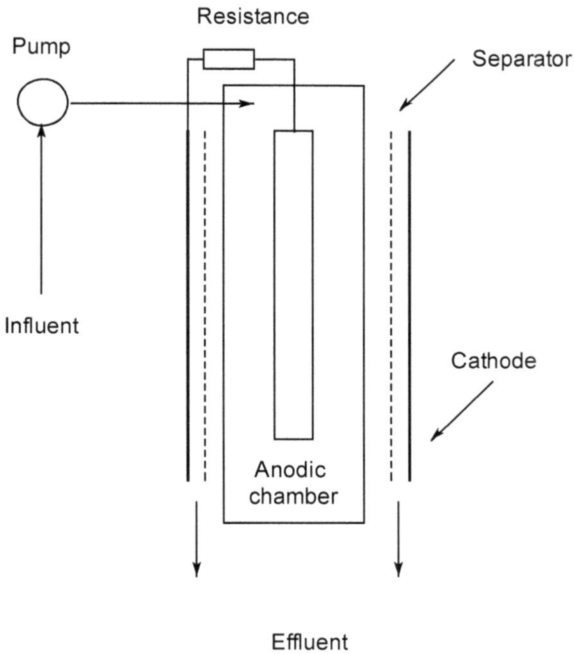

Figure 1.15 Schematic view of a bioreactor for wastewater treatment (140).

The results of this study clearly demonstrated that under optimized operating conditions, it is possible to recover net energy from wastewater, while at the same time to harvest high-quality effluent for reuse with this wastewater treatment system (140).

A bioelectrochemical membrane reactor is a promising technology, which is an integration of microbial fuel cell into a membrane bioreactor (141). It has the benefit of harvesting electricity, while biologically treating any type of wastewater to the highest extent while passing wastewater through anaerobic, aerobic, and integrated membrane compartments in a successive manner.

Various types of wastewaters have been examined as substrates for feeding bacteria in microbial fuel cells (142). The number and complexity of wastewaters have increased rapidly over the last few years, thus necessitating further documentation of this data.

In addition, various wastewater substrates that have been used in microbial fuel cells have been summarized (142, 143). The performance of different types and designs of microbial fuel cells in terms of electric current and power outputs together with the wastewater treatment efficiency in terms of chemical oxygen demand removal and coulombic efficiency have been detailed. Also, some of the challenges and future perspectives with regard to the energy recovery from wastewaters using microbial fuel cells have been discussed.

The long-term performance of a 20 *l* continuous flow microbial fuel cell for the treatment of brewery wastewater has been investigated (144).

No catalysts, Nafion or an ion exchange membrane were used. Actually, the system could be operated with brewery wastewater for nearly a year (144).

Also, a long-term investigation of an electrochemical membrane bioreactor for low-strength municipal wastewater treatment has been documented (145).

At lower temperatures below 10°C up to 15°C, the power production in the reactor was negligible. With the water temperatures over 15 to 20°C, efficient redox reactions were achieved in the reactor, which subsequently resulted in reduction of sludge of 27.3% and an alleviation of the membrane fouling process (145).

A combined approach of treating domestic wastewater using microbial fuel cell and a membrane bioreactor has been developed as a promising and reliable technology for wastewater treatment (146).

The treatment of wastewater in a single-stage microbial fuel cell is limited for achieving the required treatment efficiency and utilizing the effluent for irrigation or any other possible reuse without further treatment.

Therefore, a two-stage continuous process has been developed for the treatment of medium strength industrial wastewater combining microbial fuel cell and submerged membrane bioreactor, resulting in recovery of high quality effluent through ultrafiltration membrane (146).

Actually, the two-stage system can effectively treat medium strength organic wastewater in terms of chemical oxygen demand and removal of total suspended solids, thus producing a high-quality effluent. However, the energy demand for this treatment process is considerably high in comparison to the electrical energy produced by the microbial fuel cell (146).

1.7.11 *Hybrid Biological Fuel Cell*

1.7.11.1 *Microbial Anode for Lactate Oxidation*

A hybrid biological fuel cell with a microbial anode for lactate oxidation and an enzymatic cathode for oxygen reduction was constructed and tested in a marine environment (147).

Shewanella oneidensis DSP-10 was cultivated in a laboratory medium and then fixed on a carbon felt electrode via a silica sol-gel process in order to catalyze the anodic fuel cell processes. The cathode electrocatalyst was composed of a bilirubin oxidase, fixed to a carbon nanotube electrode using a heterobifunctional crosslinking agent, and then stabilized with a silica sol-gel coating.

The anode and cathode half-cells showed operating potentials of -0.44 *V* and 0.48 *V*, respectively, vs. Ag/AgCl. The hybrid biological fuel cell maintained a reproducible open-circuit voltage of greater then 0.7 *V* for 9 *d* under laboratory conditions and a sustained electrocatalytic activity for greater than 24 *h* in open environment tests (147).

1.7.11.2 *Hybrid Power Strip*

A flexible hybrid biofuel cell power strip has been developed for use in low power applications of less than one Watt, such as trickle charging to extend the charge of conventional batteries or to power devices such as microsensors, micropumps, and miniaturized medical devices (148).

The power strip anode contains carbon nanotubes that transfer electrons directly from the active center of the oxidation-reduction (redox) enzyme to a flexible, conductive anode substrate. This allows the building of surface architectures with pore structures customized for specific applications and enzyme substrate-containing media. The cathode comprises a catalytic layer of transition metal nanoparticle catalyst in contact with air or another source of oxygen. The flexibility of the power strip allows it to be shaped into a wide variety of conformations and applications, including attachment to or implantation within living organisms.

The anode comprises one or more redox enzymes, such as glucose oxidase or laccase alone or in combination linked to a flexible anode substrate such as carbon paper or conducting polymer sheet, through an integrated carbon nanotube/polymer network. The surfaces of the nanotubes may be functionalized with carboxylate or amine groups, which can be used to form covalent linkages with redox enzyme. The presence of background polymer backbone enhances enzyme stability and can immobilize nanotubes and redox enzyme to the flexible anode through covalent or noncovalent interactions. Exemplary polymers include charged poly(ethylene imine) or poly(*p*-phenylene ethylene) with functional side chains.

The nanotube/polymer platform can immobilize and stabilize various redox enzymes. The anode support material can be conducting support such as carbon paper, printed carbon ink on polymer, or a conducting polymer or a nonconducting polymer such as Nafion membrane polymer. If a nonconducting support such as Nafion is used, the polymer/nanotube/enzyme matrix serves as the conducting material.

The 3D pore structures of the carbon nanotube/polymer network can exhibit large surface-to-volume ratios that enhance the catalytic reaction rates. The electrode provides a direct electron transfer between the reactive center in the redox enzyme and the flexible anode substrate. This allows the biofuel cell anode to operate at negative potentials close to the redox potential of the flavin adenine dinucleotide/flavin adenine dinucleotide H2 coenzyme normally used with glucose oxidase (148). Flavin adenine dinucleotide is shown in Figure 1.16. The specific properties can be found in the literature (149).

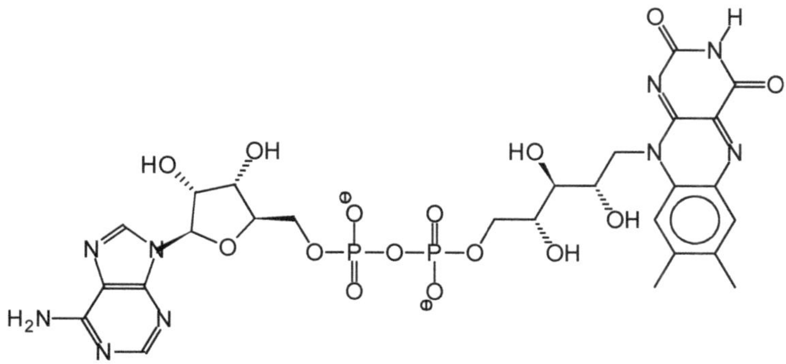

Figure 1.16 Flavin adenine dinucleotide.

A power strip prototype with an area of approximately 2 cm^2 was built and demonstrated to generate electricity from glucose using glucose oxidase as the anodic enzyme (148).

1.7.12 High Durability Fuel Cell Components with Cerium Salt Additives

A fuel cell membrane electrode assembly has been developed comprising a polymer electrolyte membrane which contains a polymer with bound anionic functional groups, wherein the polymer electrolyte membrane additionally comprises cerium cations (150).

Typically, the amount of cerium cations present is between 0.02 and 0.05 charge equivalents based on the molar amount of anionic functional groups present in the polymer electrolyte.

The distribution of cerium cations across the thickness of the polymer electrolyte membrane is uniform. Typically the cations are Ce^{3+} cations or Ce^{4+} cations (150).

It is believed that at least a portion of the cerium cations persist in the polymer electrolyte because they are exchanged with H^+ ions from the anion groups of the polymer electrolyte and become associated with those anion groups. Furthermore, it is believed that polyvalent cerium cations may form crosslinks between anion groups of the polymer electrolyte, further adding to the stability of the polymer. The membrane is a copolymer of tetrafluoroethylene and $FSO_2-CF_2CF_2CF_2CF_2-O-CF=CF_2$.

1.7.13 *Reserve Power Source*

A biological fuel cell was constructed in which the metabolism of glucose by yeast provided the electrons (151). A two-compartment plexiglass fuel cell was constructed with platinum electrodes separated by a proton-conducting membrane. One half of the cell contained yeast, *Saccharomyces cerevisiae*, glucose, and an electron mediator, methylene blue.

The other half contained an electron acceptor, potassium ferricyanide. Electrons produced during the metabolism of glucose by the yeast were captured by the methylene blue and transferred to the platinum electrode, travelled through the external circuit to the cathode compartment, and were finally accepted by the potassium ferricyanide. When yeast was added to the fuel cell, the open-circuit potential was ca. 0.5 V. The electric current was measured while holding the cell voltage at 0.3 and 0.1 V.

The electric current output was optimized for the initial concentration of yeast, temperature, glucose concentration, agitation and oxygen content. The optimum conditions for producing current within the scope of this study were obtained with agitated, partially oxygenated electrolyte at 45°C containing 0.1 M glucose (151).

1.7.14 *Performance of a Yeast-Mediated Biological Fuel Cell*

Saccharomyces cerevisiae present in common Baker's yeast was used in a microbial fuel cell in which glucose was the carbon source (152). Methylene blue was used as the electrophore in the anode compartment, while potassium ferricyanide and methylene blue were tested as electron acceptors in the cathode compartment. Methylene blue is shown in Figure 1.17.

Microbes in a mediator-free environment were used as the control. The experiment was performed in both open and closed circuit configurations under different loads ranging from 100 kO to 400 O. The eucaryotic *S. cerevisiae*-based fuel cell showed improved performance when methylene blue and ferricyanide were used as electron

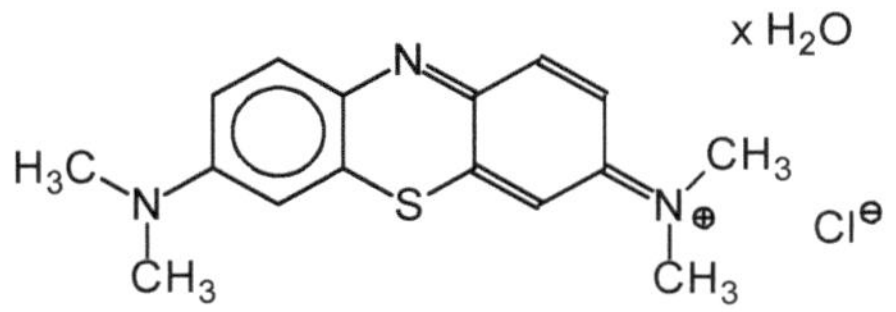

Figure 1.17 Methylene blue.

mediators, rendering a maximum power generation of 146.71 ± 7.7 mWm^{-3}. The fuel cell generated a maximum VOC of 383.6 ± 1.5 mV and recorded a maximum efficiency of 28 ± 1.8 % under 100 kO of external load (152).

1.7.15 One-Compartment Fructose/Air Biological Fuel Cell

The construction of a one-compartment fructose/air biological fuel cell based on direct electron transfer has been described (153). The biological fuel cell uses bilirubin oxidase and *D*-fructose dehydrogenase adsorbed on a cellulose-multiwall carbon nanotube matrix, reconstituted with an ionic liquid, as the biocathode and the bioanode for oxygen reduction and fructose oxidation reactions, respectively.

The performance of the bioelectrode was investigated by chronoamperometric and cyclic voltammetric techniques in a standard three-electrode cell, and the polarization and long-term stability of the biological fuel cell was tested by potentiostatic discharge. A VOC of 663 mV and a maximum power density of 126 μWcm^{-2} were obtained in buffer at pH 5.0. Using this regenerated cellulose-multiwall carbon nanotube matrix as the immobilization platform, this biological fuel cell has shown a relatively high performance and long-term stability (153).

References

1. R. O'Hayre, S.-W. Cha, W. Colella, and F.B. Prinz, *Fuel Cell Fundamentals*, John Wiley & Sons Inc, Hoboken, New Jersey, 3rd edition, 2016.
2. J. Larminie, A. Dicks, and M.S. McDonald, *Fuel Cell Systems Explained*, J. Wiley Chichester, UK, 2nd edition, 2003.

3. C.M. Branco, S. Sharma, M.M. de Camargo Forte, and R. Steinberger-Wilckens, *Journal of Power Sources*, Vol. 316, p. 139, 2016.
4. K.D. Kreuer, ed., *Fuel cells: Selected Entries from the Encyclopedia of Sustainability Science and Technology*, Springer, New York, 2013.
5. B.C. Ong, S.K. Kamarudin, and S. Basri, *International Journal of Hydrogen Energy*, Vol. 42, p. 10142, 2017.
6. B. Smitha, S. Sridhar, and A.A. Khan, *Journal of Membrane Science*, Vol. 259, p. 10, 2005.
7. M. Hotta, Sealing material for solid polymer fuel cell separator, separator seal and separator, US Patent Application 20 170 005 347, assigned to Shin-Etsu Chemical Co., Ltd., Tokyo (JP), January 5, 2017.
8. S.-G. Kim and S.-J. Lee, *Journal of Power Sources*, Vol. 230, p. 101, 2013.
9. M. Mench, *Fuel Cell Engines*, John Wiley & Sons, Hoboken, N.J, 2008.
10. T.E. Springer, T.A. Zawodzinski, and S. Gottesfeld, *Journal of the Electrochemical Society*, Vol. 138, p. 2334, 1991.
11. K. Tüber, D. Pócza, and C. Hebling, *Journal of Power Sources*, Vol. 124, p. 403, 2003.
12. X.G. Yang, F.Y. Zhang, A.L. Lubawy, and C.Y. Wang, *Electrochemical and Solid-State Letters*, Vol. 7, p. A408, 2004.
13. K. Nishida, T. Murakami, S. Tsushima, and S. Hirai, *Journal of Power Sources*, Vol. 195, p. 3365, 2010.
14. S. Tsushima, K. Teranishi, and S. Hirai, *Electrochemical and Solid-State Letters*, Vol. 7, p. A269, 2004.
15. R. Satija, D.L. Jacobson, M. Arif, and S.A. Werner, *Journal of Power Sources*, Vol. 129, p. 238, 2004.
16. T.A. Trabold, J.P. Owejan, D.L. Jacobson, M. Arif, and P.R. Huffman, *International Journal of Heat and Mass Transfer*, Vol. 49, p. 4712, 2006.
17. J.P. Owejan, T.A. Trabold, D.L. Jacobson, D.R. Baker, D.S. Hussey, and M. Arif, *International Journal of Heat and Mass Transfer*, Vol. 49, p. 4721, 2006.
18. P. Boillat, D. Kramer, B.C. Seyfang, G. Frei, E. Lehmann, G.G. Scherer, A. Wokaun, Y. Ichikawa, Y. Tasaki, and K. Shinohara, *Electrochemistry Communications*, Vol. 10, p. 546, 2008.
19. I. Manke, C. Hartnig, N. Kardjilov, H. Riesemeier, J. Goebbels, R. Kuhn, P. Krüger, and J. Banhart, *Fuel Cells*, Vol. 10, p. 26, 2010.
20. C. Hartnig, I. Manke, R. Kuhn, S. Kleinau, J. Goebbels, and J. Banhart, *Journal of Power Sources*, Vol. 188, p. 468, 2009.
21. F.T. Bacon, *Electrochimica Acta*, Vol. 14, p. 569 , 1969.
22. F.T. Bacon and T.M. Fry, *Proceedings of the Royal Society of London A: Mathematical, Physical and Engineering Sciences*, Vol. 334, p. 427, 1973.
23. Wikipedia, Alkaline fuel cell — wikipedia, the free encyclopedia, 2017. [Online; accessed 20-August-2017].
24. E. Antolini and E.R. Gonzalez, *Journal of Power Sources*, Vol. 195, p. 3431, 2010.

25. X. Li, H. Zhang, Z. Mai, H. Zhang, and I. Vankelecom, *Energy & Environmental Science*, Vol. 4, p. 1147, 2011.
26. M. Higami, I. Rozhanskii, Y. Yamakawa, N. Kanaoka, K. Fukuda, R. Takahashi, and H. Shinkai, Varnish for a solid polymer fuel cell, US Patent 8 399 148, assigned to JSR Corporation (Tokyo, JP) Honda Motor Co., Ltd. (Tokyo, JP), March 19, 2013.
27. J. Ihonen and F. Jaouen, Polymer fuel cell structure, US Patent 7 790 330, assigned to Powercell Sweden AB (SE), September 7, 2010.
28. K. Kobayashi and S. Sekino, Solid polymer fuel cell, US Patent 8 148 025, assigned to NEC Corporation (Tokyo, JP), April 3, 2012.
29. H.H. Voss, R.H. Barton, B.W. Wells, J.A. Ronne, and H.A. Nigsch, Solid polymer fuel cell system and method for humidifying and adjusting the temperature of a reactant stream, US Patent 6 783 878, assigned to Ballard Power Systems Inc. (Burnaby, B.C., CA), August 31, 2004.
30. N.W. DeLuca and Y.A. Elabd, *Journal of Polymer Science Part B: Polymer Physics*, Vol. 44, p. 2201, 2006.
31. S.S. Munjewar, S.B. Thombre, and R.K. Mallick, *Renewable and Sustainable Energy Reviews*, Vol. 67, p. 1087, 2017.
32. C. Lamy, A. Lima, V. LeRhun, F. Delime, C. Coutanceau, and J.-M. Léger, *Journal of Power Sources*, Vol. 105, p. 283, 2002. 7th Ulmer Elektrochemische Tage.
33. P.A. García-Salaberri and M. Vera, *Energy*, Vol. 113, p. 1265, 2016.
34. R.K. Mallick, S.B. Thombre, and N.K. Shrivastava, *Renewable and Sustainable Energy Reviews*, Vol. 56, p. 51, 2016.
35. T. Shimizu, T. Momma, M. Mohamedi, T. Osaka, and S. Sarangapani, *Journal of Power Sources*, Vol. 137, p. 277, 2004.
36. R. Rashidi, I. Dincer, G. Naterer, and P. Berg, *Journal of Power Sources*, Vol. 187, p. 509, 2009.
37. V. Ravi and S. Joseph, Influence of feed vapour fraction on the performance of direct methanol fuel cell in R. Mohan B., G. Srinikethan, and B.C. Meikap, eds., *Materials, Energy and Environment Engineering: Select Proceedings of ICACE 2015*, pp. 197–204. Springer Singapore, Singapore, 2017.
38. C. Weinmueller, G. Tautschnig, N. Hotz, and D. Poulikakos, *Journal of Power Sources*, Vol. 195, p. 3849, 2010.
39. A.T. Çolak, T. Eren, M.L. Yola, E. Beşli, O. Şahin, and N. Atar, *Journal of The Electrochemical Society*, Vol. 163, p. F1237, 2016.
40. Y. Cheng, P.K. Shen, and S.P. Jiang, *International Journal of Hydrogen Energy*, Vol. 41, p. 1935, 2016.
41. Y. Cao, Y. Yang, Y. Shan, and Z. Huang, *ACS Applied Materials & Interfaces*, Vol. 8, p. 5998, 2016.
42. D.E. Glass, G.A. Olah, and G.S. Prakash, *Journal of Power Sources*, Vol. 352, p. 165, 2017.

43. F. Alcaide, G. Álvarez, P.L. Cabot, R. Genova-Koleva, H.-J. Grande, and O. Miguel, *Electrochimica Acta*, Vol. 231, p. 529 , 2017.
44. H. Teller and A. Schechter, *Journal of Solid State Electrochemistry*, June 2017.
45. Q. Li, T. Wang, D. Havas, H. Zhang, P. Xu, J. Han, J. Cho, and G. Wu, *Advanced Science*, Vol. 3, p. 1600140, 2016.
46. D. Sebastián, V. Baglio, A.S. Aricò, A. Serov, and P. Atanassov, *Applied Catalysis B: Environmental*, Vol. 182, p. 297, 2016.
47. D. Sebastián, A. Serov, K. Artyushkova, P. Atanassov, A.S. Aricá, and V. Baglio, *Journal of Power Sources*, Vol. 319, p. 235, 2016.
48. Y. Liu, C. Shu, Y. Fang, Y. Chen, and Y. Liu, *Journal of Power Sources*, Vol. 361, p. 160, 2017.
49. D. Sebastián, A. Serov, K. Artyushkova, J. Gordon, P. Atanassov, A.S. Aricò, and V. Baglio, *ChemSusChem*, Vol. 9, p. 1986, 2016.
50. S. Ratso, I. Kruusenberg, A. Sarapuu, P. Rauwel, R. Saar, U. Joost, J. Aruväli, P. Kanninen, T. Kallio, and K. Tammeveski, *Journal of Power Sources*, Vol. 332, p. 129, 2016.
51. N. Radenahmad, A. Afif, P.I. Petra, S.M. Rahman, S.-G. Eriksson, and A.K. Azad, *Renewable and Sustainable Energy Reviews*, Vol. 57, p. 1347, 2016.
52. D.A. Boysen, T. Uda, C.R.I. Chisholm, and S.M. Haile, *Science*, Vol. 303, p. 68, 2004.
53. Z. Zakaria, S.K. Kamarudin, and S.N. Timmiati, *Applied Energy*, Vol. 163, p. 334, 2016.
54. S. Song, W. Zhou, Z. Zhou, L. Jiang, G. Sun, Q. Xin, V. Leontidis, S. Kontou, and P. Tsiakaras, *International Journal of Hydrogen Energy*, Vol. 30, p. 995, 2005.
55. K.S. Roelofs, T. Hirth, and T. Schiestel, *Materials Science and Engineering: B*, Vol. 176, p. 727, 2011.
56. J.P. Pereira, D.S. Falcão, V.B. Oliveira, and A.M.F.R. Pinto, *Journal of Power Sources*, Vol. 256, p. 14, 2014.
57. G. Andreadis and P. Tsiakaras, *Chemical Engineering Science*, Vol. 61, p. 7497, 2006.
58. G.M. Andreadis, A.K.M. Podias, and P.E. Tsiakaras, *Journal of Power Sources*, Vol. 194, p. 397, 2009. XIth Polish Conference on Fast Ionic Conductors 2008.
59. K.S. Roelofs, T. Hirth, and T. Schiestel, *Journal of Membrane Science*, Vol. 346, p. 215, 2010.
60. L. An and T.S. Zhao, *Journal of Power Sources*, Vol. 341, p. 199, 2017.
61. Y. Li, T. Zhao, and Z. Liang, *Journal of Power Sources*, Vol. 190, p. 223, 2009.
62. C. Bianchini and P.K. Shen, *Chemical Reviews*, Vol. 109, p. 4183, 2009.
63. T. Zhao, Y. Li, and S. Shen, *Frontiers of Energy and Power Engineering in China*, Vol. 4, p. 443, December 2010.

64. R.C. Slade, J.P. Kizewski, S.D. Poynton, R. Zeng, and J.R. Varcoe, Alkaline membrane fuel cells in K.D. Kreuer, ed., *Fuel Cells: Selected Entries from the Encyclopedia of Sustainability Science and Technology*, chapter 2, pp. 9–29. Springer, New York, 2013.
65. H. Bunazawa and Y. Yamazaki, *Journal of Power Sources*, Vol. 182, p. 48, 2008.
66. Y. Li, L.M. Wong, H. Xie, S. Wang, and P.-C. Su, *Journal of Power Sources*, Vol. 340, p. 98, 2017.
67. M.A.F. Akhairi and S.K. Kamarudin, *International Journal of Hydrogen Energy*, Vol. 41, p. 4214 , 2016.
68. Z. Zhang, L. Xin, K. Sun, and W. Li, *International Journal of Hydrogen Energy*, Vol. 36, p. 12686, 2011. 3rd Iranian Fuel Cell Seminar.
69. Y. Li and T. Zhao, *International Journal of Hydrogen Energy*, Vol. 36, p. 7707, 2011. HYSYDAYS.
70. T.S. Almeida, N.E. Sahin, P. Olivi, T.W. Napporn, G. Tremiliosi-Filho, A.R. de Andrade, and K.B. Kokoh, Direct ethanol fuel cell on carbon supported Pt based nanocatalysts in K.I. Ozoemena and S. Chen, eds., *Nanomaterials for Fuel Cell Catalysis*, pp. 435–475. Springer International Publishing, Cham, 2016.
71. P. Bert and C. Bianchini, Platinum-free electrocatalyst materials, US Patent Application 20 060 058 500, March 16, 2006.
72. L. Moraes, B. Matos, C. Radtke, E. Santiago, F. Fonseca, S. Amico, and C. Malfatti, *International Journal of Hydrogen Energy*, Vol. 41, p. 6457 , 2016.
73. C. Chaiburi, B. Cermenek, B. Pichler, C. Grimmer, A. Schenk, and V. Hacker, *Journal of New Materials for Electrochemical Systems*, Vol. 19, p. 199, 2017.
74. A. Dutta, A. Mondal, P. Broekmann, and J. Datta, *Journal of Power Sources*, Vol. 361, p. 276, 2017.
75. L. An and R. Chen, *Journal of Power Sources*, Vol. 320, p. 127, 2016.
76. N.V. Rees and R.G. Compton, *Journal of Solid State Electrochemistry*, Vol. 15, p. 2095, October 2011.
77. A. Kundu, J.H. Jang, J.H. Gil, C.R. Jung, H.R. Lee, S.-H. Kim, B. Ku, and Y. Oh, *Journal of Power Sources*, Vol. 170, p. 67, 2007.
78. S. Uhm, H.J. Lee, and J. Lee, *Physical Chemistry Chemical Physics*, Vol. 11, p. 9326, 2009.
79. C. Rice, S. Ha, R.I. Masel, and A. Wieckowski, *Journal of Power Sources*, Vol. 115, p. 229, 2003.
80. Z. Xi, D.P. Erdosy, A. Mendoza-Garcia, P.N. Duchesne, J. Li, M. Muzzio, Q. Li, P. Zhang, and S. Sun, *Nano Letters*, Vol. 17, p. 2727, 2017.
81. L. An, T.S. Zhao, Z.H. Chai, P. Tan, and L. Zeng, *International Journal of Hydrogen Energy*, Vol. 39, p. 19869, 2014.

82. X. Cheng, R. Chen, X. Zhu, Q. Liao, X. He, S. Li, and L. Li, *International Journal of Hydrogen Energy*, Vol. 41, p. 2457, 2016.
83. Y. Li, Y. He, and W. Yang, *Journal of Power Sources*, Vol. 278, p. 569, 2015.
84. L. An, T.S. Zhao, S.Y. Shen, Q.X. Wu, and R. Chen, *International Journal of Hydrogen Energy*, Vol. 35, p. 4329, 2010.
85. X. Yu and A. Manthiram, *Applied Catalysis B: Environmental*, Vol. 165, p. 63, 2015.
86. E. Kjeang, R. Michel, D.A. Harrington, D. Sinton, and N. Djilali, *Electrochimica Acta*, Vol. 54, p. 698, 2008.
87. T. Takamura and F. Mochimaru, *Electrochimica Acta*, Vol. 14, p. 111, 1969.
88. M. Rosenbaum, U. Schröder, and F. Scholz, *Journal of Solid State Electrochemistry*, Vol. 10, p. 872, October 2006.
89. K. Ohyamaa, C. Kimuraa, H. Aokia, S. Kuwabatab, and T. Suginoa, *ECS Transactions*, Vol. 11, p. 1473, 2007.
90. K. Ohyama, T. Sugino, T. Nitta, C. Kimura, and H. Aoki, *Electrical Engineering in Japan*, Vol. 174, p. 45, 2011.
91. H. Aoki, T. Nitta, S. Kuwabata, C. Kimura, and T. Sugino, *ECS Transactions*, Vol. 16, p. 849, 2008.
92. Y. Li, *International Journal of Hydrogen Energy*, Vol. 41, p. 3600, 2016.
93. Z. Fan, Y.-H. Kwon, X. Yang, W. Xu, and Z. Wu, *Energy Procedia*, Vol. 105, p. 1858, 2017. 8th International Conference on Applied Energy, ICAE2016, 8-11 October 2016, Beijing, China.
94. K. Ye, H. Zhang, L. Zhao, X. Huang, K. Cheng, G. Wang, and D. Cao, *New Journal of Chemistry*, Vol. 40, p. 8673, 2016.
95. V. Vedharathinam and G.G. Botte, ECS student achievement award of the IEEE division electrochemical oxidation of urea on nickel catalyst in alkaline medium: Investigation of the reaction mechanism, in *Meeting Abstracts*, number 10, pp. 543–543. The Electrochemical Society, 2014.
96. F. Guo, D. Cao, M. Du, K. Ye, G. Wang, W. Zhang, Y. Gao, and K. Cheng, *Journal of Power Sources*, Vol. 307, p. 697, 2016.
97. A. Yousef, M.H. El-Newehy, S.S. Al-Deyab, and N.A. Barakat, *Arabian Journal of Chemistry*, 2017. in press.
98. M. Boaro and A.S. Arico, eds., *Advances in Medium and High Temperature Solid Oxide Fuel Cell Technology*, Springer, Cham, Switzerland, 2017.
99. A. Choudhury, H. Chandra, and A. Arora, *Renewable and Sustainable Energy Reviews*, Vol. 20, p. 430, 2013.
100. N. Mahato, A. Banerjee, A. Gupta, S. Omar, and K. Balani, *Progress in Materials Science*, Vol. 72, p. 141, 2015.

101. G.D. Agnew, R.R. Moritz, O.C. Tarnowski, and M. Bozzolo, Solid oxide fuel cell system, US Patent 7 118 818, assigned to Rolls-Royce PLC (London, GB), October 10, 2006.
102. M. Bozzolo and C. Balestrino, Solid oxide fuel cell system, US Patent 9 570 766, assigned to LG Fuel Cell Systems, Inc. (Canton, OH), February 14, 2017.
103. J. Sunarso, S.S. Hashim, N. Zhu, and W. Zhou, *Progress in Energy and Combustion Science*, Vol. 61, p. 57, 2017.
104. A.B. Muñoz-García, A.M. Ritzmann, M. Pavone, J.A. Keith, and E.A. Carter, *Accounts of Chemical Research*, Vol. 47, p. 3340, 2014.
105. M. Zulfqar, M.R. Shah, and Z.S. Khan, Investigations on gadolinium doped ceria (GDC) electrolyte prepared via sol-gel and co-precipitation routes for intermediate temperature solid oxide fuel cell (IT-SOFC) applications, in *4th International Conference on Energy, Environment and Sustainable Development*, number 199, Jamshoro, Sindh, Pakistan, 2016.
106. H. Huang, J. Lin, Y. Wang, S. Wang, C. Xia, and C. Chen, *Journal of Power Sources*, Vol. 274, p. 1114, 2015.
107. S. Hong, J. Bae, B. Koo, and Y.-B. Kim, *Electrochemistry Communications*, Vol. 47, p. 1, 2014.
108. M. Boaro, A. Pappacena, C. Abate, M. Ferluga, J. Llorca, and A. Trovarelli, *Journal of Power Sources*, Vol. 270, p. 79, 2014.
109. J. An, Y.-B. Kim, J. Park, T.M. Gür, and F.B. Prinz, *Nano Letters*, Vol. 13, p. 4551, 2013.
110. A.J. Rayner, J. Briggs, R. Tremback, and R.M.C. Clemmer, *Renewable and Sustainable Energy Reviews*, Vol. 71, p. 563, 2017.
111. J. Liu, G. Cao, Z. Yang, D. Wang, D. Dubois, X. Zhou, G.L. Graff, L.R. Pederson, and J.-G. Zhang, *ChemSusChem*, Vol. 1, p. 676, 2008.
112. J.D. Baek, C.-C. Yu, and P.-C. Su, *Nano Letters*, Vol. 16, p. 2413, 2016.
113. X. Zhang, L. Liu, Z. Zhao, B. Tu, D. Ou, D. Cui, X. Wei, X. Chen, and M. Cheng, *Nano Letters*, Vol. 15, p. 1703, 2015.
114. S. Park, J.M. Vohs, and R.J. Gorte, *Nature*, Vol. 404, p. 265267, 2000.
115. J.C. Biffinger, M. Ribbens, K.H. Nealson, and B.R. Ringeisen, High-throughput biological screening assay using voltage gradients, US Patent 8 425 742, assigned to The United States of America, as represented by the Secretary of the Navy (Washington, DC), April 23, 2013.
116. R. Rao and G. Richter, Implantable fuel cell, US Patent 3 861 397, assigned to Siemens Aktiengesellschaft (Erlangen, DT), January 21, 1975.
117. H. Wang and Z.J. Ren, *Biotechnology Advances*, Vol. 31, p. 1796, 2013.
118. V.B. Oliveira, M. Simões, L. Melo, and A.M.F.R. Pinto, *Biochemical Engineering Journal*, Vol. 73, p. 53, 2013.

119. S.V. Mohan, G. Velvizhi, J.A. Modestra, and S. Srikanth, *Renewable and Sustainable Energy Reviews*, Vol. 40, p. 779 , 2014.
120. A. Heller, Biological fuel cell and method, US Patent 6 294 281, assigned to TheraSense, Inc. (Alameda, CA), September 25, 2001.
121. A. Heller, Biological fuel cell and methods, US Patent 6 531 239, assigned to TheraSense, Inc. (Alameda, CA), March 11, 2003.
122. A. Heller, N. Mano, H.-H. Kim, Y. Zhang, F. Mao, T. Chen, and S.C. Barton, Miniature biological fuel cell that is operational under physiological conditions, and associated devices and methods, US Patent 8 759 055, assigned to Abbott Diabetes Care Inc. (Alameda, CA), June 24, 2014.
123. A. Heller, Biological fuel cell and methods, US Patent 9 509 010, assigned to Abbott Diabetes Care Inc. (Alameda, CA), November 29, 2016.
124. N. Mano, F. Mao, and A. Heller, *Journal of the American Chemical Society*, Vol. 124, p. 12962, 2002.
125. N. Mano, H.-H. Kim, and A. Heller, *The Journal of Physical Chemistry B*, Vol. 106, p. 8842, 2002.
126. N. Mano, H.-H. Kim, Y. Zhang, and A. Heller, *Journal of the American Chemical Society*, Vol. 124, p. 6480, 2002.
127. P. Lv, Q. Feng, Q. Wang, D. Li, J. Zhou, and Q. Wei, *Fibers and Polymers*, Vol. 17, p. 1858, November 2016.
128. J.C. Biffinger, R. Ray, B. Little, and B.R. Ringeisen, *Environmental Science & Technology*, Vol. 41, p. 1444, 2007.
129. S. Sibbett, C. Lau, G.P.M.K. Ciniciato, and P. Atanassov, Paper-based fuel cell, US Patent 9 257 709, assigned to STC.UNM (Albuquerque, NM), February 9, 2016.
130. A.M. Sastry, M.V. Inamdar, C.W. Wang, M. Philbert, and J.A. Miller, Biological battery or fuel cell utilizing mitochondria, US Patent Application 20 080 261 085, assigned to the Regents of the University of Michigan, Ann Arbor (MI), October 23, 2008.
131. M.E. Moore, Y.M. Arias-Thode, and B.R. Goldsmith, Grafting of biomolecules onto microbial fuel cells, US Patent 9 160 024, assigned to The United States of America, as Represented by the Secretary of the Navy (Washington, DC), October 13, 2015.
132. C.L. Curchoe and S. Minteer, Biological supercapacitor structure and method for manufacturing and use of the same, US Patent Application 20 160 145 669, May 26, 2016.
133. S. Jin, P. Fallgren, J.M. Morris, A.E. Bland, P. Richards, J.D. Newcomer, and P. Colberg, Biological clean fuel processing systems and methods, US Patent Application 20 120 003 705, assigned to the University of Wyoming Research Corporation d/b/a Western Research Institute, Laramie (WY), January 5, 2012.

134. J. Danzer and S. Kerzenmacher, Filtration-active fuel cell, US Patent Application 20 160 190 627, June 30, 2016.
135. C.H. Neoh, Z.Z. Noor, N.S.A. Mutamim, and C.K. Lim, *Chemical Engineering Journal*, Vol. 283, p. 582, 2016.
136. L. Xu, Y. Zhao, L. Doherty, Y. Hu, and X. Hao, *Critical Reviews in Environmental Science and Technology*, Vol. 46, p. 60, 2016.
137. S.T. Oh, J.R. Kim, G.C. Premier, T.H. Lee, C. Kim, and W.T. Sloan, *Biotechnology Advances*, Vol. 28, p. 871 , 2010.
138. W.-W. Li, H.-Q. Yu, and Z. He, *Energy & Environmental Science*, Vol. 7, p. 911, 2014.
139. E.S. Heidrich, J. Dolfing, K. Scott, S.R. Edwards, C. Jones, and T.P. Curtis, *Applied Microbiology and Biotechnology*, Vol. 97, p. 6979, August 2013.
140. Y.-K. Wang, G.-P. Sheng, B.-J. Shi, W.-W. Li, and H.-Q. Yu, *Scientific Reports*, Vol. 3, 2013.
141. P.H. Nakhate, N.T. Joshi, and K.V. Marathe, *Reviews in Chemical Engineering*, Vol. 33, p. 143, 2017.
142. P. Pandey, V.N. Shinde, R.L. Deopurkar, S.P. Kale, S.A. Patil, and D. Pant, *Applied Energy*, Vol. 168, p. 706, 2016.
143. A. ElMekawy, S. Srikanth, S. Bajracharya, H.M. Hegab, P.S. Nigam, A. Singh, S.V. Mohan, and D. Pant, *Food Research International*, Vol. 73, p. 213, 2015.
144. M. Lu, S. Chen, S. Babanova, S. Phadke, M. Salvacion, A. Mirhosseini, S. Chan, K. Carpenter, R. Cortese, and O. Bretschger, *Journal of Power Sources*, Vol. 356, p. 274, 2017.
145. J. Ma, Z. Wang, D. He, Y. Li, and Z. Wu, *Water Research*, Vol. 78, p. 98, 2015.
146. S.G. Ray, G.D. Bhowmick, M.M. Ghangrekar, and A. Mitra, Advances in wastewater treatment by combined microbial fuel cell-membrane bioreactor, in *13th IWA Specialized Conference on Small Water and Wastewater Systems*, Athens, 2016. National Technical University of Athens.
147. G. Strack, H.R. Luckarift, S.R. Sizemore, R.K. Nichols, K.E. Farrington, P.K. Wu, P. Atanassov, J.C. Biffinger, and G.R. Johnson, *Bioresource Technology*, Vol. 128, p. 222, 2013.
148. S. Krishnamoorthy, A. Bedekar, and J. Wei, Hybrid power strip, US Patent Application 20 080 213 631, assigned to CFD Research Corporation, Huntsville (AL), September 4, 2008.
149. Wikipedia, Flavin adenine dinucleotide — wikipedia, the free encyclopedia, 2017. [Online; accessed 11-July-2017].
150. M.H. Frey, D.M. Pierpont, and S.J. Hamrock, High durability fuel cell components with cerium salt additives, US Patent 9 431 670, assigned to 3M Innovative Properties Company (Saint Paul, MN), August 30, 2016.

151. A.L. Walker and C.W. Walker, *Journal of Power Sources*, Vol. 160, p. 123 , 2006.
152. A. Gunawardena, S. Fernando, and F. To, *International Journal of Molecular Sciences*, Vol. 9, p. 1893, 2008.
153. X. Wu, F. Zhao, J.R. Varcoe, A.E. Thumser, C. Avignone-Rossa, and R.C.T. Slade, *Biosensors and Bioelectronics*, Vol. 25, p. 326, 2009.

2

Polymer Electrodes

Since the 1980s there has been a significant lowering of the platinum loading of polymer electrolyte fuel cell electrodes from about 4–10 $mgcm^{-2}$ (platinum black) to about 0.4 $mgcm^{-2}$ or even less (carbon-supported platinum), by the introduction of a ionomer liquid Nafion impregnated gas diffusion electrodes, extending the three-dimensional reaction zone (1).

Studies have been carried out to decrease the loss of performance during cell operation due both to the presence of liquid water causing flooding of the catalyst layer and mass transport limitations and to the poisoning of platinum by the use of reformed fuels. The developments in electrode configuration going from dual-layer to three-layer electrodes have been reviewed (1).

The preparation methods, the characteristics and the optimal composition of both diffusion and reactive layers of these electrodes are described. The improvement in the performance of both CO tolerant anodes and cathodes with enhanced oxygen reduction by Pt alloying has also been discussed (1).

2.1 Porous Electrode Substrate

A polymer electrolyte fuel cell is characterized by using a proton-conductive polymer electrolyte membrane, and is a device that provides electromotive force by electrochemically reacting a fuel gas, such as hydrogen, with an oxidizing gas, such as oxygen (2).

Such a polymer electrolyte fuel cell has a polymer electrolyte membrane that selectively conducts the protons. In addition, the fuel cell has two gas diffusion electrodes. The gas diffusion electrode has a catalyst layer that contains as a main component a carbon powder that supports a noble metal-based catalyst, and has a gas diffusion electrode substrate. Each of the gas diffusion electrodes is joined to the surface of the polymer electrolyte membrane with the catalyst layer facing inward.

An assembly including such a polymer electrolyte membrane and two gas diffusion electrodes is referred to as a membrane electrode assembly. In addition, on both outer sides of the membrane electrode assembly, separators are installed in which gas flow paths are formed in order to feed a fuel gas and an oxidizing gas and to discharge produced gases and excessive gases (2).

A gas diffusion electrode substrate needs mechanical strength because the gas diffusion electrode substrate is fastened by a load of several *MPa* by a separator in order to reduce electric contact resistance and suppress the leakage of a fuel gas or an oxidizing gas fed from the separator to the outside of a fuel cell.

Since the gas diffusion electrode substrate needs to mainly have the following three functions, the gas diffusion electrode substrate is usually a porous electrode substrate having a porous structure. The first function required of the gas diffusion electrode substrate is to uniformly feed the fuel gas or the oxidizing gas from the gas flow path formed in the separator, which is located on the outer side of the gas diffusion electrode substrate, to a noble metal-based catalyst in the catalyst layer. The second function is the function of discharging water produced by a reaction in the catalyst layer. Finally, the third function is the function of conducting electrons necessary for the reaction in the catalyst layer or electrons produced by the reaction in the catalyst layer to the separator (2).

Conventionally, in order to increase mechanical strength of the substrate, short carbon fibers are formed onto a paper and bound to one another by using organic polymers. Then this paper is burnt at a high temperature to carbonize the organic polymers and to produce a porous electrode substrate which is composed of carbon/carbon composites in paper shape (2).

However, the problems of this technique are that the production process is complicated and production costs are high. In addition, in order to reduce costs, a porous electrode substrate is proposed which is obtained by forming a paper from oxidized short fibers, and then firing the paper at high temperature to carbonize the oxidized short fibers. However, since the oxidized short fibers shrink during firing, the problems of the electrode substrate are its dimensional stability and surface precision.

A simple method for the production of a porous electrode substrate has been described. The porous electrode substrate is produced by a method of (2):

1. Producing a precursor sheet X-1 from short carbon fibers having a length of 2–12 *mm* and at least one fiber selected from the group consisting of short carbon fiber precursors (b) having a length of 2–20 *mm* and fibrillar carbon fiber precursors dispersed in a two-dimensional plane,
2. Subjecting the precursor sheet X-1 obtained in step 1 to entanglement treatment, thereby three-dimensionally orienting the short carbon fibers and providing a three-dimensional entangled porous electrode substrate precursor sheet, and
3. Subjecting the three-dimensional entangled porous electrode substrate precursor sheet X-2 to carbonization treatment at a temperature of 1000°C or higher, thereby producing the porous electrode substrate, wherein the entanglement treatment is carried out by a needle punching method, a water-jet punching method, or a jet stream punching method.

Monomers for their use as precursors for carbon fibers are summarized in Table 2.1. Examples of short carbon fibers include those obtained by cutting carbon fibers, such as poly(acrylonitrile) (PAN)-based carbon fibers, pitch-based carbon fibers, and rayon-based carbon fibers, to a suitable length. Taking into consideration the mechanical strength of the porous electrode substrate, PAN-based carbon fibers are preferred. The average fiber length of short carbon fibers is preferably about 2–12 *mm* from the viewpoint of dispersibility. A scanning electron micrograph of a surface of a porous electrode substrate is shown in Figure 2.1.

The gas permeability of the porous electrode substrate is preferably 500–30000 $ml\, hr^{-1} cm^{-2} mmAq^{-1}$.

Table 2.1 Monomers for precursors for carbon fibers (3).

Monomer	Monomer
Methyl acrylate	Hydroxypropyl methacrylate
Ethyl acrylate	Diethylaminoethyl methacrylate
Isopropyl acrylate	Acrylic acid
n-Butyl acrylate	Methacrylic acid
2-Ethylhexyl acrylate	Maleic acid
2-Hydroxyethyl acrylate	Itaconic acid
Hydroxypropyl acrylate	Acrylamide
Methyl methacrylate	*N*-Methylolacrylamide
Ethyl methacrylate	Diacetone acrylamide
Isopropyl methacrylate	Styrene
n-Butyl methacrylate	Vinyl toluene
Isobutyl methacrylate	Vinyl acetate
tert-Butyl methacrylate	Vinyl chloride
n-Hexyl methacrylate	Vinylidene chloride
Cyclohexyl methacrylate	Vinylidene bromide
Lauryl methacrylate	Vinyl fluoride
2-Hydroxyethyl methacrylate	Vinylidene fluoride

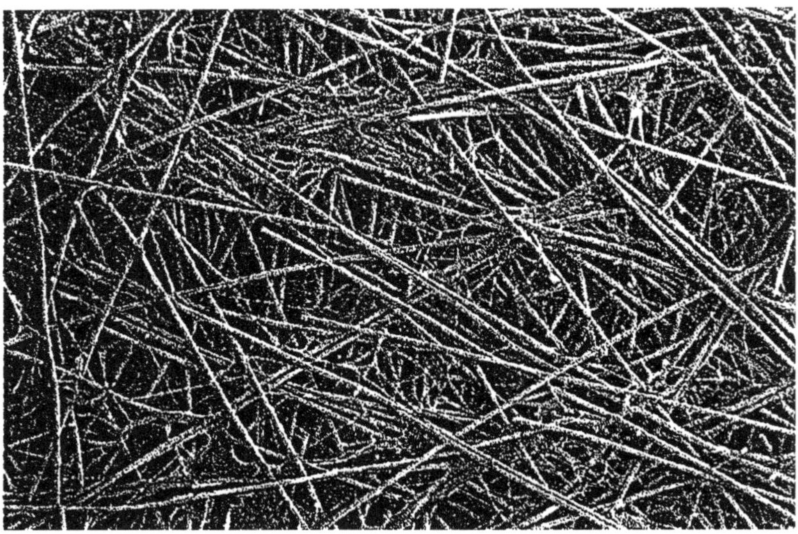

Figure 2.1 Scanning electron micrograph of a surface of a porous electrode substrate (2).

2.2 Electrode Assembly for Solid Polymer Fuel Cell

A membrane electrode assembly for a polymer electrolyte fuel cell has been described that has a laminate with a polymer electrolyte membrane (4). Catalyst layers are on both sides. Gas diffusion layers hold the polymer electrolyte membrane between the gas diffusion layers. Further, a first plastic film is present that covers a rim portion of the polymer electrolyte membrane, the catalyst layers and the gas diffusion layers. Metal porous bodies are disposed on both entire faces of the laminate, and a second plastic film is there that further covers a rim portion of the laminate and the metal porous bodies that are laminated together. Rim portions of the metal porous bodies are held between the first plastic film and the second plastic film (4).

The polymer electrolyte membrane may be a perfluorosulfonic acid electrolyte membrane or a hydrocarbon electrolyte membrane. Such perfluorosulfonic acid electrolyte membranes include, for example, perfluorocarbon sulfonic acid polymers such as Nafion®, Aciplex®, and Flemion®, and also perfluorocarbon phosphonic acid polymers, trifluorostyrene sulfonic acid polymers, ethylene tetrafluoroethylene-*g*-styrene sulfonic acid polymers, ethylene tetrafluoroethylene copolymer, and poly(vinylidene fluoride)-perfluorocarbon sulfonic acid polymers.

In the membrane electrode assembly, the metal porous bodies are made of a metal mesh. In addition to a metal mesh, materials that may be used include, metal foam, expanded metal, punching metal, etching plate, precision-pressed plate, metal mesh, sintered metal fiber, or metal nonwoven devices (4).

2.3 Electrode for Fuel Cell

An electrode for fuel cell has been described that comprises a catalyst carrier that is an electrically conductive carrier with a catalyst supported thereon, a first electrolyte resin, and a second electrolyte resin (5).

The first electrolyte resin has oxygen permeability of less than $2.2 \times 10^{-14}\ molm^{-1}s^{-1}Pa^{-1}$ in an environment with a temperature of 80°C and a relative humidity of 50%. The second electrolyte resin has oxygen permeability of not less than 2.2×10^{-14} $molm^{-1}s^{-1}Pa^{-1}$ in an environment with a temperature of 80°C and a relative humidity of 50%. The electrode is manufactured by the following steps (5):

1. Preparing a first catalyst ink by dispersing a catalyst carrier that is an electrically conductive carrier having at least a catalyst supported thereon and a first electrolyte resin in a solvent,
2. Preparing a second catalyst ink by additionally dispersing a second electrolyte resin in the first catalyst ink,
3. Applying the second catalyst ink on an electrode substrate and evaporating at least part of the solvent included in the second catalyst ink, wherein the first electrolyte resin has oxygen permeability of less than 2.2×10^{-14} $molm^{-1}s^{-1}Pa^{-1}$ in an environment having a temperature of 80°C and relative humidity of 50%, and
4. The second electrolyte resin with oxygen permeability of not less than 2.2×10^{-14} $molm^{-1}s^{-1}Pa^{-1}$ in an environment having a temperature of 80°C and a relative humidity of 50%; the step of preparing the first catalyst ink or the step of preparing the second catalyst ink controls a mass fraction of the first electrolyte resin so that it is not less than 2% and not greater than 50% relative to a total mass of the first electrolyte resin and the second electrolyte resin.

2.4 Flow-Field Plate

The role of the flow-field plate is of major importance in determining the performance of a polymer electrolyte fuel cell (6). The flow-field plate constitutes the largest volumetric and gravimetric proportion of the fuel cell stack and has a strong bearing on the cost and efficiency of the system.

The materials being used to make flow-field plates and the methods used to characterize the materials properties and performance have been detailed (6).

2.5 Catalyst for Fuel Electrode

A catalyst for a fuel electrode of a solid polymer fuel cell has been developed, wherein the catalyst comprises fine precious metal particles loaded on a support composed of an electrically conductive material, and wherein the weight ratio of the fine precious metal particles and the support is composed of an electrically conductive material. These are fine precious metal particles: Electrically conductive material and fine precious metal particles. These materials satisfy the following conditions (7):

1. The fine precious metal particles contain platinum and ruthenium, and the mixing ratio thereof (platinum:ruthenium) is within a range between 1:1 and 1:3 in terms of molar ratio,
2. The fine precious metal particles have an average particle diameter of 3 to 10 *nm*, and
3. The fine precious metal particles contain oxygen, and the weight ratio of the fine precious metal particles and oxygen (fine precious metal particles:oxygen) is 86:14 to 96:4.

2.6 Electrode Catalyst and Solid Polymer Fuel Cell

In the case of the chelate catalyst that is a complex of a macrocyclic compound, such as a porphyrin derivative, cf. (8), a salt of an unsupported transition metal functions as a *foaming agent* for a nitrogen-containing organic transition metal complex. Thus, it is thought that a carbon matrix becomes porous and thus the activity surface area is extended, contributing to an improvement in catalyst activity (8).

However, a chelate catalyst comprising a complex of a macrocyclic compound, such as a porphyrin derivative, is problematic, because a foaming agent cannot be completely removed, and the pore size is not optimized. Therefore, further improvement in the activity catalyst should be necessary (9).

The catalyst performance of a chelate catalyst using a complex of a macrocyclic compound such as a porphyrin derivative can be improved.

A particularly simple and process-efficient method of producing a platinum-free chelate catalyst material for the selective reduction of oxygen with at least one unsupported transition metal, a nitrogen and a carbon component structured as a porous conductive carbon matrix into which are bonded the unsupported transition metal as an electron donor and transition metal coordinated by the nitrogen as a catalysis center, provides for the following method steps (9):

1. Mixing of a transition metal salt as precursor compound for the unsupported transition metal with the nitrogen-containing organo-metallic transition complex and the organic chalcogen compound,
2. Heating the mixture to a pyrolysis temperature in the range of 450°C during a period of a several hours,
3. Cooling the polymerized mixture and mixing with an acid,
4. Boiling the acid mixture during a period of a few minutes and subsequent cooling,
5. Removal of the resultant powder by suction and washing with deionized water, and
6. Drying of the powdered chelate catalyst material.

During the production of the chelate catalyst material, a spongy transition metal containing a carbon matrix is formed by a fine transition metal salt which is initially covered with the nitrogen-containing organo-metallic transition complex and the organic chalcogen compound by mixing. The mixture is then subjected to pyrolysis at a moderate temperature range of 450°C. This initially causes the evaporation of the crystal water bound in the transition metal salt.

Thereafter, the organic chalcogen compound decomposes, and the nitrogen-containing organo-metallic transition complex melts. The latter begins to polymerize causing a strongly crosslinked and, hence, very stable carbon matrix to be formed. During this process, decomposition of at least one unsupported transition metal salt commences simultaneously. This causes formation, with the generation of a gas, of nanocrystals from the unsupported transition metal. However, a fraction of the transition metal is also firmly bonded to the carbon matrix (9).

The carbon matrix formed from the polymerizing nitrogen-containing organo-metallic transition complex deposits around the nanocrystals from at least one transition metal. At the selected moderate process temperature, the coordination sphere for the MeN_4 cores is substantially maintained. The chalcogen from the organic chalcogen compound is bonded into the carbon matrix as electrically conductive connecting bridges between the unsupported transition metal and the chelate cores. The formed nanocrystals are then washed out in a subsequent step which is entirely novel in the context of such methods of synthesis, and a conductive, highly porous carbon matrix with nano and micro structures and containing transition metals, chalcogen and nitrogen remains.

The thus formed highly porous carbon matrix is already of excellent stability and activity for the selective oxygen reduction (9). However, the activity can be further improved by a process step to be executed before or after the process step of boiling the acid mixture, i.e., heating the powdered chelate catalyst material under a protective atmosphere to a high temperature in the range of 850°C for one hour or more (9).

2.7 Membrane Electrode Assembly

A membrane electrode assembly, based on a poly(oxometalate)-modified low-Pt loading cathode and a sulfated titania ($S{-}TiO_2$)-doped Nafion membrane, has been evaluated in a polymer electrolyte membrane fuel cell (10).

The modification of fuel cell cathode with $Cs_3HPMo_{11}VO_{40}$ poly(oxometalate) has been performed to enhance the dispersion of the particles and to increase the active area, so allowing a low Pt loading while maintaining the performance. The high surface acidity of the poly(oxometalate) favors the kinetics of oxygen reduction reaction.

The mesoporous features of poly(oxometalate) allow the embedding of Pt inside the micro-mesopores, avoiding the Pt aggregation during fuel cell operation and delaying the aging process, with a consequent increase of lifetime.

On the other hand, when commercial Nafion is modified with superacidic sulfated titanium oxide nanoparticles, the operation at low relative humidity and controlled polarization of the membrane electrode assembly is allowed. Also, membrane electrode assemblies, formed from an unmodified Nafion membrane and the poly-

(oxometalate)-based cathode, as well as sulfated titanium-added Nafion and commercial Pt-based electrodes, have been used for comparison. The cell performances have been studied by polarization, electrochemical impedance spectroscopy, Tafel plot analysis and high frequency resistance measurements.

Also, the dependence of cell performances on relative humidity has been studied. The catalytic and transport properties can be improved using the coupled system, despite the reduced Pt loading, thanks to a rich proton environment provided by cathode and membrane (10).

References

1. E. Antolini, *Journal of Applied Electrochemistry*, Vol. 34, p. 563, 2004.
2. K. Sumioka and Y. Sako, Porous electrode substrate, method for producing the same, precursor sheet, membrane electrode assembly, and polymer electrolyte fuel cell, US Patent 9 343 751, assigned to Mitsubishi Rayon Co., Ltd. (Tokyo, JP), May 17, 2016.
3. H. Tatsuno, K. Sumioka, and T. Samejima, Porous electrode substrate, method for manufacturing same, precursor sheet, membrane electrode assembly, and polymer electrolyte fuel cell, US Patent 9 705 137, assigned to Mitsubishi Rayon Co., Ltd. (Tokyo, JP), July 11, 2017.
4. N. Horibe, Electrode assembly for solid polymer fuel cell, US Patent 9 496 562, assigned to Nisson Motor Co., Ltd. (Kanagawa, JP), November 15, 2016.
5. M. Aimu, R.L. Perry, M.G. Roelofs, R.C. Wheland, and R.M. Aten, Electrode for fuel cell, manufacturing method of electrode for fuel cell, polymer electrolyte fuel cell and catalyst ink, US Patent 9 461 312, assigned to Toyota Jidosha Kabushiki Kaisha (Toyota-shi, JP), E.I. Dupont de Nemours and Company (Wilmington, DE), October 4, 2016.
6. D.J.L. Brett and N.P. Brandon, *Journal of Fuel Cell Science and Technology*, Vol. 4, p. 29, 2007.
7. T. Tada, M. Inoue, and K. Matsutani, Catalyst for fuel electrode of solid polymer fuel cell, US Patent 7 335 619, assigned to Tanaka Kikinzoku K.K. (Tokyo, JP), February 26, 2008.
8. M. Hilgendorff, I. Dorbandt, H. Schulenburg, M. Bron, S. Fiechter, P. Bogdanoff, and H. Tributsch, Platinum-free chelate-catalyst material for the selective reduction of oxygen and method for production thereof, US Patent 7 534 739, assigned to Helmholtz-Zentrum Berlin Fuer Materialien und Energie (Berlin, DE), May 19, 2009.

9. N. Iwata, H. Takahashi, P. Bogdanoff, S. Fiechter, I. Herrmann-Geppert, and U. Kramm, Method for preparing fuel cell electrode catalyst and solid polymer fuel cell, US Patent 8 455 384, assigned to Toyota Jidosha Kabushiki Kaisha (Toyota-shi, Aichi-Ken, JP) Helmholtz-Zentrum Berlin Fuer Materialien und Energie GmbH (Berlin, DE), June 4, 2013.
10. M. Renzi, M. Agostini, M.A. Navarra, and F. Nobili, *International Journal of Hydrogen Energy*, Vol. 42, p. 16686, 2017.

3

Polymer Membranes

Fuel cells represent a clean alternative to the technologies for utilizing hydrocarbon fuel resources (1). Polymer electrolyte membrane fuel cells have acquired an importance as they are best suited for applications where a quick startup is required such as in automobiles.

The major requirements of fuel cell membranes are high proton conductivity, low methanol permeability and water permeability, good mechanical and thermal stability and a moderate price.

Membranes and the operating parameters together have a profound influence on performance of polymer electrolyte membrane fuel cells. Perfluorinated ionomers, hydrocarbon and aromatic polymers and acid-base complexes have been reviewed (1).

The performance of this special class of polymers, considering their structure-property relationship and the state of art involving their applicability in fuel cell systems, has been presented. Modifications made to Nafion membranes, the conceptual design of substitutes for perfluorosulfonic acid materials and modifications made to aromatic membranes to render them suitable for this application have been summarized (1).

3.1 History

In 1839 the fuel cell was discovered by Sir William Grove (2).

Proton exchange membrane fuel cells were first used by NASA in the 1960s for the Gemini and Apollo space program (3, 4). This fuel cell used pure hydrogen and oxygen as reactant gases.

The first proton exchange membrane used in a fuel cell system was sulfonated poly(styrene) (PS) membrane. This type was developed by General Electric for NASA in the early 1960s, as an onboard power source (5). NASA was also interested in future development of fuel cells because of the energy crisis in 1973.

The performance of the fuel cell was investigated by the fundamental model of polymer electrolyte membrane fuel cell, which was developed in the 1990s by Springer (6,7).

The first hydrogen fuel cell automobile was developed by Roger Billings (8,9).

In a polymer electrolyte membrane fuel cell an ion exchange membrane, i.e., fluorinated sulfonic acid polymer, is used as an electrolyte. The membrane is an excellent proton conductor. Water management is the critical problem in polymer electrolyte membrane fuel cell because the conductivity of membrane is highly dependent on the water content, the membrane must be hydrated for an efficient performance of the fuel cell, which depends on the reactant stream humidification, flow field of the gas diffusion layer and the wetting property of the gas diffusion layer and the polymer membrane (4).

3.2 Desired Properties of Membranes

In order to achieve a high efficiency, a membrane should exhibit the following properties (1):

1. A high proton conductivity to support high currents with minimal resistive losses and zero electronic conductivity,
2. An adequate mechanical strength and stability,
3. Chemical and electrochemical stability under the specific operating conditions,
4. Moisture control in stack,
5. Extremely low fuel or oxygen bypass to maximize its coulombic efficiency, and
6. Low production costs.

The performance of a membrane is dependent on the proton conductivity. This depends on prevailing levels of hydration. A higher conductivity is supported by higher levels of hydration. However, for operations with wet membranes, there is a possibility of the cathode being flooded, which slows down the oxidation reaction. This is particularly a problem with Nafion, because of a phenomenon known as electro-osmotic drag. The electro-osmotic drag coefficient is a quantitative measure of hydration. This is defined as the number of water molecules that are transported per proton.

The electro-osmotic drag has been detailed (10). Here, the water transport numbers for protons in a variety of available poly(perfluorosulfonic acid) membranes have been studied as a function of the water content. The data indicated that for membranes equilibrated with water vapor, a water drag coefficient of unity could be observed (10).

The water drag or water crossover can be avoided by a reduction of the membrane thickness. This results in an improvement of the fuel cell performance. Other advantages of reduced thickness are a lower membrane resistance, lower cost and rapid hydration (1).

3.2.1 *Permeation and Diffusion*

Hydrogen permeation data and diffusion parameters at elevated temperatures are important for the selection and development of new materials for fuel cells that are operating at lower temperatures.

A radiotracer method has been used to collect and analyze hydrogen permeation data across polymer membranes (11). Initially, poly(tetrafluoroethylene) (PTFE) and poly(ethylene) were tested. The permeation and diffusion of hydrogen in polymers was measured using tritium as a radiotracer (12). The permeation and diffusion coefficients and their respective activation energies are determined using the time lag method for Viton, Teflon, EPDM, Santoprene and Noryl.

3.2.2 *Water Transport in Polymer Electrolyte Membrane Fuel Cells*

Polymer electrolyte membrane fuel cells have been identified as a promising zero-emission power source for portable, mobile and stationary applications (13).

To ensure both a high membrane proton conductivity and sufficient reactant delivery to reaction sites, the management of water has become one of the most important issues for the commercialization of a polymer electrolyte membrane fuel cell.

The proper water management requires a good understanding of the water transport in different components of polymer electrolyte membrane fuel cell.

The knowledge of the water transport in a polymer electrolyte membrane fuel cell has been reviewed (13). The state and transport mechanism of water in different components have been detailed. It has been found that in fact experimental techniques have been developed to predict the distribution of water, gas species, temperature and other parameters in polymer electrolyte membrane fuel cell. However, certain difficulties are still present for simultaneous measurements of multiple parameters, and the cell and system design modifications required by measurements need to be minimized.

Different models concerning the water transport in polymer electrolyte membrane fuel cell have been adopted for different purposes and all together they can provide a comprehensive view of water transport in polymer electrolyte membrane fuel cell. With the development of computational power, application of lower length scale methods to higher length scales for more accurate and comprehensive results is feasible in the future.

Research related to cold start, i.e., startup from subzero temperatures and high-temperature polymer electrolyte membrane fuel cell, i.e., operating at the temperatures higher than 100°C, also have been described (13).

Ice formation that hinders the delivery of the reactant and damages cell materials is the major issue for a polymer electrolyte membrane fuel cell cold start. Enhancing the water absorption by the membrane electrolyte and external heating have been identified as the most effective ways to reduce the formation of ice and accelerate temperature increment.

A high-temperature polymer electrolyte membrane fuel cell that can operate without liquid water formation and membrane hydration greatly simplifies the strategy of the water management (13).

3.2.3 *Water Management System for Solid Polymer Electrolyte Fuel Cell Power Plants*

A simplified solid polymer electrolyte fuel cell power plant may utilize porous conductive separator plates having central passages which are filled with circulating coolant water (14). The coolant water passes through a heat exchanger which rejects heat generated in the power plant.

Water appearing on the cathode side of each cell membrane is pumped into the water circulation passages through the porous oxidant reactant flow-field plates by a positive ΔP created between the cathode reactant flow field of each cell and the coolant water circulation passages between each cell. In order to create the desired ΔP, at least one of the reactant gas streams will be referenced to the coolant water loop so as to create a coolant loop pressure which is less than the referenced reactant gas stream pressure.

Excess water is removed from the coolant water stream. The system can operate at ambient or at elevated pressures. Each cell in the power plant is individually cooled on demand, and the power plant does not require a separate cooling section or reactant stream humidifying devices (14).

3.2.4 *Accelerated Conditioning*

A newly fabricated polymer electrolyte membrane fuel cell usually needs a so-called break-in/conditioning/incubation period to activate it and reach its best performance (15).

Typically, during this activation period the cell performance increases gradually, and then reaches a plateau without further increase. Depending on the membrane electrode assemblies, this process can take hours and even days to complete, which consumes a considerable amount of hydrogen fuel, leading to a higher operating cost.

To provide for accelerated conditioning techniques that can complete the process in a short time period, established conditioning protocols and reported methods to condition polymer electrolyte membrane single cells and stacks have been reviewed, in an attempt to summarize available information on polymer electrolyte membrane fuel cell conditioning and the underlying mechanisms.

The techniques can be arranged into two categories (15):

1. On-line conditioning, and
2. Off-line conditioning.

For each technique, the experimental procedure and outcomes have been detailed. Also, the weaknesses of the currently used conditioning techniques are indicated and further research efforts were proposed (15).

3.2.5 *Working Principle of a Polymer Exchange Membrane*

The working principle of a polymer exchange membrane fuel cell has been reviewed (4).

Also, the water management problem in polymer exchange membrane fuel cell has been detailed. The discussions are based on elimination of the water management problem by proper design of fuel cell.

The various types of efficiency, polarization characteristics and power characteristics have been elucidated. Also, the various parameters, such as pressure, temperature, stoichiometry ratio and humidity have been described, which affect the performance of a fuel cell, and the optimum range in which fuel cell operates safely and efficiently.

The performance of a fuel cell is increased by a proper water management on the membrane. The basic parameters which enhance the fuel cell performance are relative humidity, flow-field design, temperature, and the stoichiometric ratio.

It has been observed that the fuel cell performance is improved by increasing the relative humidity, temperature, pressure, stoichiometric ratio and using the split serpentine flow field instead of single serpentine flow field (4).

3.2.6 *Membranes for Direct Methanol Fuel Cells*

The literature on composites and multilayer membranes for polymer electrolyte fuel cell applications, including intermediate-temperature polymer electrolyte fuel cells and direct methanol fuel cell systems, has been reviewed (16).

A direct methanol fuel cell system has a tremendous potential for energy converters due to the simplicity and low temperature of its operation (17). However, the weaknesses of commercial polymer electrolyte membrane of the cell, perfluorinated ionomer membrane, such as methanol crossover, limited operating temperature, susceptibility to osmotic swelling and high costs are among the factors hindering the commercialization of direct methanol fuel cell.

A number of studies that have been performed in order to overcome the weaknesses have been reviewed. The membrane development is classified into three different branches, namely (17):

1. The modification of perfluorinated ionomer membranes,
2. The development of other fluoropolymer membranes, and
3. The development of non-fluorinated polymer membranes.

In a direct methanol fuel cell, methanol at the anode is oxidized to an hydrogen ion and an electron, cf. Eq. 3.1.

The electrons released flow through an electrical circuit that extends from the anode to the cathode. The hydrogen ions travel simultaneously to the cathode through the electrolyte membrane. At the cathode, the electron and hydrogen ion will react with oxygen to form water, cf. Eq. 3.2.

$$\mathrm{CH3OH} + \mathrm{H_2O} \rightarrow \mathrm{CO_2} + 6\mathrm{H^+}6\mathrm{e^-} \tag{3.1}$$

$$\frac{3}{2}\mathrm{O_2} + 6\mathrm{H^+} \rightarrow 3\mathrm{H_2O} \tag{3.2}$$

The technology of a direct methanol fuel cell membrane is very similar to a proton exchange fuel cell membrane (17).

3.2.6.1 *Anion Exchange Membranes*

A series of anion exchange membranes was prepared from the copolymer of 1-vinyl imidazole and *N*-vinyl carbazole for direct methanol fuel cells (18). The structure of the membranes was studied using 1H nuclear magnetic resonance, scanning electron microscope (SEM), transmission electron microscopy, atomic force microscopy (AFM), and small angle X-ray scattering.

The thermal stability of the membranes was characterized by thermogravimetric analysis. Also, the ion conductivity, methanol permeability, ionic exchange capacity, water uptake, swelling ratio, and alkaline stability of the membranes were investigated.

It has been found that the ion conductivity of the membranes varied from 0.0934 to 0.2028 Scm^{-1} in deionized water and the methanol permeability varied from 4.5×10^{-8} to 12.3×10^{-8} $cm^2 s^{-1}$ at 30°C. All the prepared membranes are stable in a 1.0 M KOH solution at 60°C for 1400 h due to the polyolefinic backbone. A methanol/oxygen single-cell evaluation exhibited a open-circuit voltage of 0.93 V and a peak power density of 125.8 $mW\,cm^{-2}$. Thus, these membranes have a great potential for application in alkaline fuel cells (18).

3.2.6.2 *Polymeric Nano-sieve Nafion Composite Membrane*

A poly(amide) hyperbranched macromolecular proton conductor with end-capped –COOH has been used as a bifunctional polymeric nano-sieve in composite Nafion membranes to simultaneously improve the proton conductivity and suppress the methanol permeation (19). The method of synthesis has been detailed in a previous paper (20).

The incorporation in an amount of 1–5% of the bifunctional polymeric nano-sieve into the composite Nafion membrane was found to improve both the proton conductivity and the methanol permeation resistivity. Also, a stronger mechanical strength was obtained compared to a pure Nafion membrane (19).

A membrane with a 5% bifunctional polymeric nano-sieve content gives an optimal performance and the composite membrane is well suited for applications in direct methanol fuel cells.

The performance of the membrane used in a direct methanol fuel cell was found to be more than 60% better than the performance of a recast pure Nafion membrane (19).

3.2.6.3 *Graphene-Nafion Sandwich Membrane*

Methanol crossover due to the low selectivity of proton exchange membranes is a long-standing issue in the technology of direct methanol fuel cells (21). A composite membrane fabricated by sandwiching a monolayer graphene between two thin Nafion membranes to take advantage of monolayer graphene's selective permeability to only protons has been developed.

The methanol permeability of the present membrane could be demonstrated to have a 68.6% decrease in comparison to that of a pristine Nafion membrane. The test in a passive direct methanol fuel cell showed that the designed membrane retains a high proton conductivity, while substantially suppressing the methanol crossover. As a result, the present membrane enables the passive direct methanol fuel cell to exhibit a decent performance even at a methanol concentration as high as 10.0 *M* (21).

3.2.6.4 Carbon-Based Materials

The diffusion layer is an important structure in the membrane electrode assembly of direct methanol fuel cells that provides a support layer for catalysts, electronic channels, and gas-liquid mass transport channels. Three types of carbon-based materials were used to fabricate anode diffusion layers (22):

1. Carbon black Vulcan®,
2. M-15 grade graphene nanosheets, and
3. C-500 grade graphene nanosheets.

Carbon black Vulcan consists of nanosized carbon particles, while both M-15 grade graphene nanosheets and C-500 grade graphene nanosheets are made of stacks of graphene sheets with flaky structures that increase catalyst utilization.

The microporous layers of cathodes were constructed with carbon black Vulcan. A carbon-based microporous layer with a 2 $mg\,cm^{-2}$ loading was coated onto a PTFE-pretreated carbon cloth, while a Nafion-117 membrane was applied as the electrolyte to the direct methanol fuel cells.

Pt-Ru black and Pt black were used as anode and cathode electrode catalysts, each with loadings of 8 $mg\,cm^{-2}$ and 4 $mg\,cm^{-2}$, respectively. All tests were conducted using membrane electrode assemblies with active areas of 4 cm^2 and air was supplied to single cells by passive modes.

Performance tests of the direct methanol fuel cells were conducted using a potentiostat that generated polarization curves. The highest peak power density of 13.7 $mW\,cm^{-2}$ was obtained with the C-500 grade graphene nanosheets anode diffusion layer using 3 *M* methanol as fuel. The energy efficiency of the passive direct methanol fuel cells was approximately 10% with a specific energy of approximately 610 $Wh\,kg^{-1}$, which is higher than that of conventional lithium-ion batteries (22).

The high power densities obtained by both graphene-based materials, M-15 grade graphene nanosheets and C-500 grade graphene nanosheets, demonstrate that graphene is a material other than the state-of-the-art carbon black that has the potential to be used as a direct methanol fuel cell anode support material (22).

3.2.6.5 *Hybrid Membranes*

Graphene oxide sheets have been functionalized by histidine molecules and incorporated into sulfonated poly(ether ether ketone) matrix to fabricate hybrid polymer electrolyte membranes for direct methanol fuel cells (23). Histidine is shown in Figure 3.1.

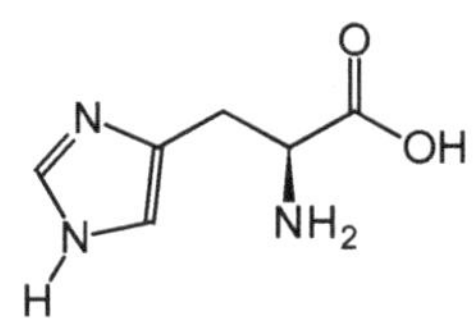

Figure 3.1 *L*-Histidine.

The loading of the functionalized graphene oxide has been varied to investigate its influence on cross sectional morphology, crystalline structure, polymer chain stiffness, thermal stability, and fractional free volume of the membrane.

The acidic $-SO_3H$ groups, the proton donors in sulfonated poly(ether ether ketone) and basic imidazole groups, the proton acceptors in the histidine molecules form acid-base pairs and transport protons synergistically, thus yielding efficient proton channels inside the hybrid membranes.

The maximum proton conductivity at 100% relative humidity of the hybrid membranes is elevated by 30.2% in comparison to a plain sulfonated poly(ether ether ketone) membrane at room temperature. The functionalized graphene oxide flakes also effect a low methanol permeability in the range of 1.32×10^{-7} to 3.91×10^{-7} cm^2s^{-1}. With the filler content of 4%, the hybrid membrane shows a superior selectivity of 5.14×10^5 $S\,s\,cm^{-3}$ and its maximum power density of single direct methanol fuel cell of 43.0 $mW\,cm^{-2}$ is 80.7% higher than that of a plain sulfonated poly(ether ether ketone) membrane (23).

3.2.6.6 Organically Modified Metal Oxide Nanoparticles

Organic-inorganic composite proton exchange membranes of sulfonated poly(arylene ether sulfone) and organically modified metal oxide nanoparticles have been synthesized (24).

Sulfonated poly(arylene ether sulfone) ionomers with different degrees of sulfonation were synthesized by condensation polymerization. The monomers used for the condensation polymerization are shown in Figure 3.2.

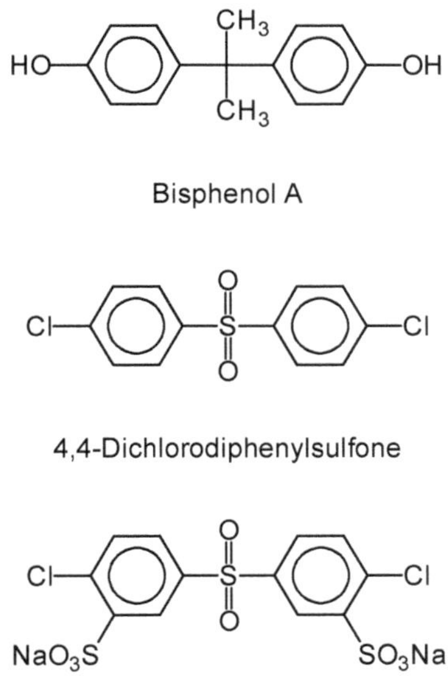

Figure 3.2 Monomers used for the condensation polymerization (24).

Nanocrystalline titania and zirconia particles were prepared by sol-gel reactions catalyzed by *p*-toluene sulfonic acid in the presence of acetylacetone as an organic surface modifier. Acetylacetone is shown in Figure 3.3.

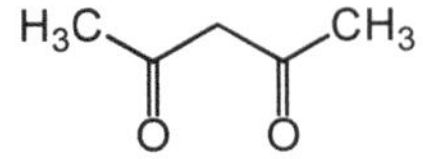

Figure 3.3 Acetylacetone.

The transparent composite membranes with 1% nanoparticle content were obtained by simply mixing the sulfonated poly(arylene ether sulfone) and the nanoparticles in dimethyl sulfoxide followed by membrane casting.

A posttreatment in aqueous sulfuric acid resulted in composite membranes exhibiting reduced proton conductivities and highly improved methanol permeabilities and water uptakes in comparison to pristine sulfonated poly(arylene ether sulfone) membranes.

The zirconia-containing sulfonated poly(arylene ether sulfone) with a degree of sulfonation of 48% composite membrane exhibited the best proton exchange property and also the best power density.

The improved properties of these composite membranes can be attributed to the effective barrier effect of both titania and zirconia nanoparticles provided by their small particle sizes of smaller than 10 *nm* without significant aggregation within the sulfonated poly-(arylene ether sulfone) matrix (24).

3.2.6.7 Sulfonated Polymer Membranes

A series of tetra-sulfonated poly(*p*-phenylene-*co*-aryl ether ketone) membranes with microblock moieties have been synthesized by a nickel catalytic coupling copolymerization (25). The materials show a good dimensional stability. This compound is shown in Figure 3.4. Here, the sulfonic acid groups are located on the short aromatic side chains. The side chains have been synthesized from 2,5-dichloro-4′-(bromopropyl)benzophenone and 4-(triphenylmethyl) phenol by methods reported in the literature (26, 27). These compounds are shown in Figure 3.5

In comparison to mono-sulfonated poly(*p*-phenylene-*co*-aryl ether ketone) membranes the power density is higher. The valuable properties of the membranes can be attributed to the synchronous introduction of locally and densely sulfonated hydrophilic units and

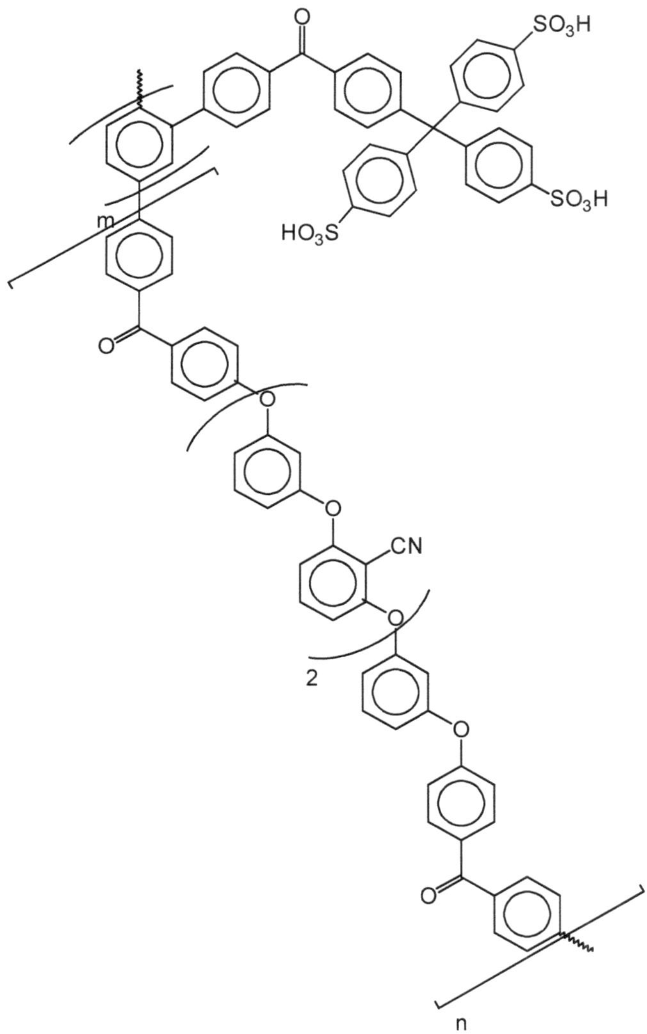

Figure 3.4 Tetra-sulfonated poly(*p*-phenylene-*co*-aryl ether ketone).

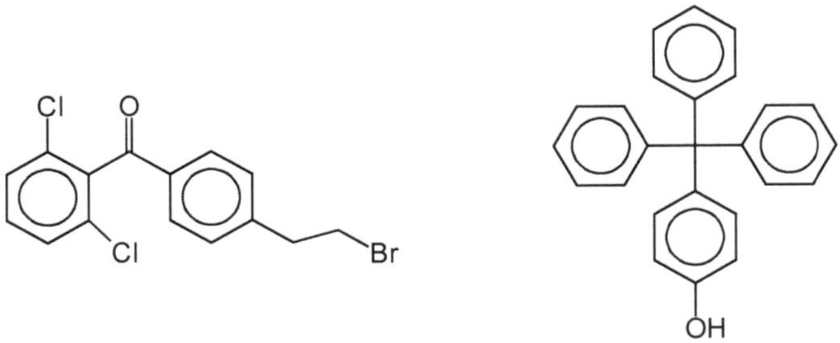

2,5-Dichloro-4′-(bromopropyl)benzophenone 4-(Triphenylmethyl) phenol

Figure 3.5 Side chains.

hydrophobic microblock moieties in the membrane structure, resulting in the formation of connected proton transport channels (25).

3.2.6.8 Quaternized Poly(phenylene oxide) Anion Exchange Membrane

A series of anion exchange membrane electrolytes with quaternary ammonium moiety have been fabricated from poly(phenylene oxide) (PPO) for application in alkaline direct methanol fuel cells (28).

In the first step, poly(2,6-dimethyl-1,4-phenylene oxide) is chloromethylated by substituting the chloromethyl groups in the aryl position of polymer (29,30). In the second step, the chloromethylated PPO is further homogeneously quaternized and ion exchanged to form an anion exchange membrane. The reaction scheme is shown in Figure 3.6.

Then, several anion exchange membranes are prepared by changing the mole ratio of amine in relation to chloromethylated PPO. The presence of quaternary ammonium group in the membrane was confirmed by elemental analysis. The fabricated membranes have been subjected to cell polarization studies in alkaline direct methanol fuel cells, wherein a membrane from quaternized poly(2,6-dimethyl-1,4-phenylene oxide) in a ratio of chloromethylated PPO to amine of 1:8 exhibits higher peak power density of 3.5 $mWcm^{-2}$ when compared with the other ratios of chloromethylated PPO:amine in the absence of the KOH solution (28).

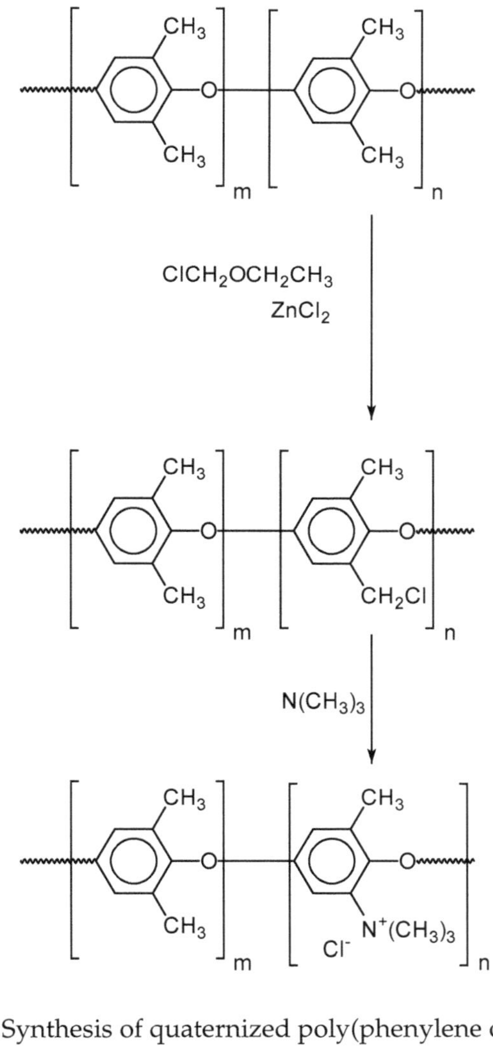

Figure 3.6 Synthesis of quaternized poly(phenylene oxide) (29).

3.2.6.9 *Acid-Base Polyion Complex Membrane*

An acid-base polyion complex membrane was synthesized by blending a poly(amide-imide) (Torlon®), cf. Figure 3.7, with a sulfonated poly(ethersulfone) (31).

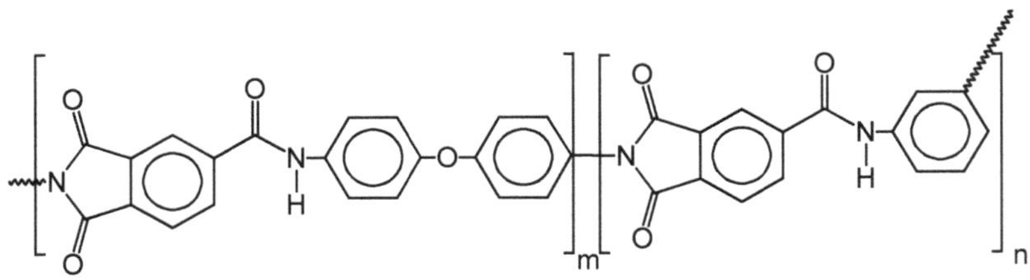

Figure 3.7 Torlon® (32).

A robust proton-conducting electrolyte for portable fuel cells was fabricated (31). The chemical interactions between Torlon and the sulfonated poly(ethersulfone) enabled the formation of ionic clusters that are useful for facilitating the proton conduction and the water sorption with prevention of fuel bypass.

The complex exhibited high mechanical, thermal and oxidative stability with a low methanol permeability. Sorption experiments showed that the membrane possesses a moderate affinity toward water with preferably low methanol uptake. Also, the blend membrane exhibited a high proton conductivity of 0.13 $S\,cm^{-1}$ at low humidity and high-temperature conditions (31).

3.2.6.10 *Membranes from Polymer Composites*

A vinyl group-modified montmorillonite clay, vinyl group-modified graphene oxide, and a vinyl group-modified multiwalled carbon nanotube were prepared by the ion exchange reaction of 1-[(4-ethylphenyl)methyl]-3-butyl-imidazolium chloride, cf. Figure 3.8. The materials were used for the protection against methanol crossover in a direct methanol fuel cell membrane (33).

Then polymeric nanocomposite membranes using these compounds were prepared by the solvent casting method after a radiation-induced polymerization of vinyl monomers in a mixture

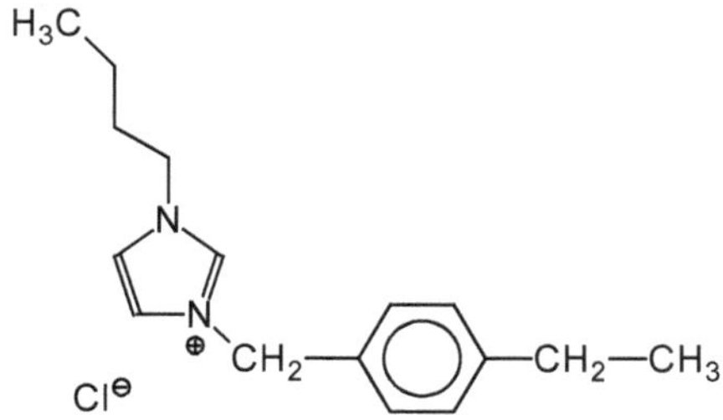

Figure 3.8 1-[(4-Ethylphenyl)methyl]-3-butyl-imidazolium chloride.

of water and methanol as solvent (33). The method of radiation-induced graft polymerization has been detailed elsewhere (34). As vinyl monomers, styrene, sodium styrene sulfonate, 2-hydroxyethyl methacrylate, and acrylic acid were used.

Ionic polymer membranes of different thicknesses of 50–450 μm) based on poly(vinylpyrolidone), poly(vinyl alcohol) (PVA), sulfosuccinic acid and silicotungstic acid have been synthesized for polymer electrolyte membrane fuel cells (35). Silicotungstic acid is shown in Figure 3.9.

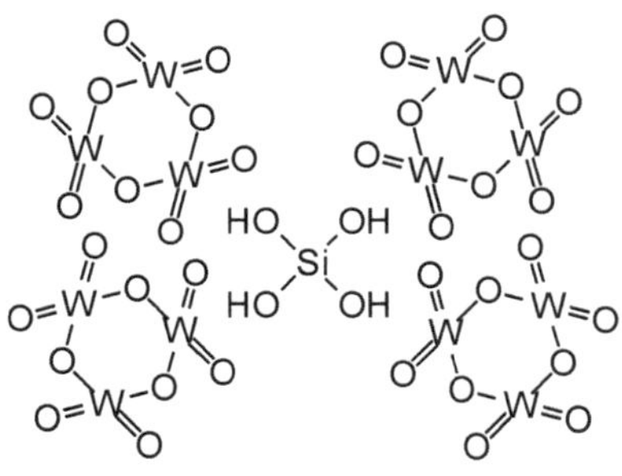

Figure 3.9 Silicotungstic acid.

The water uptake of these membranes ranged from 35% to 75%. The ionic conductivities of these membranes ranged between $1.025\times 10^{-3}\ S\ cm^{-1}$ to $7.55\times 10^{-3}\ S\ cm^{-1}$.

The best water uptake and ionic conductivity were those of the membrane based on PVA, poly(vinylpyrolidone), sulfosuccinic acid, and 10.3% silicotungstic acid (35).

3.2.6.11 *Sulfonated Poly(vinylidene fluoride and Sulfonated Poly(ethersulfone)*

Sulfonated poly(vinylidene fluoride-*co*-hexafluoropropylene)/sulfonated poly(ethersulfone) blend polymer electrolyte membranes (PEMs) were fabricated effectively as an alternative polymer electrolyte membrane for direct methanol fuel cell applications (36).

In order to prepare polymer electrolyte membranes with an improved proton conductivity, poly(vinylidene fluoride-*co*-hexafluoropropylene) and poly(ethersulfone) were sulfonated using chlorosulfonic acid and sulfuric acid, respectively.

The influential characteristics of the polymer electrolyte membranes, such as water uptake, swelling ratio, ion exchange capacity, proton conductivity, methanol crossover and selectivity ratio, were elucidated.

The tensile strength and elongation at break slightly decreases by the addition of the hydrophilic sulfonated poly(ethersulfone). The water uptake and the proton conductivity of the sulfonated poly(vinylidene fluoride-*co*-hexafluoropropylene)/sulfonated poly-(ethersulfone) blend membranes were increased and found to be higher than that of the pure sulfonated poly(vinylidene fluoride-*co*-hexafluoropropylene) (36).

3.2.6.12 *Comb-like Ionomers*

A poly(2,6-dimethyl-1,4-phenylene oxide)-based comb-like ionomer, 3.10, has been synthesized. The physical and electrochemical properties of this ionomer have been investigated.

The ionomer consists of a PPO backbone and a partially fluorinated cationic side chain. In comparison to an imidazolium functionalized PPO ionomer, the comb-like ionomer showed a higher stability regarding ionic conductivity and ion exchange capacity in alkaline media.

Also, a low swelling ratio for 4 *M* methanol anodic fuel was found for the ionomer. This property makes it a suitable candidate for an application in the anodic catalyst layer in anion exchange membrane direct methanol fuel cells.

Thermogravimetric analysis coupled with a mass spectrometer proved the ionomer to be thermally stable in anion exchange mem-

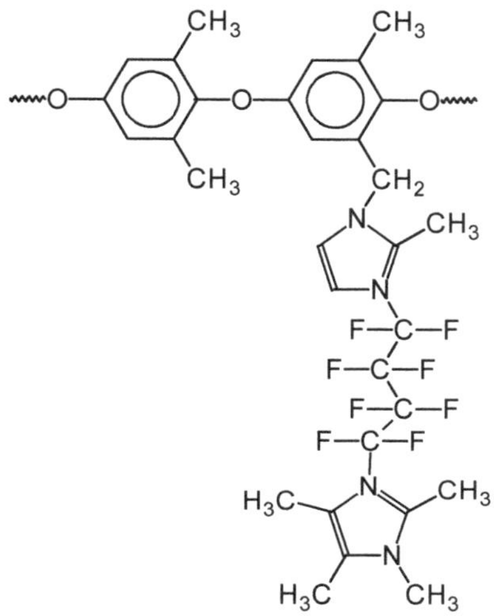

Figure 3.10 Comb-like ionomer (37).

brane direct methanol fuel cell working conditions. Therefore, the comb-like ionomer was implemented in single cells as a catalyst binder. A single cell with an ionomer content of 25% showed a 2.75 times higher power output compared to a single cell with PTFE as anode catalyst binder when run with KOH-free anodic fuel (37).

3.2.7 *Membranes for Direct Ethanol Fuel Cells*

The electrolyte membrane is an important component of a fuel cell. An excellent electrolyte membrane should have a high proton conductivity, low electron conductivity, prevention of oxidation, low fuel crossover, good mechanical stability, long-term chemical and thermal stability and water management (38).

Currently, two types of electrolyte membranes are commonly used in direct ethanol fuel cells: Proton exchange membranes and anion exchange membranes, typically used in alkaline cells (39).

Proton exchange membranes and alkaline exchange membranes for direct ethanol fuel cells have been summarized (38). Current problems and advancements in direct ethanol fuel cell membranes are reviewed. Also, specifications and performances of the membranes used in direct ethanol fuel cells have been described.

3.2.7.1 *Nafion Membranes*

Perfluorinated sulfonic acid electrolyte membranes (Nafion®, manufactured by DuPont) are commonly used for proton exchange membranes due to their excellent chemical and electrochemical properties as well as mechanical stabilities with high proton conductivity (38).

The drawback of Nafion membrane arises from its high production costs and high permeability for fuels inside the membranes. This leads to a swelling problem and causes the loss of fuel.

One of the main reasons for the drawback is the performance drop of the membrane at elevated temperature above 80°C. This arises due to the dehydration of the membrane that results in adverse effects in the proton conductivity and the mechanical stability (38).

3.2.7.2 *Poly(vinyl alcohol) Functionalized Carbon Nanotubes*

The application of a PVA functionalized carbon nanotubes composite in alkaline direct ethanol fuel cells has been investigated. The carbon nanotubes are functionalized with PVA using the ozone mediation method (40).

The ozone mediation method for the preparation of PVA functionalized carbon nanotubes runs as (40):

Preparation 3–1: First 1 *g* of PVA was dissolved in 30 *ml* of water at 70°C and the PVA solution was placed in a 100 *ml* flask with a stirrer. The PVA solution was purged with ozone gas for 15 min at an ozone gas flow rate of 6 $l\,min^{-1}$, resulting in an ozone concentration of 28 $mg\,l^{-1}$. The solution was then purged with argon gas for another 15 *min* to remove free peroxide groups. Then, 0.5 *g* of carbon nanotubes was rapidly added to the PVA solution. The mixture was stirred at 80°C for 3 *h* to graft the PVA polymer chains onto the carbon nanotubes. After the reaction was completed, the functionalized carbon nanotubes (referred to as an m-carbon nanotube) and the solution were separated using a centrifuge, and the m-carbon nanotube was washed with hot water until the solution was clear. The m-carbon nanotube was collected using filtration and dried overnight

Further, the PVA/carbon nanotube composite is prepared as (40):

Preparation 3–2: A small amount of 0.0075 *mg* of m-carbon nanotube is suspended in a beaker containing 10 *ml* of deionized water by using ultrasonication at room temperature. Then 15 *g* of PVA was dissolved in 50 *ml* of deionized water to form a polymer solution. The m-carbon nanotube suspension was mixed into the PVA solution. Another 75 *ml* of deionized water was used to rinse the beaker wall and remove any remaining m-carbon nanotube.

The rinse solution was then combined with the m-carbon nanotube and PVA solution. The solution with a total volume of 135 *ml* was heated to 90°C under ultrasonication and stirred at 250 *rpm* for 6 *h* to obtain a homogeneous suspension. The suspension was cast on a glass plate with an application knife (model 3580, Elcometer Instruments Ltd., Edge Lane, England). A membrane of uniform thickness was obtained after the cast film was dried in vacuum at 60°C for 6 *h*. The resulting PVA composite consisted of 0.05% of m-carbon nanotube. The thickness of the dried composite membrane was 130–180 μm. The PVA and PVA/m-carbon nanotube composites were immersed in KOH solutions of various concentrations for at least 24 *h* prior to conductivity and fuel cell tests.

The addition of the carbon nanotubes into the PVA matrix enhances the alkaline uptake and the ionic conductivity of the KOH-doped electrolyte.

The carbon nanotube containing membrane exhibited a lower swelling ratio and suppressed ethanol permeability compared to the pristine PVA film. The optimal conditions for alkaline direct ethanol fuel cells were determined to be under operation at an anode feed of 3 *M* ethanol in a 5 *M* KOH solution at a flow rate of 5 $cm^3\ min^{-1}$ with a cathode feed of moisturized oxygen with a flow rate of 100 $cm^3\ min^{-1}$ and the KOH-doped PVA/carbon nanotube electrolyte.

A peak power density value of 65 $mW\ cm^{-2}$ at 60°C was achieved, which is the highest among the alkaline direct ethanol fuel cells literature data and several times higher than the proton exchange direct ethanol fuel cells using sulfonated membrane electrolytes (40). Therefore, the KOH-doped PVA/carbon nanotube electrolyte is a suitable solid electrolyte for alkaline direct ethanol fuel cells and has the potential for commercialization in alkaline fuel cell applications.

3.2.8 High-Temperature Polymer Electrolyte Membrane Fuel Cell

The issue of auxiliary power units with enhanced reformate tolerance for high-temperature polymer electrolyte membrane fuel cells has been reviewed (41).

The developments in diesel reforming for fuel cells as auxiliary power units, single fuel cells and stacks and systems have been outlined in detail and the key findings have been presented.

A summary of cooling high-temperature polymer electrolyte membrane fuel cell stacks using a classic schematic diagram of a 24-cell high-temperature polymer electrolyte membrane fuel cell stack, with a cooling plate for every third cell, has been presented as part of a stack analysis. Also, a summary of CO tolerances for fuel cells has been given, along with the effects of different CO volume fractions on polarization curves, the fraction of CO coverage, hydrogen coverage, anode overpotential and cell potential (41).

3.2.9 *Functionalized Microporous Zeolite-13X Membrane*

The impact of a modified hydrophilic microporous zeolite, i.e., zeolite-13X, by introducing organo-sulfonic acid groups through silane condensation has been investigated (42).

The zeolite is dispersed in a sulfosuccinic acid-sulfonated poly(ether ether ketone) to form a mixed matrix membrane. This material has been tested for its application in direct methanol fuel cells.

Organo-sulfonic acid groups present in modified zeolite-13X serve to restrict the methanol crossover and also provide additional ion-conducting groups for the overall improvement of the performance. The crosslinking of the poly(ether ether ketone) with sulfosuccinic acid has been shown to be beneficial in providing stability to the matrix and also helps in enhancing the ionic conductivity (42).

3.2.10 *Nanoporous Carbon-Nafion Hybrid Membranes*

In order to improve the efficiency of a direct methanol fuel cell an alternative membrane with a reduced methanol crossover has been developed (43). A nanoporous carbon Nafion hybrid membrane reduces the methanol crossover by 50% compared to a pristine Nafion membrane.

Nanoporous carbon was synthesized using a surfactant template route with sodium dodecyl sulfate in order to get a well-established pore geometry in the nanoporous carbon during synthesis. Nanoporous carbon acts as effective filler in Nafion polymer matrix by restricting the methanol crossover in a hybrid membrane and thus helps to enhance the direct methanol fuel cell output power density.

The Nafion nanoporous carbon hybrid membrane delivers a peak power density of 171 $mW\,cm^{-2}$ at 70°C under ambient pressure, which is about three times higher than a pristine Nafion® membrane under identical operating conditions (43).

3.2.11 *Proton Exchange Membranes*

Proton exchange membranes that operate at temperatures above 120°C are needed to avoid catalyst poisoning. They enhance electrochemical reactions, simplify the design and reduce the cost of fuel cells (44). The developments in proton exchange membranes have been reviewed.

In order to design new membranes for elevated temperature operation, the chemistry, morphology and dynamics of protons and water molecules in existing membranes must be understood.

The integration of experiments with modeling and simulation can shed light on the hierarchical structure of the membrane and dynamical processes associated with molecular transport.

Based on such a fundamental understanding, membranes can be modified by controlling the polymer chemistry and architecture or adding inorganic fillers that can retain water under low relative humidity conditions.

The development of anhydrous membranes based on phosphoric acid-doped polymers, ionic liquid-infused polymer gels and solid acids can enable fuel cell operation above 150°C (44).

3.2.12 *Catalyst Degradation and Starvation*

In proton exchange membrane fuel cells, cost, reliability and durability are important issues that must be solved (45). The decrease in their performance during operation has been attributed, among other things, to the loss of electrochemical surface area occurring during long-term aging, after transients or after an incident of faulty operation. These losses are mainly due to catalyst metal degradation and carbon-support corrosion, which are continuous irreversible processes that can dramatically reduce the fuel cell lifetime.

The phenomena linked to catalyst and carbon-support degradation have been reviewed, focusing on those caused by fuel and oxidant starvation, since these faulty conditions are amongst the most critical for fuel cell durability (45).

The reactions potentially involved in the catalyst degradation associated with thermodynamic and kinetic considerations related to fuel cell operation have been reviewed.

This information can be used to interpret the experimental results presented in the literature. An analysis of the reverse-current decay mechanism has been done and an alternative mechanism has been suggested.

Also, some characterization methods or mitigation strategies have been elucidated and an illustrative fault tree has been built, pointing out the relationship between the causes and the symptoms in the catalyst degradation (45).

3.2.13 Durability Test Protocols

Durability is one of the major barriers to polymer electrolyte membrane fuel cells being accepted as a commercially viable product (46). It is therefore important to understand their degradation phenomena and analyze degradation mechanisms from the component level to the cell and stack level so that novel component materials can be developed and novel designs for cells/stacks can be achieved to mitigate insufficient fuel cell durability.

It is generally impractical and costly to operate a fuel cell under its normal conditions for several thousand hours, so accelerated test methods are preferred to facilitate rapid learning about key durability issues.

Based on the U.S. Department of Energy and U.S. Fuel Cell Council accelerated test protocols, as well as degradation tests performed by researchers and published in the literature, degradation test protocols have been reviewed at both component and cell/stack levels (driving cycles), with the aim of gathering the available information on accelerated test methods and degradation test protocols for polymer electrolyte membrane fuel cells, and thereby providing practitioners with a useful toolbox to study durability issues.

These protocols help prevent the prolonged test periods and high costs associated with real lifetime tests, assess the performance and durability of polymer electrolyte membrane fuel cell components, and ensure that the generated data can be compared (46).

3.2.13.1 *Stack Testing*

An overview of polymer electrolyte membrane fuel cell stack testing has been presented (47). Stack testing is critical for evaluating and demonstrating the viability and durability required for commercial applications. Single-cell performance cannot be employed alone to fully derive the expected performance of polymer electrolyte membrane fuel cell stacks, due to the non-uniformity in potential, temperature, and reactant and product flow distributions observed in stacks.

The main topics of investigation have been discussed, including single cell vs. stack level performance, cell voltage uniformity, influence of operating conditions, durability and degradation, dynamic operation, and stack demonstrations.

Also, opportunities have been presented for future work, including the need to verify the impact of stack size and cell voltage uniformity on performance, determine operating conditions for achieving a balance between electrical efficiency and flooding/dry-out, meet lifetime requirements through endurance testing, and develop a stronger understanding of degradation (47).

3.2.14 Nanoscale Properties

The properties of the components of a membrane electrode assembly in a polymer electrolyte fuel cell determine its efficiency and its performance (48). The importance of nanoscale properties of polymer electrolyte fuel cell membranes and electrodes has been discussed.

The nanostructure and conductivity of freshly prepared, as well as artificially degraded Nafion membranes and Pt/C electrodes, have been investigated by contact AFM, conductive AFM, pulsed force mode AFM, *in-situ* scanning tunneling microscopy, and SEM. The different techniques can provide complementary information on structure and conductivity. With *in-situ* scanning tunneling microscopy on Pt catalyst covered graphite, a layer of very small Pt particles between the catalyst particles is imaged, which is probably not visible with TEM and can explain a systematic discrepancy between TEM and XRD in particle size distribution. Conductive AFM is used to investigate the conductivity of Nafion.

The images show a quite inhomogeneous distribution of current at the surface. The percentage of conductive surface increases with humidity, but regions without any current still present up to 80% of relative humidity.

The comparison with PFM-AFM images, where the differences in the adhesion forces can be measured, indicates that hydrophobic regions are present at the surface with comparable dimensions, which are attributed to a nonconductive PTFE-like polymer backbone. The changes in hydrophilic and hydrophobic parts after artificial degradation by plasma etching in air plasma can be imaged by PFM.

High-resolution current images of the membrane were used to directly compare the measured nanostructure of the single conductive channels with model predictions from the literature. Recent models in the literature propose the formation of water-filled inverted micelles with a mean diameter of 2.4 *nm*, and their agglomeration into clusters agrees well with the current images (48).

3.3 Types of Membrane Materials

The types of membrane materials are summarized in Table 3.1.

The structures of some polymeric membrane materials are shown in Figure 3.11

3.3.1 Biological Fuel Cells with Nanoporous Membranes

A fuel cell has been described that consists of an anode chamber, a cathode chamber, and a nanoporous membrane between the anode chamber and the cathode chamber (49).

The use of nanoporous membranes in biological fuel cells will lead to inexpensive designs, realistic power generation in real world scenarios, and increased coulombic efficiencies without relying on creating stable biofilms on the anodes.

The nanoporous membrane sequesters and isolates a microbe in the anode chamber. Also, the nanoporous membrane allows nutrients to flow actively or passively from the cathode chamber to

Table 3.1 Types of Membrane Materials (1).

Material Type	Examples
Perfluorinated ionomers	Perfluorosulfonic acid, Perfluorocarboxylic acid, Bis(perfluoroalkylsulfonyl)imide
Partially fluorinated polymers	α,β,β-Trifluorostyrene grafted onto PTFE with post sulfonation, Styrene grated on sulfonated poly(vinylidiene fluoride)
Non-fluorinated membranes with aromatic backbone	Naphthalenic poly(imide), Ballard advance material of third generation membrane, Sulfonated poly(ether ether ketone), Sulfonated poly(4-phenoxy benzoyl-1,4-phenylene), Methyl benzensulfonated poly(benzimidazole)s
Non-fluorinated hydrocarbons	
Acid-base blends	Sulfonated poly(ether ether ketone)/Polybenzimidazole, Sulfonated polysulfone/Poly-(ethylene imine), Poly(vinyl alcohol)/H_3PO_4

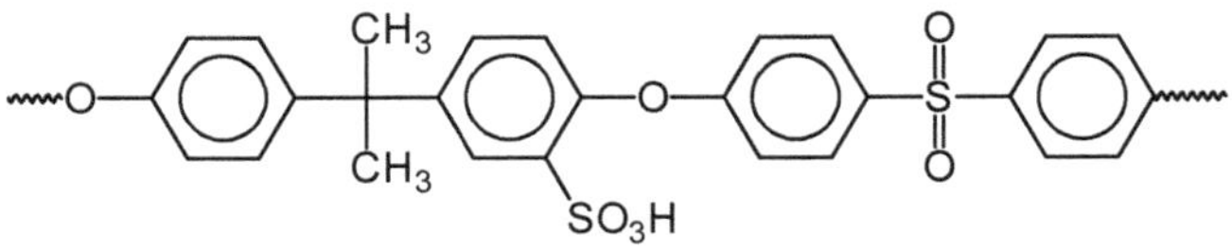

SPSU

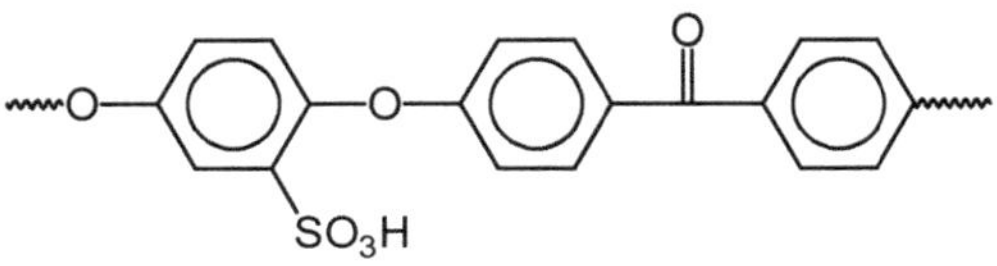

SPEEK

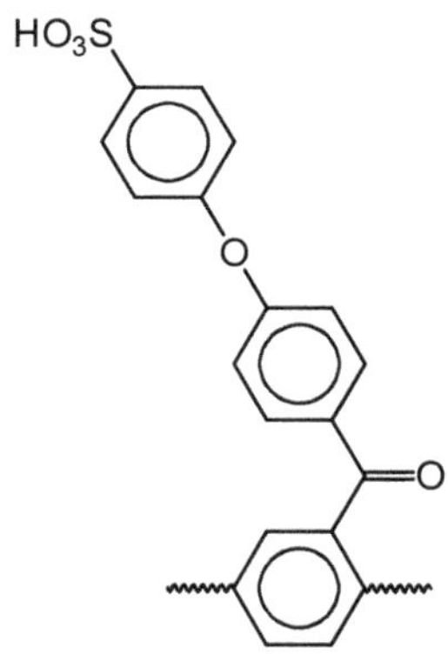

SPPBP

Figure 3.11 Sulfonated poly(sulfone) (SPSU), Sulfonated poly(ether ether ketone) (SPEEK), Sulfonated poly(4-phenoxy benzoyl-1,4-phenylene) (SPPBP).

the anode chamber and can be modified by a thin-film composite (TFC) to create a thin-film composite nanofiltration membrane. The nanoporous membrane can have a pore size from about 100 *nm* to about 1000 *nm*.

The basic design of a macroscopic microbial fuel cell includes the following (49):

1. An anaerobic anode chamber with a volume of 200–2000 *ml* that contains a solution of bacteria and possibly electron shuttles/mediators as well as a conductive anode with either enzymes attached or microbial biofilm formation,
2. A cathode chamber with an equal volume that is oxygen rich, contains a conductive cathode, and biocatalysts that promote oxidation reactions, and
3. A proton exchange membrane, usually Nafion that is placed in a channel that separates the anode and cathode chamber.

There are many variations on these devices that include (49): an air-exposed cathode, a mediator-less anode chamber that utilizes metal-reducing bacteria like *Geobacter sulfurreducens*, *Shewanella putrefaciens*, *Shewanella oneidensis*, *Geobacter metallireducens*, and *Rhodoferax ferrireducens*. Further variations are electrically conducting polymers coated onto the anode for protection and electron shuttling, Fe and Mn-traced anodes that eliminate the need for solution-bourne electron shuttles, seafloor devices that eliminate the need for the proton exchange membrane by placing the anode in sediment and the cathode in open ocean water, devices run off of sewage sludge for both delivery of nutrients and bacteria, and single-chamber devices with an air cathode.

Several examples of prototypes for the construction of such cells have been described in detail (49).

3.3.2 *Proton-Selective Membrane for Solid Polymer Fuel Cells*

A proton-selective membrane has been developed using a solid polymer electrolyte membrane for fuel cells that selectively allows only protons to pass through it (50).

The solid polymer electrolyte membrane can be used in solid polymer electrolyte fuel cells, which are also known as proton exchange membrane fuel cells, ion exchange membrane fuel cells, or polymer electrolyte membrane fuel cells.

The proton-selective membrane can be produced from one or more template molecules, providing one or more functional monomers to interact with the template molecules, providing an initiating agent to start a chemical reaction which results in an imprinted polymer, providing at least one crosslinking agent to covalently bond polymer chains created with the template molecules and functional monomers by polymerization, and removing the template molecules from the imprinted polymer to create a proton-selective membrane.

An example of a proton-selective membrane includes proton-conducting template molecules, vinylpyridine as the functional monomer, at least one of ethylene dimethacrylate, trimethylolpropane trimethacrylate, acrylamide and divinylbenzene as a crosslinking agent. As initiating agent, 2,2-azobis-(2-methylpropionitrile), dibenzoyl peroxide, Irgacure® 1800, 2,2′-azobis(2,4-dimethyl-valeronitrile) may be used (50).

The structures of some initiators are shown in Figure 3.12.

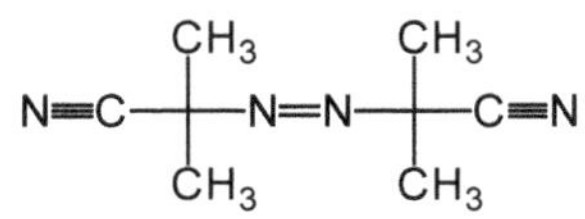

2,2-Azobis-(2-methylpropionitrile)

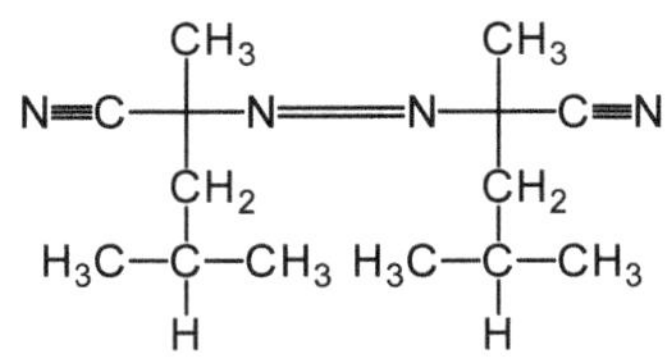

2,2′-Azobis(2,4-dimethyl-valeronitrile)

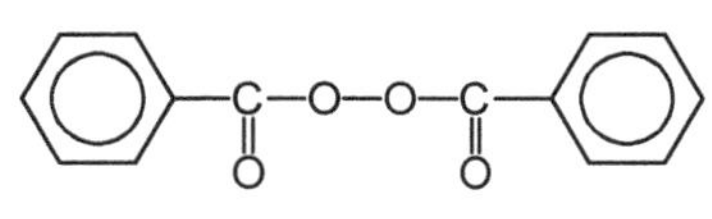

Dibenzoyl peroxide

Figure 3.12 Initiators.

Another example of a proton-selective membrane may include any of the above listed proton-conducting template molecules, vinylpyridine, methacrylic acid, acrylic acid, acrylamide, or the combination of vinylpyridine and acrylamide as the functional monomers, at least one of ethylene glycol dimethacrylate, trimethylolpropane trimethacrylate, acrylamide and divinylbenzene as a crosslinking agent, and at least one of 2,2′-azobis-(2-methylpropionitrile), dibenzoyl peroxide, Irgacure 1800, 1,4-divinylbenzene, 2,2-dimethoxy-2-phenylacetophenone, cf. Figure 3.13, and 2,2′-azobis(2,4-dimethyl-valeronitrile) as an initiating agent (50).

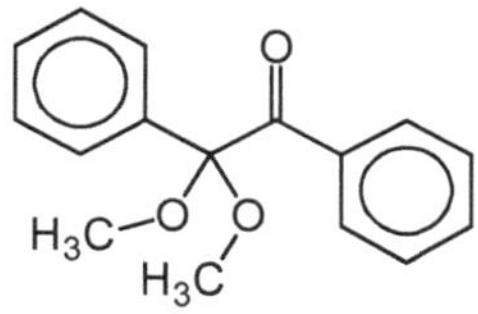

Figure 3.13 2,2-Dimethoxy-2-phenylacetophenone.

The structures of some vinyl monomers are shown in Figure 3.14.

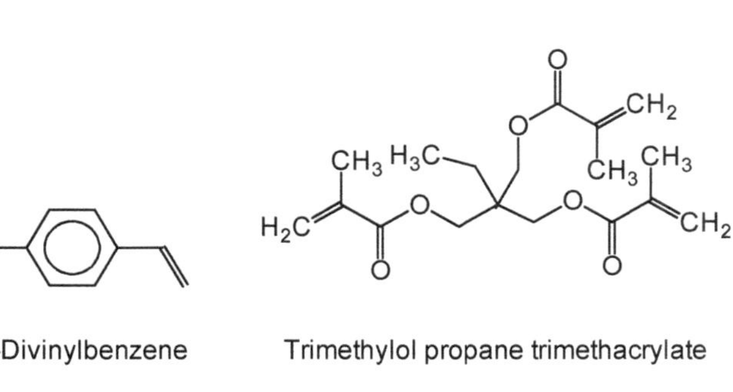

Figure 3.14 Vinyl monomers.

3.3.3 *Polymer Electrolyte Membranes for Direct Methanol Fuel Cells*

Numerous publications document the synthesis and characterization of new polymer electrolyte membranes for the direct methanol fuel cell. This research has been reviewed, as well as transport phenomena in polymer electrolyte membranes, and experimental techniques used to evaluate new polymer electrolyte membranes for a direct methanol fuel cell.

A series of materials for polymer electrolyte membranes have been developed for direct methanol fuel cells. A few of these materials are summarized in Table 3.2

Although many polymer electrolyte membranes do not show significant improvements over Nafion, the benchmark polymer electrolyte membrane in direct methanol fuel cells, experimental results show that several new polymer electrolyte membranes exhibit lower methanol crossover at similar proton conductivities and/or higher direct methanol fuel cell power densities (77).

3.3.3.1 *Graphene Oxide*

Graphene oxide has been investigated intensively because of its excellent electrical properties, unique two-dimensional structure and large specific surface (78–81).

Reduced Graphene Oxide. Octahedral Fe_3O_4/reduced graphene oxide composites with sandwich-like structures were synthesized through ultrasonic and thermal reduction process (81).

The preparation of graphene oxide runs as (81):

Preparation 3–3: First 3 *g* of graphite was dispersed in 360 *mL* H_2SO_4 and 40 *ml* H_3PO_4 and 18 *g* $KMnO_4$ was slowly added. Then the reaction was heated to 50°C and stirred for 12 *h*. After cooling to room temperature, 200 *ml* of deionized water and 30% H_2O_2 solution was added and stirred until the color of the mixture changed to bright yellow. In order to further purify the mixture it was centrifuged and the solid remained. Then it was washed with deionized water, 30% HCl and ethanol until the pH was nearly 6. The diameter of the so-prepared graphene oxide was 10–20 μm.

Octahedral Fe_3O_4 could be prepared according to the following method (81):

Table 3.2 Materials for Polymer Electrolyte Membranes (77).

Material Type	Reference
Blends of sulfonated poly[bis(phenoxy)phosphazene] and poly(benzimidazole)	(51)
Nafion/montmorillonite nanocomposite	(52)
Crosslinked poly(vinyl alcohol)/poly(acrylic acid)/silica hybrid	(53)
poly(vinylidene fluoride-hexafluoropropylene) copolymer/Nafion® blend	(54)
Nitrile-functional, disulfonated poly(arylene ether sulfone)	(55)
Nafion/ORMOSILS composite	(56)
Sulfonated poly(ether ether ketone ketone)	(57)
Sulfonated poly(styrene-*b*-ethylene-*r*-butadiene-*b*-styrene) block copolymer	(58)
Sulfonated PS/PTFE composite	(59)
Sulfonated co-poly(imide)	(60)
4-Dodecylbenzene sulfonic acid-doped polyethylene glycol/silica hybrid	(61)
Sulfonated poly(ethersulfone)-Cardo	(62)
Sulfonated poly[(aryloxy)phosphazene]	(63)
Sulfonated PS	(64)
Sputter-coated palladium on Nafion	(65)
Phosphotungstic acid/poly(vinyl alcohol) composite	(66)
IonClad® R-1010	(67)
Nano-silica layered Nafion composite	(68)
Sulfonated poly(ether ether ketone)/zirconium oxide composite	(69)
Palladium deposited on Nafion	(70)
4-Dodecylbenzene sulfonic acid-doped poly(ethylene glycol)/silica hybrid	(71)
Nafion/H-substituted montmorillonite composite	(72)
Polypropylene-g-poly(styrene sulfonic acid)/Nafion® laminate	(73)
Sulfonated poly(phthalazinone ether sulfone ketone)/silica hybrid	(74)
IPN of crosslinked poly(2-acrylamido-2-methyl-1-propanesulfonic acid) and Nafion	(75)
Sulfonated naphthalene dianhydride-based poly(imide) copolymer	(76)

Preparation 3–4: First 4 *g* poly(ethylene glycol), 5.4 *g* $FeCl_3 \times 6H_2O$ and 4 *g* NaCl were dispersed in 160 *ml* glycol solvent with a mechanical stirrer for 30 *min*, then 20 *g* NaOH was added. After stirring again for a few minutes, the mixture was sealed in a Teflon-lined stainless steel autoclave at 200°C for 12 *h*. Finally, the products were washed with distilled water and ethanol several times and dried at 60°C overnight.

The octahedral Fe_3O_4 nanoparticles were incorporated into the reduced graphene oxide by coordination bonding, which was confirmed by Fourier transform infrared spectroscopy and SEM. Compared with octahedral Fe_3O_4, the obtained composites exhibited an obviously enhanced microwave absorption property which was attributed to the complementarities between the dielectric loss and the magnetic loss (81).

Sulfonated Graphene Oxide. Proton exchange membranes consisting of sulfonated poly(arylene ether nitrile) have been successfully prepared by incorporating a different amount of sulfonated graphene oxide (82).

The incorporation of sulfonated graphene oxide can improve proton conductivity and reduce the methanol permeability. Also, the existence of the intermolecular interactions between sulfonated poly(arylene ether nitrile) and sulfonated graphene oxide may improve the interfacial compatibility between filler and matrix.

The composite membranes show better mechanical properties, proton conductivity and a lower methanol permeability in comparison to pure sulfonated poly(arylene ether nitrile). The composite membrane with 1% of sulfonated graphene oxide has a good interfacial compatibility, exhibits excellent proton conductivity of 0.109 $S\,cm^{-1}$ at 20°C and 0.265 $S\,cm^{-1}$ at 80 °C and a low methanol permeability of 0.17×10^{-6} cm^2s^{-1} at 20°C. The highest selectivity is about 14 times higher than that of Nafion® 117. These data indicate that the sulfonated poly(arylene ether nitrile)/sulfonated graphene oxide composite membranes have a good potential for applications in direct methanol fuel cells (82).

3.3.4 *Nafion*

Copolymers of tetrafluoroethylene and a comonomer according to the formula $FSO_2–CF_2–CF_2–O–CF(CF_3)–CF_2–O–CF–CF_2$ are known and sold in sulfonic acid form, i.e., with the FSO_2- end group hydrolyzed to HSO_3^-, under the trade name Nafion® by DuPont Chemical Company, Wilmington, Del. Nafion is commonly used in making polymer electrolyte membranes for use in fuel cells (83).

Also, copolymers of tetrafluoroethylene and a comonomer according to the formula $FSO_2-CF_2-CF_2-O-CF-CF_2$ are known and used in sulfonic acid form, i.e., with the FSO_2- end group hydrolyzed to HSO_3-, in making polymer electrolyte membranes for use in fuel cells.

3.3.4.1 *Model for Nafion Membranes*

Transport is a major source of the pollution in cities. As a result, the development of cars and buses which generate a low or negligible level of greenhouse gas emissions is an environmental priority. Two promising technologies compete for this niche: Batteries and fuel cells (84).

Among the few established fuel cell designs, those based on a polymer electrolyte membrane and di-hydrogen are promising candidates as power sources for cars as they function in the appropriate operating temperature range of 80°C to 120°C. The best performing polymer electrolyte membranes in hydrogen/oxygen fuel cells have been composed of Nafion, a perfluoro-sulfonated copolymer developed by DuPont in the 1960s.

The structure of Nafion is responsible for its good properties in polymer electrolyte membranes. A newly proposed model indicates the nanoscale arrangement that could explain the excellent transport properties of this material. X-ray scattering measurements indicate the tubular structure of Nafion. A number of other studies demonstrate that the Nafion membrane exhibits a bicontinuous nanostructure involving a hydrophobic matrix and ionic domains that swell upon hydration.

Strong molecular interactions between the polymeric backbones make the cylindrical walls stiff and stable. In addition, this matrix is able to swell perpendicular to the bundle direction when water is sorbed. The ions can thus diffuse easily in this tubular nanostructure (84).

3.3.5 *Fuel Cell Polymer Electrolyte Membrane Containing Manganese Oxide*

Fuel cell polymer electrolyte membranes that contain manganese oxides show an increased durability (83).

A fuel cell membrane electrode assembly has been described that is a polymer electrolyte membrane which contains a highly fluorinated polymer electrolyte and at least one manganese oxide, wherein the distribution of the manganese oxide across the thickness of the polymer electrolyte membrane is uniform.

Typically, the highly fluorinated polymer electrolyte is perfluorinated. The manganese oxide is present in an amount of between 0.2% and 0.3% In particular, the manganese oxide may be MnO_2 or Mn_2O_3.

The method of making a fuel cell polymer electrolyte membrane consists of the following steps (83):

1. Providing a highly fluorinated polymer electrolyte comprising acidic functional groups,
2. Adding at least one manganese oxide compound in an amount of 0.2% and 0.3% of the total weight of the polymer electrolyte membrane, and
3. Afterwards forming a polymer electrolyte membrane containing the polymer electrolyte, wherein the distribution of each manganese oxide across the thickness of said polymer electrolyte membrane is uniform.

The lifetime using the same ionomer casting solution can be increased from 59 *h* by adding manganese oxides up to 177 *h* (83).

3.3.6 *High-Temperature Polymer Electrolyte Membrane Fuel Cells*

One possible solution of combating issues posed by climate change is the use of the high-temperature polymer electrolyte membrane fuel cell in some applications (85).

Their typical operating temperatures are in the range of 100–200°C which allows the generation of both heat and power, high tolerance to fuel impurities and a simpler system design. The literature concerning the high-temperature polymer electrolyte membrane fuel cell, ranging from cell materials to stack and stack testing has been reviewed (85).

Only acid-doped membranes meet the U.S. Department of Energy targets for high temperature membranes operating under no humidification on both anode and cathode sides, thus barring the durability. This eliminates the stringent requirement for humidity; however, they have many potential drawbacks, including increased degradation, leaching of acid and incompatibility with current state-of-the-art fuel cell materials.

In this type of fuel cell, the choice of membrane material determines the other fuel cell component material composition. For example, when using an acid-doped system, the flow-field plate material must be carefully selected to take into account the advanced degradation (85).

3.3.7 *Fluorinated High-Performance Polymers*

The introduction of fluorine exhibits dramatic improvements in several properties of the polymers (86). Polymers containing fluorinated groups are endowed with solubility in organic solvents, lower dielectric constant and water uptake, higher thermal and thermooxidative stability, better optical transparencies along with higher gas permeability and flame resistance in comparison to their non-fluorinated counterparts.

The introduction of trifluoromethyl ($-CF_3$) groups into polymers has been one of the most widely used strategies for the structural modification which leads to a substantial property enhancement. High-performance polymers, e.g., poly(arylene ether)s and aromatic poly(imide)s (PIs) containing $-CF_3$ substituents, have been shown to possess a combination of excellent thermal, mechanical, solubility, processability, optical and electrical properties, rendering them suitable for a wide range of applications, e.g., as low-dielectric materials, in optical devices, as well as membranes for gas and solvent separation, and fuel cells.

The presence of $-CF_3$ substitution in aromatic groups enables the facile synthesis of poly(arylene ether)s by activating the leaving group towards nucleophilic displacement reaction during the polymerization reaction. Most of these polymers have been synthesized by solution polycondensation of the corresponding $-CF_3$-substituted monomer.

A lot of research has been focused towards the synthesis of new $-CF_3$-substituted monomers and their polymerization, followed by property evaluations of the resulting polymers that has eventually enabled an understanding of the structure-property correlation in these polymers (86).

A comprehensive presentation of $-CF_3$-substituted aromatic PIs and poly(arylene ether)s developed in the last decade has been done. The research on $-CF_3$-substituted poly(aryl ether ketone)s and poly(aryl ether sulfone)s, especially with respect to proton exchange membranes for fuel cell applications, has been detailed. The main focus has been devoted to the synthesis of the polymers from the corresponding $-CF_3$-substituted monomers, and the consequent property advantages brought about in the polymer (86).

3.3.8 Fluor-Containing Copolymers for Polymer Membranes

Fluor-containing ionic copolymer systems were synthesized and studied to investigate the role of polymer architecture on the morphology and the properties of solid polymer electrolytes. Two types of compositionally similar but architecturally distinct copolymers were investigated (87):

1. P(VDF-*co*-CTFE)-*g*-SPS graft copolymers, comprising a hydrophobic fluorous backbone and sulfonated styrene side chains, and
2. P(VDF-*co*-HFP)-*b*-SPS diblock copolymers, comprising a hydrophobic fluorous segment linearly connected to a sulfonated styrenic segment.

The above-mentioned compounds are shown in Figure 3.15.

It was found that the macromolecular structure plays an important role in the membrane morphology. Grafted membranes possess a small ionic cluster morphology. On the other hand, diblock membranes possess a lamellar-like morphology. These differences in the morphology affect the threshold of ionic percolation, water sorption, proton mobility and concentration, proton conductivity, and anisotropy of ion conduction (87).

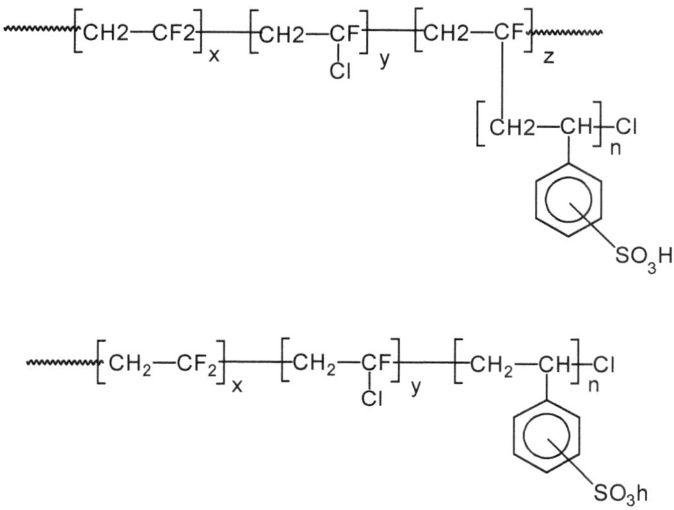

Figure 3.15 Fluor-Containing Copolymers.

3.3.9 *Solid Electrolyte Membrane*

Organic polymer materials having sulfonic acid groups, carboxylic groups, or phosphoric groups are used as solid electrolyte membranes of fuel cells (88). Solid electrolyte membranes are indispensable materials for electrochemical elements such as solid polymer fuel cells, temperature sensors, gas sensors, and electrochromic devices. When a solid electrolyte membrane is used for a fuel cell, it is often called a proton conductive membrane, since it plays a role in conducting protons.

A high proton conductivity is provided by sulfonic acid groups connected to the benzene rings. The reduction of the methanol crossover can be realized by the introduction of a rigid structure with aromatic rings, or a combination of a rigid structure with aromatic rings and a three-dimensional crosslinked structure.

However, the problem with these membranes is that although they have excellent proton conductivity, there is a strong tendency for the methanol, which has a high affinity for water, to permeate from the anode side to the cathode side (methanol crossover), when they are used as solid electrolyte membranes. When a methanol crossover occurs, the supplied fuel, i.e., methanol, directly reacts with oxygen at the cathode, thus making it unable to output energy as electricity (88).

3.3.9.1 *Low Methanol Crossover*

An electrolyte composition has been described that shows a low methanol crossover and exhibits a high proton conductivity when used as a solid electrolyte for solid polymer fuel cells has been developed.

An electrolyte composition has been described that can furnish a good adhesion to perfluorinated resins such as Nafion, that are used in the binders of electrode layers of fuel cells, and shows excellent resistance to acids and oxidative conditions, low methanol crossover, and high proton conductivity, when used as solid electrolytes for solid polymer fuel cells. The synthesis of several suitable monomers has been detailed. These monomers are listed in Table 3.3. Some of these monomers are shown in Figures 3.16 and 3.17.

Table 3.3 Monomers (88).

Monomers
2,4-Dichloro-6-(4-fluorophenyl)-1,3,5-triazine
2,4-Bis(4-trifluorovinyloxyphenyl)-6-(4-fluorophenyl)-1,3,5-triazine
Potassium 2,4-bis[4-(trifluorovinyloxy)phenyl]-6-[4-[4-(sulfonatephenoxy)]phenyl]-1,3,5-triazine
3-(2-Bromo)tetrafluoroethoxy-6-fluorobenzotrifluoride
3-(Trifluorovinyloxy)-6-fluorobenzotrifluoride
Potassium 2,5-bis[(2-trifluoromethyl-4-trifluorovinyloxy)phenoxy]-benzenesulfonate
2,4,6-Tris(4-trifluorovinyloxyphenyl)-1,3,5-triazine
1,1,1-Tris(4-trifluorovinyloxyphenyl)ethane
1,3,5-Tris(4-acetylphenoxy)benzene
1,3,5-Tris(4-hydroxyphenoxy)benzene
1,3,5-Tris(4-trifluorovinyloxyphenyl)benzene

An electrolyte composition that shows only a low methanol crossover and exhibits high proton conductivity when used as a solid electrolyte for solid polymer fuel cells has been described (89).

The electrolyte composition is a perfluorocyclobutane-containing polymer. High proton conductivity is provided by sulfonic acid

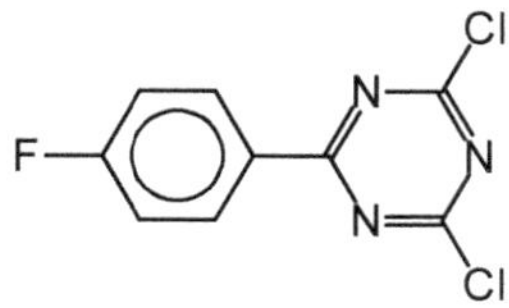

2,4-Dichloro-6-(4-fluorophenyl)-1,3,5-triazine

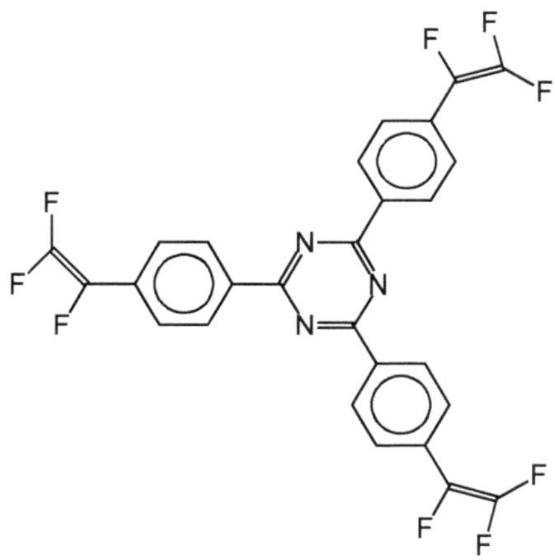

2,4,6-Tris(4-trifluorovinyloxyphenyl)-1,3,5-triazine

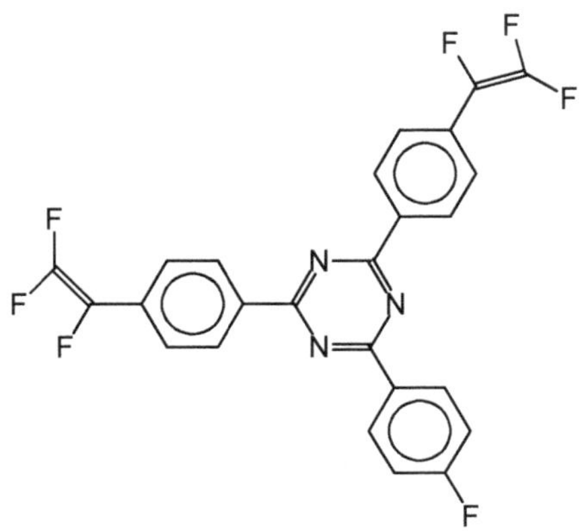

2,4-Bis(4-trifluorovinyloxyphenyl)-6-(4-fluorophenyl)-1,3,5-triazine

Figure 3.16 Triazine monomers.

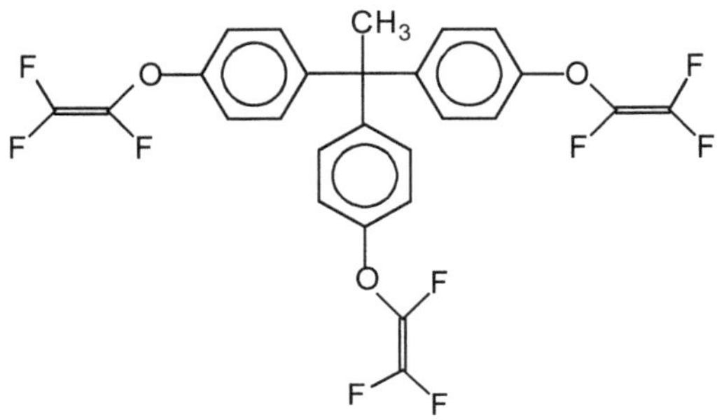

1,1,1-Tris(4-trifluorovinyloxyphenyl)ethane

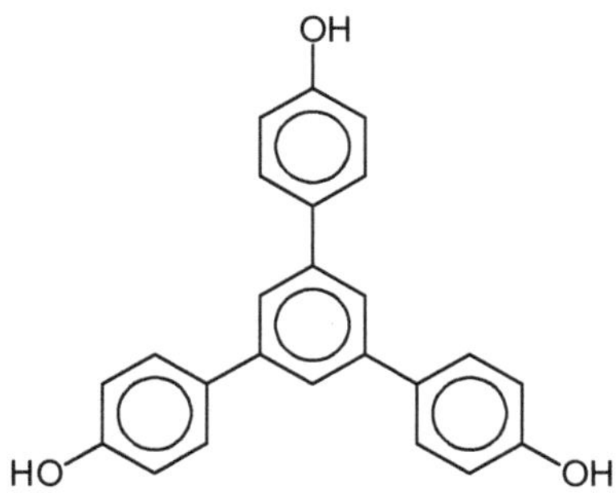

1,3,5-Tris(4-hydroxyphenoxy)benzene

Figure 3.17 Other monomers.

groups connected to the benzene rings. The reduction of methanol crossover is realized by the introduction of a rigid structure with aromatic rings, or a combination of a rigid structure with aromatic rings and a three-dimensional crosslinked structure.

The composition contains a perfluorocyclobutane-containing polymer, and also, for example, potassium 2,4-bis[4-(trifluorovinyloxy)phenyl]-6-[4-[4-(sulfonatephenoxy)]phenyl]-1,3,5-triazine. A perfluorocyclobutane-containing polymer is shown in Figure 3.18.

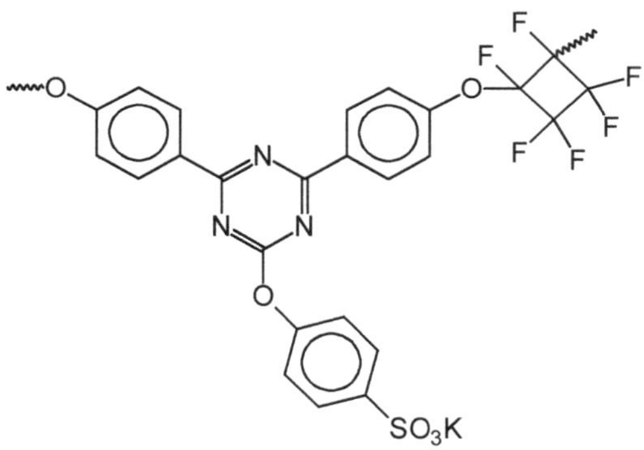

Figure 3.18 Perfluorocyclobutane-containing polymer (89).

3.3.10 *Triazine Polymer for Fuel Cell Membrane*

A disadvantage of the polymers of the Nafion type in operation in the cell, is their relatively limited chemical stability. This arises because perfluoro polymers are known to absorb large amounts of water responsible for repeated dimensional changes and swellings of the membrane: repeated cycles of drying and humidification, during successive shutdowns and startups of the fuel cell.

This results in an increased permeability to gases such as hydrogen and oxygen. The increased permeability is responsible for the formation of hydrogen peroxide and free radicals (OH·). So many mechanisms are operating, which can result in a rapid degradation in a membrane and in the premature end of life of the fuel cell. In order to limit these dimensional changes and to thus improve the endurance of the membranes, it has been proposed in particular to add, as reinforcing polymer, a second fluoropolymer, in particular a PTFE of the expanded microporous type, and to thus form tougher composite membranes (90).

Another major disadvantage of the polymers of the Nafion type is the cost of their synthesis (91). It has been proposed to replace the polymers with aromatic polymers, which are lower in cost and which furthermore have the advantage of exhibiting a reduced permeability to the gases. Examples of such polymers are, for example, poly(arylene-ether-sulfone)s or poly(ether-ether-ketone)s (91). These aromatic polymers, once sulfonated, still do not make it possible today to achieve the compromise in performance and in cost offered with the fluorinated aliphatic polymers of the Nafion type.

Special inexpensive monomers that can be prepared via a simple and economical synthesis process have been developed (91). These are based on triphenyl-1,3,5-triazine, cf. Figure 3.19. Examples are shown in Table 3.4.

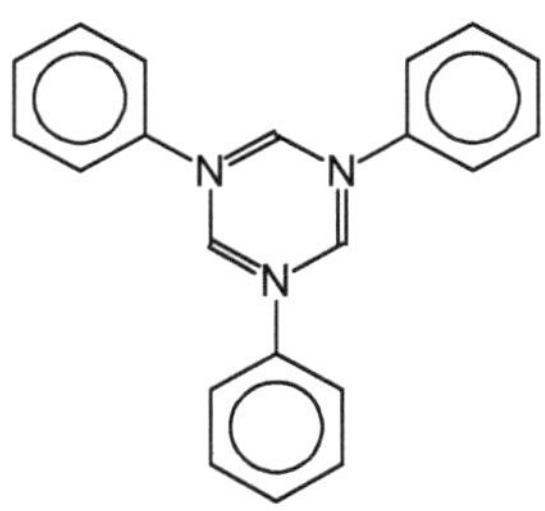

Figure 3.19 Triphenyl-1,3,5-triazine.

Table 3.4 Triazine monomers (91).

Monomer
2,4-Bis(*p*-fluorophenyl)-6-phenyl-1,3,5-triazine
2,4-[4(4-Hydroxyphenylsulfonyl)phenyl]-6-phenyl-1,3,5-triazine
2,4-[4-Hydroxyphenylsulfanyl)phenyl]-6-phenyl-1,3,5-triazine

3.3.11 Polymer-Nanocomposite Electrolyte Membranes

Proton exchange membrane fuel cells are promising for the generation of power because of their high efficiency compared to the coal combustion engine and eco-environment (92).

Among the various components found in the fuel cell systems, proton exchange membranes are pivotal. Currently, the polymer electrolyte membrane fuel cells are based on perfluorosulfonic acid membranes such as Nafion and Flemion, which have certain drawbacks such as high fuel crossover and cost.

Consequently, researchers have focused on making proton exchange membranes with high proton conductivity, durability, thermal stability, maximum power density and low fuel crossover, and low cost.

In recent years, the hybrid organic-inorganic composite membrane has emerged as an interesting alternative. It provides a unique combination of organic and inorganic properties, and overcomes the limitations of the pure polymeric membranes. Several alternatives have been reviewed for the fabrication and evaluation of polymer electrolyte and composite membranes for fuel cell applications (92).

3.4 Fabrication

3.4.1 *Low-Pressure Plasmas*

The use of low-pressure plasmas has been reported for elaborating materials at the heart of solid polymer fuel cells, in particular electrodes and the membrane electrolyte (93).

Electrodes can be formed using plasma sputtering techniques while the ion-conducting membranes are built up using plasma polymerization. The fuel cell performance can be improved by these approaches. The electrode catalyst profile is optimized while the membrane working temperature is increased and the methanol crossover is lowered compared to conventional polymer electrolyte membrane fuel cells (93).

3.4.2 *Electrospinning*

A proton exchange membrane is an electrolyte which behaves as an important indicator for the performance of a fuel cell (94).

Electrospinning is a promising technique owing to its more widespread dispersion of inorganic filler within the polymer matrix, which can reduce the size of the filler up to nanoscale dimensions.

The issues regarding an electrospun sulfonated poly(ether ether ketone)/inorganic nanocomposite fiber have been addressed (94).

The properties of several electrospun fiber polymer-based membranes for fuel cell application have been detailed (95).

Table 3.5 Findings on electrospun fiber polymer-based membranes for fuel cell application.

Polymer	Filler or Carrier Polymer	Proton Conductivity
Poly(vinyl alcohol)	Nafion	22
Poly(vinylidene fluoride)	Nafion	2
Sulfonated poly(ethersulfone)	Nafion	85
Sulfonated random co-poly(imide)	Sulfonated poly(imide)	370

3.5 Degradation

3.5.1 *Mechanical Degradation*

Mechanical degradation is caused by the repetition of expansion and contraction associated with changes in wet and dry conditions. Long-term durability studies under various conditions have been reported in order to understand the performance decrease mechanism of perfluorosulfonic acid under critical operating conditions (96,97).

Pozio *et al.* reported that the long-term operation at low humidification led to a decrease of the three-dimensional reaction zone due to ionomer degradation by dehydration of the membranes (98).

Schmittinger and Vahidi pointed out the importance of water management in membranes (99). In order to carefully analyze the water in the membrane, observation techniques of liquid water in the membrane have been proposed that use time-resolved neutron radiography and high-resolution dynamics in-plane neutron imaging (100, 101).

Furthermore, the water distribution in the membrane could be analyzed by computational fluid dynamics (102, 103).

3.5.2 *Thermal Degradation*

The phenomenon of thermal degradation is caused at both freezing and high temperatures (104–107). The most favorable working temperature of a perfluorosulfonic acid membrane is usually around 80°C to maintain a highly efficient operation. However, a wide temperature range operation is required to use a polymer electrolyte fuel cell in various environments.

Membrane degradation at subfreezing temperature is one of the critical issues. It has been observed that freezing water on a perfluorosulfonic acid membrane results in degradation due to the different densities of water and ice.

In addition, high-temperature operation above 100°C has been targeted for faster electrochemical kinetics, easier water management, and for the improvement of CO tolerance. The development of high durable and proton conductive membrane is one of the most important research fields.

Various kinds of membranes with blends, such as poly(arylene ether sulfonate ketone)s, sulfonated poly(imide) membrane containing a triazole group, and sulfonated poly(ethersulfone), have been proposed for high durable membranes for thermal degradation (108–110)

3.5.3 *Chemical Degradation*

The chemical degradation of perfluorosulfonic acid membrane is one of the most serious problems for stable and long-term operations of the polymer electrolyte fuel cell (111).

The chemical degradation is caused by the chemical reaction between the perfluorosulfonic acid membrane and certain chemical species, such as free radicals. Although chemical degradation of the perfluorosulfonic acid membrane has been studied by various experimental techniques, the mechanism of chemical degradation relies much on speculations from *ex-situ* observations.

It is believed that the degradation of a perfluorosulfonic acid membrane is caused by the attack of free radicals from hydrogen peroxide (112)

Recent activities applying theoretical methods such as density functional theory, *in-situ* experimental observation, and mechanistic study by using simplified model compound systems have led to a gradual clarification of the atomistic details of the chemical degradation mechanism. The recent reports on the chemical degradation mechanism of the perfluorosulfonic acid membrane from an atomistic point of view have been summarized (111).

References

1. B. Smitha, S. Sridhar, and A.A. Khan, *Journal of Membrane Science*, Vol. 259, p. 10, 2005.
2. Wikipedia, Fuel cell — wikipedia, the free encyclopedia, 2017. [Online; accessed 3-June-2017].
3. D.W. Sheibley, J.D. Denais, and L.S. Murgia, NASA fuel cell application for space, in *National Fuel Cell Seminar*, p. 107, 1983.
4. S. Bhatt, B. Gupta, V.K. Sethi, and M. Pandey, *International Journal of Current Engineering and Technology*, Vol. 2, p. 219, 2012.
5. S.M.J. Zaidi, *Development of Proton Conducting Composite Membranes For Fuel Cell Applications*. Ph.D thesis, Laval University, Québec City, Canada, 2000.
6. T.E. Springer, T.A. Zawodzinski, and S. Gottesfeld, *Journal of the Electrochemical Society*, Vol. 138, p. 2334, 1991.
7. T.E. Springer, M.S. Wilson, and S. Gottesfeld, *Journal of the Electrochemical Society*, Vol. 140, p. 3513, 1993.
8. R.E. Billings, R.L. Woolley, and V.R. Anderson, Hydrogen fuel systems, US Patent 4 253 428, March 3, 1981.
9. R. Billings, *The Hydrogen World View*, American Academy of Science, Independence, Mo., 1991.
10. T.A. Zawodzinski, J. Davey, J. Valerio, and S. Gottesfeld, *Electrochimica Acta*, Vol. 40, p. 297 , 1995.
11. H. Miyake, M. Matsuyama, K. Ashida, and K. Watanabe, *Journal of Vacuum Science & Technology A: Vacuum, Surfaces, and Films*, Vol. 1, p. 1447, 1983.
12. D.O. Stodilka, N.P. Kherani, W.T. Shmayda, and S.J. Thorpe, *International Journal of Hydrogen Energy*, Vol. 25, p. 1129, 2000.
13. K. Jiao and X. Li, *Progress in Energy and Combustion Science*, Vol. 37, p. 221, 2011.
14. A.P. Meyer, G.W. Scheffler, and P.R. Margiott, Water management system for solid polymer electrolyte fuel cell power plants, US Patent 5 503 944, assigned to International Fuel Cells Corp. (South Windsor, CT), April 2, 1996.
15. X.-Z. Yuan, S. Zhang, J.C. Sun, and H. Wang, *Journal of Power Sources*, Vol. 196, p. 9097, 2011.
16. C.M. Branco, S. Sharma, M.M. de Camargo Forte, and R. Steinberger-Wilckens, *Journal of Power Sources*, Vol. 316, p. 139, 2016.
17. M.H.D. Othman, A.F. Ismail, and A. Mustafa, *Malaysian Polym J.*, Vol. 5, p. 1, 2010.

18. A.N. Lai, K. Zhou, Y.Z. Zhuo, Q.G. Zhang, A.M. Zhu, M.L. Ye, and Q.L. Liu, *Journal of Membrane Science*, Vol. 497, p. 99, 2016.
19. W. Cai, K. Fan, J. Li, L. Ma, G. Xu, S. Xu, L. Ma, and H. Cheng, *International Journal of Hydrogen Energy*, Vol. 41, p. 17102, 2016.
20. J. Li, W. Cai, L. Ma, Y. Zhang, Z. Chen, and H. Cheng, *Chemical Communications*, Vol. 51, p. 6556, 2015.
21. X. Yan, R. Wu, J. Xu, Z. Luo, and T. Zhao, *Journal of Power Sources*, Vol. 311, p. 188, 2016.
22. B.C. Ong, S.K. Kamarudin, M.S. Masdar, and U.A. Hasran, *International Journal of Hydrogen Energy*, Vol. 42, p. 9252, 2017. Special Issue on Sustainable Fuel Cell and Hydrogen Technologies: The 5th International Conference on Fuel Cell and Hydrogen Technology (ICFCHT 2015), 1-3 September 2015, Kuala Lumpur, Malaysia.
23. Y. Yin, H. Wang, L. Cao, Z. Li, Z. Li, M. Gang, C. Wang, H. Wu, Z. Jiang, and P. Zhang, *Electrochimica Acta*, Vol. 203, p. 178, 2016.
24. W. Lee, S.C. Gil, H. Kim, K. Han, and H. Lee, *Composites Science and Technology*, Vol. 129, p. 101, 2016.
25. J. Zheng, W. Bi, X. Dong, J. Zhu, H. Mao, S. Li, and S. Zhang, *Journal of Membrane Science*, Vol. 517, p. 47, 2016.
26. S. Seesukphronrarak and A. Ohira, *Chemical Communications*, pp. 4744–4746, 2009.
27. Y. Takagi, K. Ohta, S. Shimosugi, T. Fujii, and E. Itoh, *Journal of Materials Chemistry*, Vol. 22, p. 14418, 2012.
28. K.H. Gopi, S.D. Bhat, A.K. Sahu, and P. Sridhar, *Journal of Applied Polymer Science*, Vol. 133, p. n/a, 2016.
29. K.H. Gopi, S.G. Peera, S. Bhat, P. Sridhar, and S. Pitchumani, *International Journal of Hydrogen Energy*, Vol. 39, p. 2659, 2014.
30. K.H. Gopi, S.G. Peera, S.D. Bhat, P. Sridhar, and S. Pitchumani, *Bulletin of Materials Science*, Vol. 37, p. 877, 2014.
31. H. Nagar, V.V. Basava Rao, and S. Sridhar, *Journal of Materials Science*, Vol. 52, p. 8052, July 2017.
32. M.R. Kosuri and W.J. Koros, *Journal of Membrane Science*, Vol. 320, p. 65 , 2008.
33. Y.-S. Kim, K.-S. Seo, and S.-H. Choi, *Radiation Physics and Chemistry*, Vol. 118, p. 35, 2016. Ionizing Radiation and Polymers Symposium, IRaP 2014.
34. K.-I. Kim, S.-H. Oh, H.-D. Kwen, and S.-H. Choi, *Journal of Applied Polymer Science*, Vol. 126, p. E64, 2012.
35. S. Maarouf, B. Tazi, and F. Guenoun, *Journal of Materials and Environmental Sciences*, Vol. 8, p. 2870, 2017.
36. A.U. Devi, A. Muthumeenal, R.M. Sabarathinam, and A. Nagendran, *Renewable Energy*, Vol. 102, p. 258, 2017.
37. T. Jurzinsky, R. Bär, N. Heppe, C. Cremers, and J. Tübke, *Solid State Ionics*, Vol. 303, p. 1, 2017.

38. Z. Zakaria, S.K. Kamarudin, and S.N. Timmiati, *Applied Energy*, Vol. 163, p. 334, 2016.
39. Y. Li, T. Zhao, and Z. Liang, *Journal of Power Sources*, Vol. 187, p. 387, 2009.
40. C.-Y. Huang, J.-S. Lin, W.-H. Pan, C.-M. Shih, Y.-L. Liu, and S.J. Lue, *Journal of Power Sources*, Vol. 303, p. 267, 2016.
41. Y. Liu, W. Lehnert, H. Janßen, R.C. Samsun, and D. Stolten, *Journal of Power Sources*, Vol. 311, p. 91, 2016.
42. S. Sasikala, K.H. Gopi, and S.D. Bhat, *Microporous and Mesoporous Materials*, Vol. 236, p. 38, 2016.
43. V. Parthiban, S. Akula, and A. Sahu, *Journal of Membrane Science*, Vol. 541, p. 127, 2017.
44. R. Devanathan, *Energy & Environmental Science*, Vol. 1, p. 101, 2008.
45. N. Yousfi-Steiner, P. Moçotéguy, D. Candusso, and D. Hissel, *Journal of Power Sources*, Vol. 194, p. 130, 2009.
46. X.-Z. Yuan, H. Li, S. Zhang, J. Martin, and H. Wang, *Journal of Power Sources*, Vol. 196, p. 9107, 2011.
47. M. Miller and A. Bazylak, *Journal of Power Sources*, Vol. 196, p. 601, 2011.
48. R. Hiesgen, I. Wehl, E. Aleksandrova, E. Roduner, A. Bauder, and K.A. Friedrich, *International Journal of Energy Research*, Vol. 34, p. 1223, 2010.
49. B.R. Ringeisen and J.C. Biffinger, Biological fuel cells with nanoporous membranes, US Patent 8 048 547, assigned to The United States of America, as represented by the Secretary of the Navy (Washington, DC), November 1, 2011.
50. Y. Zhou, Proton selective membrane for solid polymer fuel cells, US Patent 8 835 078, September 16, 2014.
51. R. Wycisk, J.K. Lee, and P.N. Pintauro, *Journal of the Electrochemical Society*, Vol. 152, p. A892, 2005.
52. J.-M. Thomassin, C. Pagnoulle, D. Bizzari, G. Caldarella, A. Germain, and R. Jérôme, *e-Polymers*, Vol. 4, p. 182, 2004.
53. D.S. Kim, H.B. Park, J.W. Rhim, and Y.M. Lee, *Solid State Ionics*, Vol. 176, p. 117, 2005.
54. K.-Y. Cho, J.-Y. Eom, H.-Y. Jung, N.-S. Choi, Y.M. Lee, J.-K. Park, J.-H. Choi, K.-W. Park, and Y.-E. Sung, *Electrochimica Acta*, Vol. 50, p. 583, 2004. Polymer Batteries and Fuel Cells: Selection of Papers from First International Conference.
55. M.J. Sumner, W.L. Harrison, R.M. Weyers, Y.S. Kim, J.E. McGrath, J.S. Riffle, A. Brink, and M.H. Brink, *Journal of Membrane Science*, Vol. 239, p. 199, 2004.
56. Y.J. Kim, W.C. Choi, S.I. Woo, and W.H. Hong, *Journal of Membrane Science*, Vol. 238, p. 213, 2004.

57. X. Li, C. Zhao, H. Lu, Z. Wang, and H. Na, *Polymer*, Vol. 46, p. 5820, 2005.
58. B. Kim, J. Kim, and B. Jung, *Journal of Membrane Science*, Vol. 250, p. 175, 2005.
59. J.-P. Shin, B.-J. Chang, J.-H. Kim, S.-B. Lee, and D.H. Suh, *Journal of Membrane Science*, Vol. 251, p. 247, 2005.
60. K.-I. Okamoto, Y. Yin, O. Yamada, M.N. Islam, T. Honda, T. Mishima, Y. Suto, K. Tanaka, and H. Kita, *Journal of Membrane Science*, Vol. 258, p. 115, 2005.
61. R. Thangamuthu and C.W. Lin, *Solid State Ionics*, Vol. 176, p. 531, 2005.
62. L. Li and Y. Wang, *Journal of Membrane Science*, Vol. 246, p. 167, 2005.
63. X. Zhou, J. Weston, E. Chalkova, M.A. Hofmann, C.M. Ambler, H.R. Allcock, and S.N. Lvov, *Electrochimica Acta*, Vol. 48, p. 2173, 2003. Eighth International Symposium on Polymer Electrolytes.
64. N. Carretta, V. .Tricoli, and F. Picchioni, *Journal of Membrane Science*, Vol. 166, p. 189 , 2000.
65. S. Yoon, G. Hwang, W. Cho, I.-H. Oh, S.-A. Hong, and H. Ha, *Journal of Power Sources*, Vol. 106, p. 215, 2002. Proceedings of the Seventh Grove Fuel Cell Symposium.
66. L. Li, L. Xu, and Y. Wang, *Materials Letters*, Vol. 57, p. 1406, 2003.
67. V. Tricoli, N. Carretta, and M. Bartolozzi, *Journal of the Electrochemical Society*, Vol. 147, p. 1286, 2000.
68. D. Kim, M.A. Scibioh, S. Kwak, I.-H. Oh, and H.Y. Ha, *Electrochemistry Communications*, Vol. 6, p. 1069, 2004.
69. L. Li, J. Zhang, and Y. Wang, *Journal of Membrane Science*, Vol. 226, p. 159, 2003.
70. Y.-M. Kim, K.-W. Park, J.-H. Choi, I.-S. Park, and Y.-E. Sung, *Electrochemistry Communications*, Vol. 5, p. 571, 2003.
71. H. Chang and C. Lin, *Journal of Membrane Science*, Vol. 218, p. 295, 2003.
72. J.-M. Thomassin, C. Pagnoulle, G. Caldarella, A. Germain, and R. Jerome, *Polymer*, Vol. 46, p. 11389, 2005.
73. J. Sauk, J. Byun, Y. Kang, and H. Kim, *Korean Journal of Chemical Engineering*, Vol. 22, p. 605, July 2005.
74. D.S. Kim, K.H. Shin, H.B. Park, and Y.M. Lee, *Macromolecular Research*, Vol. 12, p. 413, August 2004.
75. K.-Y. Cho, H.-Y. Jung, S.-S. Shin, N.-S. Choi, S.-J. Sung, J.-K. Park, J.-H. Choi, K.-W. Park, and Y.-E. Sung, *Electrochimica Acta*, Vol. 50, p. 588 , 2004. Polymer Batteries and Fuel Cells: Selection of Papers from First International Conference.
76. B.R. Einsla, Y.S. Kim, M.A. Hickner, Y.-T. Hong, M.L. Hill, B.S. Pivovar, and J.E. McGrath, *Journal of Membrane Science*, Vol. 255, p. 141, 2005.

77. N.W. DeLuca and Y.A. Elabd, *Journal of Polymer Science Part B: Polymer Physics*, Vol. 44, p. 2201, 2006.
78. H. Yu, T. Wang, B. Wen, M. Lu, Z. Xu, C. Zhu, Y. Chen, X. Xue, C. Sun, and M. Cao, *Journal of Materials Chemistry*, Vol. 22, p. 21679, 2012.
79. Y. Zhan, X. Yang, H. Guo, J. Yang, F. Meng, and X. Liu, *Journal of Materials Chemistry*, Vol. 22, p. 5602, 2012.
80. Y. Zhan, J. Yang, Y. Zhou, X. Yang, F. Meng, and X. Liu, *Materials Letters*, Vol. 78, p. 88, 2012.
81. Y. Huang, Q. Qi, H. Pan, X. Lei, and X. Liu, *Journal of Materials Science: Materials in Electronics*, Vol. 27, p. 9577, September 2016.
82. T. Cheng, M. Feng, Y. Huang, and X. Liu, *Ionics*, March 2017.
83. M.H. Frey, S.J. Hamrock, G.M. Haugen, and P.T. Pham, Method of making a fuel cell polymer electrolyte membrane comprising manganese oxide, US Patent 8 092 954, assigned to 3M Innovative Properties Company (St. Paul, MN), January 10, 2012.
84. O. Diat and G. Gebel, *Nature Materials*, Vol. 7, p. 13, January 2008.
85. A. Chandan, M. Hattenberger, A. El-Kharouf, S. Du, A. Dhir, V. Self, B.G. Pollet, A. Ingram, and W. Bujalski, *Journal of Power Sources*, Vol. 231, p. 264, 2013.
86. M.G. Dhara and S. Banerjee, *Progress in Polymer Science*, Vol. 35, p. 1022, 2010.
87. E.M.W. Tsang, Z. Zhang, Z. Shi, T. Soboleva, and S. Holdcroft, *Journal of the American Chemical Society*, Vol. 129, p. 15106, 2007.
88. N.F. Cooray, F. Takei, and M. Tomoi, Electrolyte composition, solid electrolyte membrane, solid polymer fuel cell and manufacturing method for solid electrolyte membrane, US Patent 7 037 614, assigned to Fujitsu Limited (Kawasaki, JP), May 2, 2006.
89. N.F. Cooray, F. Takei, and M. Tomoi, Electrolyte composition, solid electrolyte membrane, solid polymer fuel cell and manufacturing method for solid electrolyte membrane, US Patent 8 906 526, assigned to Fujitsu Limited (Kawasaki, JP), December 9, 2014.
90. A.J. Cisar, Process of making a composite membrane, US Patent 6 495 209, assigned to Lynntech, Inc. (College Station, TX), December 17, 2002.
91. M. Fedurco and A. Delfino, Triazine polymer that can be used as membrane in a fuel cell, US Patent 8 889 817, assigned to Compagnie Compagnie Générale des Établissements Michelin (Clermont-Ferrand, FR) Michelin Recherche et Technique S.A. (Granges-Paccot, CH), November 18, 2014.
92. D.J. Kim, M.J. Jo, and S.Y. Nam, *Journal of Industrial and Engineering Chemistry*, Vol. 21, p. 36, 2015.
93. P. Brault, S. Roualdes, A. Caillard, A.-L. Thomann, J. Mathias, J. Durand, C. Coutanceau, J.-M. Léger, C. Charles, and R. Boswell, *The European Physical Journal Applied Physics*, Vol. 34, p. 151, 2006.

94. H. Junoh, J. Jaafar, M.N.A.M. Norddin, A.F. Ismail, M.H.D. Othman, M.A. Rahman, N. Yusof, W.N.W. Salleh, and H. Ilbeygi, *Journal of Nanomaterials*, Vol. 2015, p. 4:4, January 2015.
95. H. Junoh, J. Jaafar, M.H.D. Othman, and M.A. Rahman, *Jurnal Teknologi*, Vol. 69, p. 77, 2014.
96. C. Hartnig and T.J. Schmidt, *Journal of Power Sources*, Vol. 196, p. 5564, 2011.
97. J. Scholta, J. Pawlik, N. Chmielewski, and L. Jörissen, *Journal of Power Sources*, Vol. 196, p. 5264, 2011.
98. A. Pozio, A. Cemmi, F. Mura, A. Masci, E. Serra, and R.F. Silva, *Journal of Solid State Electrochemistry*, Vol. 15, p. 1209, 2011.
99. W. Schmittinger and A. Vahidi, *Journal of Power Sources*, Vol. 180, p. 1, 2008.
100. J. Yu, T. Matsuura, Y. Yoshikawa, M.N. Islam, and M. Hori, *Electrochemical and Solid-State Letters*, Vol. 8, p. A156, 2005.
101. M.A. Hickner, N.P. Siegel, K.S. Chen, D.S. Hussey, and D.L. Jacobson, *Journal of The Electrochemical Society*, Vol. 157, p. B32, 2010.
102. S. He and M.M. Mench, *Journal of The Electrochemical Society*, Vol. 153, p. A1724, 2006.
103. M.F. Serincan and U. Pasaogullari, *Journal of Power Sources*, Vol. 196, p. 1303, 2011.
104. S. Kim and M.M. Mench, *Journal of Power Sources*, Vol. 174, p. 206, 2007.
105. X.G. Yang, Y. Tabuchi, F. Kagami, and C.-Y. Wang, *Journal of The Electrochemical Society*, Vol. 155, p. B752, 2008.
106. G.-G. Park, S.-J. Lim, J.-S. Park, S.-D. Yim, S.-H. Park, T.-H. Yang, Y.-G. Yoon, and C.-S. Kim, *Current Applied Physics*, Vol. 10, p. S62, 2010. The Proceedings of the International Renewable Energy Conference and Exhibition 2008 (RE2008).
107. A. Carbone, A. Saccà, C. Busacca, P. Frontera, P.L. Antonucci, and E. Passalacqua, *Journal of Nanoscience and Nanotechnology*, Vol. 11, p. 8768, 2011.
108. T. Yamaki, J. Tsukada, M. Asano, R. Katakai, and M. Yoshida, *Journal of Fuel Cell Science and Technology*, Vol. 4, p. 56, 2007.
109. A. Kabasawa, J. Saito, K. Miyatake, H. Uchida, and M. Watanabe, *Electrochimica Acta*, Vol. 54, p. 2754, 2009.
110. T. Okanishi, Y. Tsuji, Y. Sakiyama, S. Matsuno, B. Bae, K. Miyatake, M. Uchida, and M. Watanabe, *Electrochimica Acta*, Vol. 56, p. 8989, 2011.
111. T. Ishimoto and M. Koyama, *Membranes*, Vol. 2, p. 395, 2012.
112. L. Gubler and W.H. Koppenol, *Journal of The Electrochemical Society*, Vol. 159, p. B211, 2011.

4

Solar Cells

There are monographs concerning the issues of solar cells. The physics of solar cells concerning basic principles up to advanced concepts has been described in detail (1). This text contains the recent knowledge on the mechanisms of solar energy conversion.

A comparison of solar cell materials has been presented, including both new materials based on organics, nanostructures and inorganics and the developments in more traditional photovoltaic materials (2).

The materials and the trends in this field have been presented, including third generation solar cells, i.e., multiple energy level cells, thermal approaches and the modification of the solar spectrum, and the use of abundant nontoxic materials.

The current status of semiconductor materials for conversion of sunlight to electricity has been reviewed, also the advances in both basic science and manufacturing (3). The full range of semiconductor materials for solar-to-electricity conversion, from crystalline silicon and amorphous silicon to cadmium telluride, copper indium gallium sulfide selenides, dye-sensitized solar cells, organic solar cells, and environmentally friendly copper zinc tin sulfide selenides have been described. Also, the most recent methods for synthesis and characterization of solar cell materials have been described, together with techniques for measuring the efficiency of solar cells.

The art of organic solar cell technology has been detailed (4,5). Active layer, interfacial, and transparent electrode materials have been discussed. Also, how to relate synthesis parameters to morphology of the photoactive layer using molecular dynamics simulations have been shown.

New emerging technologies, such as organic and hybrid solar cells, have the potential to decrease the price of solar energy drastically (6). An introduction to these new types of solar cells have been given. Also, the fabrication, different architectures and their device physics have been discussed. Also, a comparison with conventional solar cells has been be given and the specialties of organic solar cells were emphasized.

The Solar Electricity Handbook is a practical guide for using electric solar panels and for the design and installation of photovoltaic systems (7).

The fundamental issues of organometal perovskite materials and their photovoltaics, including materials preparation and device fabrications have been reviewed (8,9). Special emphasis has been given to halide perovskites. The optoelectronic properties of perovskite materials and the recent progress in perovskite in the field of solar cells have been described.

The rapidly expanding field of polymer and organic solar cells has been reviewed in the context of materials, processes and devices (10). In particular, devices have been described that significantly deviate from the standard approach which involves rigid glass substrates, indium tin oxide electrodes, spin-coated layers of conjugated polymer/fullerene mixtures and evaporated metal electrodes in a flat multilayer geometry.

4.1 History

The history of solar cells have been described in detail (11). The establishment of current solar power is no more than 60 years old. However, the inventions that resulted in the solar cell started nearly 200 years ago. A timeline summarizing the most important events is shown in Table 4.1.

Edmond Becquerel, was a French physicist who studied the solar spectrum, magnetism, electricity and optics (12). He discovered the photovoltaic effect, the operating principle of the solar cell, in 1839. Silver chloride was placed in an acidic solution and illuminated,

Table 4.1 Important events in the use of solar cells (11).

Incident	Year
Discovery of the photovoltaic effect	1839
Discovery of photoconductivity of Se	1873–1876
Creation of the first solar cell	1883
Discovery of the photoelectric effect	1887
Commercial production of silicon solar cells	1953–1956
Solar energy used in space	1958
Creation of the first solar parks	1982
Creation of retractable RV solar panels	1995
Do it yourself solar panels become popular	2005
Flexible printed solar panels on the market	2015
Discovery of sunless solar power	2016

while connected to platinum electrodes, generated electric voltage and electric current (13).

Willoughby Smith discovered the photoconductivity of selenium (14). A few years later, Adams and Day found that selenium could produce electricity simply from light (15). The photoelectric effect, where light is used to free electrons from a solid surface, was first observed by Heinrich Hertz in 1887.

4.2 Types of Solar Cells

4.2.1 *Inorganic-Organic Hybrid Perovskite Solar Cells*

Inorganic-organic hybrid structures have become innovative alternatives for dye-sensitized solar cells because they combine the advantages of both systems (16). Methylammonium lead halide perovskites have been identified as promising absorbers for solar cells (17). The performance of perovskite-based solar cells could be rapidly improved to reach efficiencies as high as 15%.

The reported high-efficiency perovskite solar cells make use of a mesoscopic metal oxide, such as Al_2O_3, TiO_2 or ZrO_2, which requires a high-temperature sintering process (17). It could be demonstrated that methylammonium lead iodide perovskite layers, when sandwiched between two thin organic charge transporting layers, also lead to solar cells with high power conversion efficiencies of 12%.

To ensure a high purity, the perovskite layers have been prepared by sublimation in a high-vacuum chamber. This simple planar device structure and the room-temperature deposition processes are suitable for many conducting substrates, including plastic and textiles (17).

A layered sandwich-type architecture has been evaluated (16). The core of consists of a bicontinuous three-dimensional nanocomposite of mesoporous TiO_2, with $CH_3NH_3PbI_3$ perovskite as light harvester, as well as a polymeric hole conductor. This structure creates new opportunities for the development of low-cost, solution processed, high-efficiency solar cells.

The use of a polymeric hole conductor, especially poly(triarylamine), substantially improves the open-circuit voltage (VOC) and fill factor of the cells. Solar cells based on these inorganic-organic hybrids exhibit a short-circuit current density (J_{SC}) of 16.5 $mAcm^{-2}$, a VOC of 0.997 V and fill factor of 0.727. They can yield a power conversion efficiency (PCE) of 12.0% under standard AM 1.5 conditions (16).

Organolead trihalide perovskite materials have been successfully used as light absorbers in efficient photovoltaic cells (18). Two different cell structures based on mesoscopic metal oxides and planar heterojunctions have demonstrated very impressive advances in performance.

A bilayer architecture comprising the key features of mesoscopic and planar structures obtained by a fully solution-based process has been reported. This is $CH_3NH_3Pb(I_{1-x}Br_x)3$, $x = 0.1 - -0.15$ as the absorbing layer and poly(triarylamine) as the hole-transporting material.

The use of a mixed solvent of γ-butyrolactone and dimethyl sulfoxide followed by toluene drop-casting results in extremely uniform and dense perovskite layers via a $CH_3NH_3I{-}PbI_2$ dimethyl sulfoxide intermediate phase, and allows the fabrication of remarkably improved solar cells with a certified power conversion efficiency of 16.2% with no hysteresis. These results constitute an important progress towards the understanding of the role of solution processing in the realization of low-cost and highly efficient perovskite solar cells (18).

4.2.1.1 *Lead-free Solid-State Organic-Inorganic Halide Perovskite Solar Cells*

Lead-free solution processed solid-state photovoltaic devices based on methylammonium tin iodide ($CH_3NH_3SnI_3$) perovskite semiconductor as the light harvester have been developed (19). Featuring an optical bandgap of 1.3 *eV*, the $CH_3NH_3SnI_3$ perovskite material can be incorporated into devices with the organic hole-transport layer spiro-OMeTAD and show an absorption onset at 950 *nm*, which is significantly red-shifted compared with the benchmark $CH_3NH_3PbI_3$ counterpart (1.55 *eV*). Bandgap engineering was implemented by chemical substitution in the form of $CH_3NH_3SnI_{3-x}Br_x$ solid solutions, which can be controllably tuned to cover much of the visible spectrum, thus enabling the realization of lead-free solar cells with an initial PCE of 5.73% under simulated full sunlight.

Further efficiency enhancements are expected following optimization and a better fundamental understanding of the internal electron dynamics and corresponding interfacial engineering. The reported $CH_3NH_3SnI_{3-x}Br_x$ perovskite solar cells represent a step towards the realization of low-cost, environmentally friendly solid-state solar cells (19).

4.2.1.2 *Ultrathin Air-Stable Perovskite Solar Cells for Powering Unmanned Aircraft*

It has been demonstrated that ultrathin (3 μm), highly flexible perovskite solar cells that have stabilized 12% efficiency and a power-per-weight value as high as 23 $W\,g^{-1}$ can be used for aircraft applications (20).

To realize these devices, 1 μm thick plastic foils have been used as substrates and pinhole-free perovskite films at high yield could be processed from solution at low temperature.

A perfect growth of tightly packed perovskite crystallites was achieved by treating the transparent polymer electrode with dimethyl sulfoxide. In addition, a chromium oxide-chromium interlayer was introduced, which can effectively protect the metal top contacts from reacting with the perovskite, to facilitate an air-stable operation.

For the device, the transparent conducting electrode and the absorber layer are processed from solution, and the electron-selective metal top contacts are thermally evaporated.

The devices were tested using a model airplane powered by the perovskite solar cell (20).

4.2.2 *Solar Powered Biological Fuel Cell*

Sun powered photosynthetically-driven biological fuel cells were already described in 1968 (21). There, a device is described in which an electrical fuel cell is formed by using two chambers, one placed in sunlight and supplied with nutrients and microorganisms which transfer light energy or photons into chemical energy in the form of algae or carbohydrate, and the other placed in the dark where the chemical energy is released by reducing bacteria which produces compounds which release electrons. A bridge is included in the device to provide a pathway for cations and anions without a transfer of material between chambers. Electrons are released to an anode of the device by sulfites generated from sulfates by bacterial action. The energy of this action is derived from the sun and stored as bacterial metabolites, these being fed to the bacteria to drive the reduction reactions generating compounds which, in turn, give up electrons to an electrode element.

A solar powered biological fuel cell has been constructed which is capable of generating a direct electric current in response to incident solar energy (22). This cell includes a suspension of mesophyll cells isolated from *Digitaria sanguinalis* (crabgrass), malic enzyme, a nicotinamide adenine dinucleotide, cf., Figure 4.1, a xanthine oxidase enzyme, a potential mediator such as benzyl viologen or methylene blue, and a catalyst such as pyruvate in an aqueous solution. Benzyl viologen and methylene blue are shown in Figure 4.2.

Investigations in the field of plant physiology have demonstrated that mesophyll cells have the possibility of producing extracellular reducing equivalents at the level of malate, which can be transported through a series of oxidation and reduction reactions to an inert electrode. A suspension of mesophyll cells isolated from the leaves of these species export malate and absorb pyruvate and CO_2. The oxygen produced from the water-splitting activity in the photosynthesis process can be used to accept electrons at a cathode.

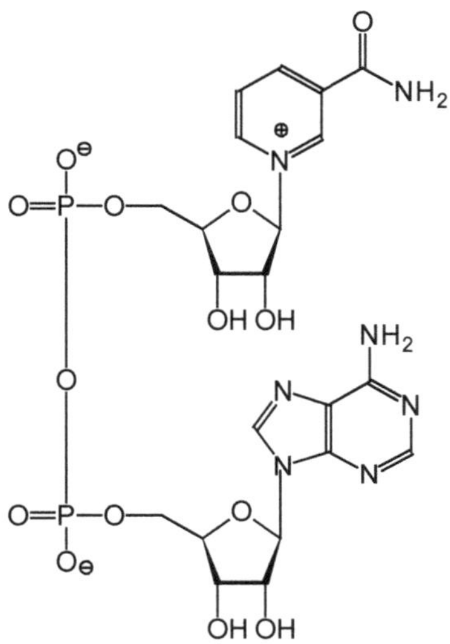

Figure 4.1 Nicotinamide adenine dinucleotide.

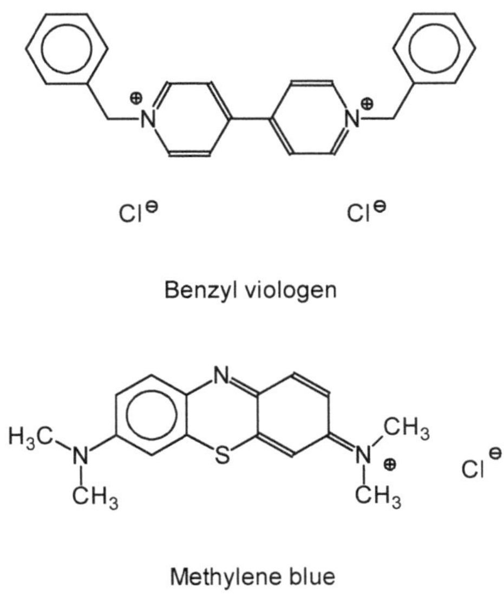

Figure 4.2 Mediators.

The optimal condition for a photosynthetically-driven fuel cell would be one in which the cells collecting sunlight had as their genetic-based biochemical directive that most of the photonic energy captured within the chloroplasts of the cells, assuming eucaryotic cells are used rather than photosynthetic bacteria or blue-green algae, would be exported from within the living cells to outside of the cell organism, where it could be acted upon without further catabolism by any other organism to produce electrons with a negative standard reduction potential as close as possible to hydrogen (22).

4.2.3 *Conjugated Polymer-Based Organic Solar Cells*

Conjugated polymer/fullerene bulk heterojunction solar cells have been reviewed (23). These are mainly poly(phenylene vinylene) derivatives, (1-(3-methoxycarbonyl) propyl-1-phenyl[6,6]C 61) fullerene derivatives, and poly(3-hexylthiophene) (P3HT) systems.

The blending of conjugated polymers with electron acceptors, such as fullerenes, is an efficient way to break apart photoexcited excitons into free charge carriers. Ultrafast photophysical studies showed that the photoinduced charge transfer in such blends happens on a timescale of 45 fs. This is much faster than other competing relaxation processes. For example, photoluminescence usually occurs around 1 ns (23).

Also, comparative data of the charge carrier mobility of organic semiconductors have been presented (24). The most common commonly used organic dielectrics are collected in Table 4.2.

Table 4.2 Organic dielectrics (24).

Compound	Acronym
Poly(4-vinyl phenol)	PVP
Poly(styrene)	PS
Poly(methyl methacrylate)	PMMA
Poly(vinyl alcohol)	PVA
Poly(vinyl chloride)	PVC,
Poly(vinylidene fluoride)	PVDF
Poly(α-methylstyrene)	PaMS
Cyano ethylpullulan	CYEPL
Divinyltetramethyldisiloxane-bis(benzocyclobutene)	BCB

Divinyltetramethyldisiloxane-bis(benzocyclobutene) is shown in Figure 4.3. The synthesis starts with the pyrolysis of α-chloro-*o*-xylene to get benzocyclobutene. This compound is then brominated and reacted with divinyltetramethylsiloxane (25).

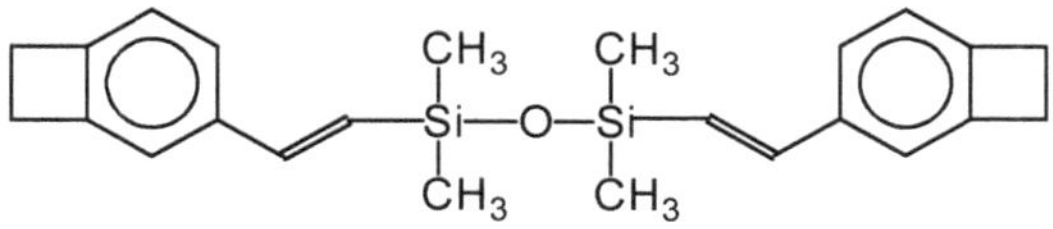

Figure 4.3 Divinyltetramethyldisiloxane-bis(benzocyclobutene).

Also, commonly used *p*-type and *n*-type organic semiconductors are collected in Tables 4.3 and 4.4. Some of these compounds are shown in Figures 4.4 to 4.5.

Table 4.3 *p*-Type organic semiconductors (24).

Compound	Acronym
Poly[9,9′-dioctyl- fluorene-*co*-bithiophene]	F8T2
Poly[2-methoxy-5-(3,7-dimethyloctyloxy)]-1,4-phenylene vinylene	MDMO-PPV
Regioregular poly[3-hexylthiophene]	P3HT
Poly(triarylamine)	PTAA
Poly-[2,5-thienylene vinylene]	PVT
α, ω-Dihexylquinquethiophene	DH-5T
α, ω-Dihexylsexithiophene	DH-6T
Phthalocyanine	
Pentacene	
α-Sexithiophene	a-6T

Quinquethiophene and sexithiophene are oligomeric thiophene compounds that contain five and six thiophene units, respectively.

Pullulan is a polysaccharide polymer that contains maltotriose units (26). Three glucose units in the maltotriose are connected by an α-1,4 glycosidic bond, whereas consecutive maltotriose units are connected to each other by an α-1,6 glycosidic bond. Pullulan is shown in Figure 4.6.

In the case of cyano ethylpullulan, most of the hydroxy units shown in Figure 4.6 are replaced by $-O - CH_2 - CH_2 - CN$ groups.

Table 4.4 *n*-Type organic semiconductors (24).

Compound	Acronym
Naphthalene diimide	NDI
Perfluorocopperphthalocyanine	F 16 CuPc
Perylene	
3,4,9,10-Perylene-tetracarboxylic dianhydride	PTCDA
N,N'-Dimethyl 3,4,9,10- perylene tetracarboxylicdiimide	PDI
C60 Fullerene	
Methanofullerene [6,6]-phenyl C61-butyric acid methyl ester	PCBM

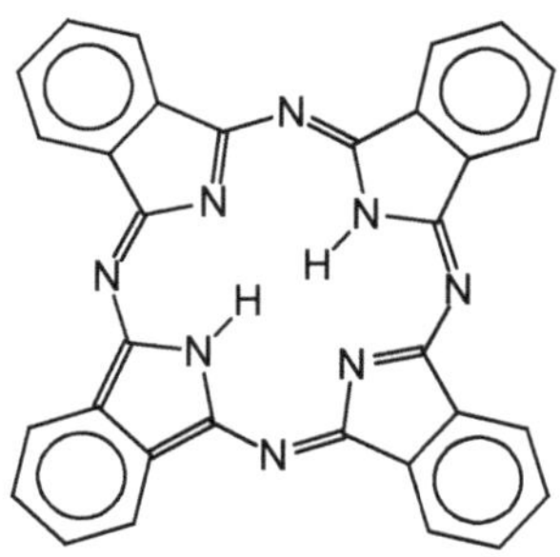

Figure 4.4 Phthalocyanine.

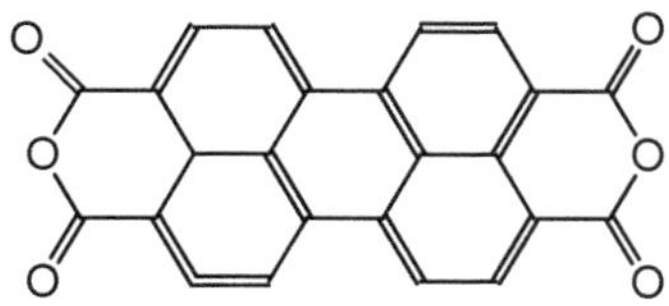

3,4,9,10-Perylene-tetracarboxylic dianhydride

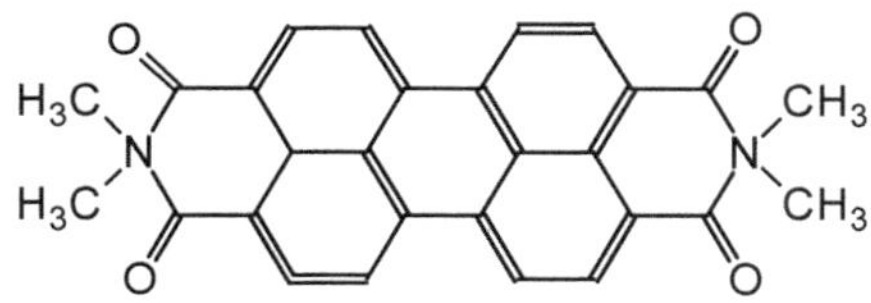

N,*N*'-Dimethyl 3,4,9,10- perylene tetracarboxylicdiimide

Figure 4.5 3,4,9,10-Perylene-tetracarboxylic dianhydride, *N*,*N*′-Dimethyl 3,4,9,10-perylene tetracarboxylicdiimide.

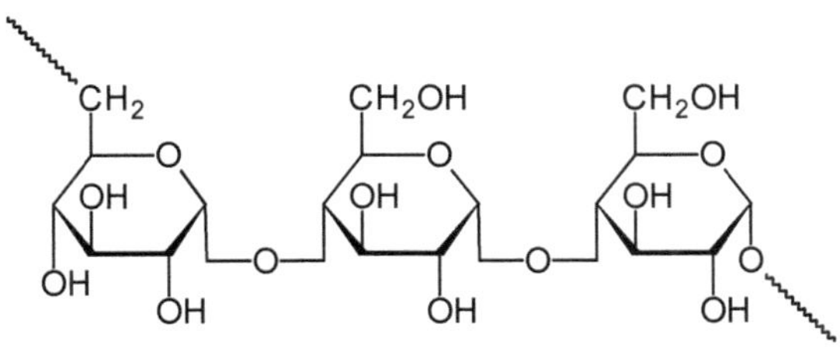

Figure 4.6 Pullulan.

Pullulan can be readily cyanoethylated by the reaction with acrylonitrile in the presence of an alkali catalyst such as sodium hydroxide (27,28).

4.2.4 *Heterojunction Polymer Solar Cell*

A highly efficient inverted bulk heterojunction polymer solar cell has been developed, which is based on regioregular P3HT:[6,6]-phenyl C61 butyric acid methyl ester with a low temperature annealed interfacial buffer layer, cesium carbonate (Cs_2CO_3) (29).

This approach improves the PCE of the inverted cell from 2.3% to 4.2%, with short-circuit current of 11.17 $mA\,cm^{-2}$, VOC of 0.59 V, and fill factor of 63% under AM 1.5G, 100 $mW\,cm^{-2}$ irradiation.

This result is comparable to the previous regular structure device on the same system. Ultraviolet photoelectron spectroscopy shows that the work function of annealed Cs_2CO_3 layer decreases from 3.45 to 3.06 eV.

Furthermore, X-ray photoelectron spectroscopy (XPS) results reveal that Cs_2CO_3 can decompose into low work function, doped cesium oxide Cs_2O upon annealing, which is accountable for the work function reduction and device efficiency improvement (29).

4.2.4.1 *Gold Nanoclusters*

The effect of the insertion of gold nanoclusters with various thickness on the PCE in bulk heterojunction polymer solar cells has been investigated (30).

The polymer solar cells were based on blended P3HT:[6,6]-phenyl C61 butyric acid methyl ester.

The gold nanoclusters were vacuum deposited on pre-cleaned indium tin oxide substrates prior to the deposition of a poly(3,4-ethylene dioxythiophene:poly(styrene sulfonate) (PSS) buffer layer. 3,4-Ethylene dioxythiophene is shown in Figure 4.7.

It has been found that both the J_{SC} and the PCE increased after the incorporation of the gold nanoclusters between the indium tin oxide/poly(3,4-ethylene dioxythiophene:PSS interface (30).

The enhancement of the PCE has been attributed to a localized surface plasmonic excitation (32).

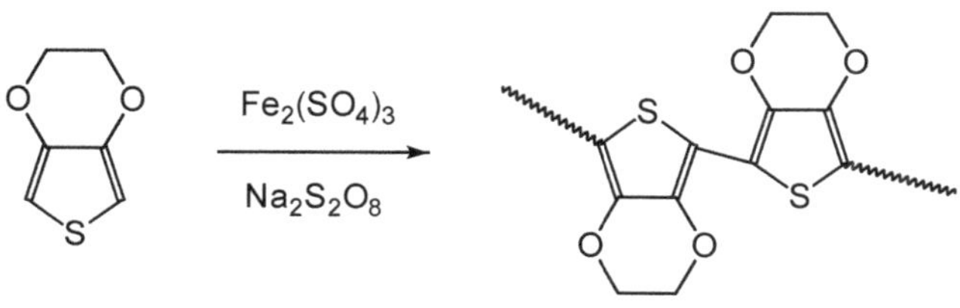

Figure 4.7 Polymerization of 3,4-ethylene dioxythiophene (31).

4.2.5 *Hybrid Bulk Heterojunction Type Solar Cells*

A hybrid architecture has been introduced containing a P3HT nanowire and CdSe nanotetrapod as bicontinuous charge channels for holes and electrons, respectively (33). The P3HT nanowires were synthesized using a self-assembly method. The CdSe tetrapods were synthesized using cetyltrimethylammonium bromide and heat transfer fluids (34).

In comparison to the traditionally applied P3HT molecules, the well-crystallized P3HT nanowires allow an enhanced light absorption at the long wavelength as well as strengthened charge carrier transport in the hybrid active layer (33).

Based on the efficient dissociation of photogenerated excitons, the interpercolation of these two nano-building blocks allows a photovoltaic conversion efficiency of 1.7% in the hybrid solar cell, up to 42% enhancement compared to the reference solar cell with traditional P3HT molecules as electron donor (33).

4.2.6 *Triple-Junction Polymer Solar Cell*

Tandem solar cells have the potential to improve photon conversion efficiencies beyond the limits of single-junction devices (35). A triple-junction tandem design has been designed by employing three distinct organic donor materials having bandgap energies ranging from 1.4 to 1.9 eV. Through optical modeling, balanced photon absorption rates can be achieved and thereby the photocurrents are matched among the three subcells. Thus, an efficient triple-junction tandem organic solar cell can exhibit a high photon conversion efficiency of 11.5% (35).

4.2.7 *Amorphous Silicon Multijunction Solar Cells*

Highly efficient hybrid multijunction solar cells have been constructed with a wide bandgap amorphous silicon for the front subcell and a low bandgap polymer for the back subcell (36).

Power conversion efficiencies of 11.6% could be achieved in tandem-junction configurations and power conversion efficiencies of 13.2% triple-junction configurations. These high efficiencies are enabled by deploying effective optical management and by using photoactive materials with complementary absorption (36).

4.2.8 *Multijunction Polymer Solar Cells*

Wide bandgap benzodithiophene-benzothiadiazole copolymers have been described for their use in highly efficient multijunction polymer solar cells (37).

These devices exhibit efficiencies exceeding 6.5% for active layer thicknesses between 90 and 250 *nm*, with a highest efficiency of 7.7% at 100 and 250 *nm*. This enables the construction of tandem polymer solar cells with an efficiency of 8.9% (37).

4.2.9 *Wide Bandgap Photovoltaic Polymers*

In the past decade significant advances in the field of organic solar cells have occurred (38). Ongoing improvements in the PCE of organic solar cells have been achieved, which were mainly attributed to the design and synthesis of novel conjugated polymers with different architectures and functional moieties.

Among various conjugated polymers, the development of wide bandgap polymers has received less attention than that of low bandgap and medium bandgap polymers.

The recent advances in wide bandgap polymers and their applications in organic photovoltaic devices have been summarized (38). These applications include tandem, ternary, and nonfullerene solar cells.

Also, the application of high VOC tandem solar cells in photovoltaic-driven electrochemical water dissociation has been discussed. The molecular design strategies, the structure-property correlations, and the photovoltaic performance of these wide bandgap polymers have been detailed (38).

4.2.10 *Low Bandgap Polymer*

An effective way to improve polymer solar cell efficiency is to use a tandem structure, as a broader part of the spectrum of solar radiation is used and the thermalization loss of photon energy is minimized (39).

In the past, the lack of high-performance low bandgap polymers was the major limiting factor for achieving high-performance tandem solar cell. The development of a high-performance low bandgap polymer has been reported with a bandgap of less than 1.4 *eV*. Polymers, shown in Figure 4.8, have been used.

The polymer is poly[2,7-(5,5-bis-(3,7-dimethyloctyl)-5H-dithieno [3,2-b:2′,3′-d] pyran)-*alt*-4,7-(5,6-difluoro-2,1,3-benzothiadiazole)] (PCPDTBT) with a bandgap of 1.38 *eV*, high mobility, deep highest occupied molecular orbital.

Two strong electron-withdrawing fluoroine atoms on the benzothiadiazole unit have been introduced to form the difluorobenzothiadiazole (DFBT), cf. Figure 4.8.

By adding two fluor atoms onto the BT unit, the absorption spectrum of the polymer PCPDT-DFBT shows a blue shift of around 30 *nm* (bandgap of around 1.51 *eV*). But the addition of fluor atoms did not affect the absorption spectrum of other polymer systems.

To further lower the bandgap to match a P3HT-based wide bandgap cell in a tandem structure, a strong electron-donating oxygen atom is introduced into the CPDT unit to form the DTP unit. By copolymerizing with the strong electron-withdrawing DFBT unit, the polymer PDTP-DFBT shows a significantly lower bandgap. The absorption spectrum of PDTP-DFBT is ca. 80 *nm* red-shifted in comparison to PCPDT-DFBT and the bandgap is calculated to be 1.38 *eV*.

Single-junction photovoltaic cells based on these three polymers were fabricated in an inverted device structure (40–44). All polymers showed molecular weight of around 20 *kDa* and a polydispersity index of around 2.5.

As a result, a single-junction device shows high external quantum efficiency of more than 60% and spectral response that extends to 900 *nm*, with a PCE of 7.9%. The polymer enables a solution processed tandem solar cell with certified 10.6% PCE under standard reporting conditions of 25°C, 1,000 Wm^{-2} (39).

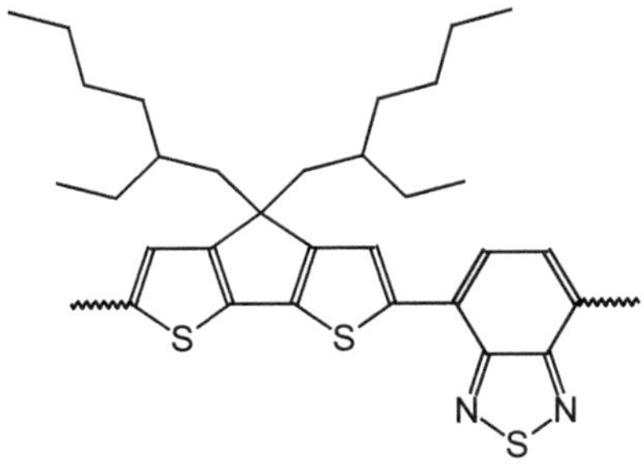

PCPDT-BT

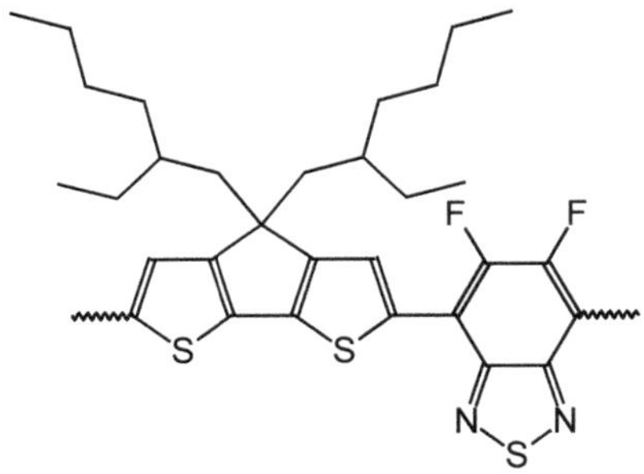

PCPDT-DFBT

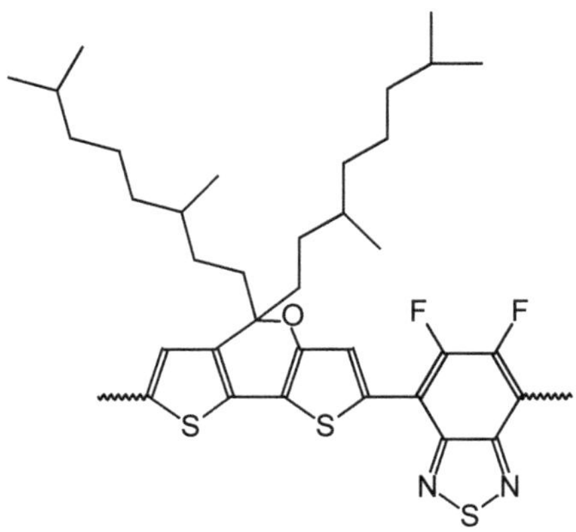

PDTP-DFBT

Figure 4.8 Polymers.

Due to the insertion of the electron-donating oxygen atom, the PDTP-DFBT-based devices show a significantly enhanced J_{SC} of 17–18 $mA\,cm^{-2}$, which is among the highest reported J_{SC} in photovoltaic cells.

4.2.11 *Fluorinated Benzothiadiazole*

A fluorinated benzothiadiazole was built in a polymer which was used in high-performance solar cells (45). The polymer exhibits lower HOMO-energy and LUMO-energy in comparison to the non-fluorinated analogues. The fluorinated system has a conversion efficiency of energy of 7.2%, but the non-fluorinated system has a conversion efficiency of energy of 7.2% (45). The polymer is shown in Figure 4.9.

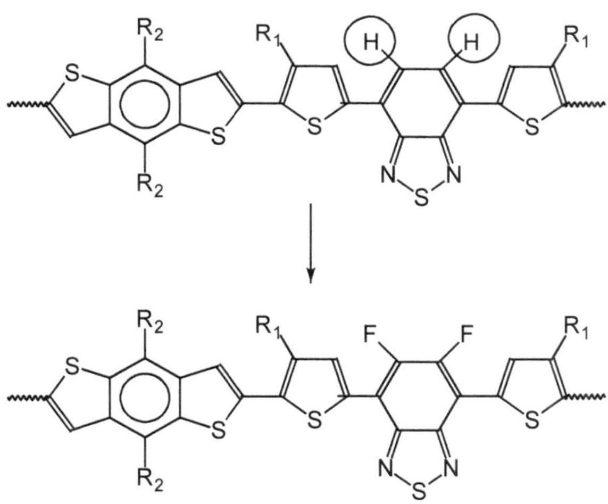

Figure 4.9 Fluorinated benzothiadiazole-containing polymer.

4.2.12 *Indene C_{60} Bisadduct*

Polymer solar cells are commonly composed of a blend film of a conjugated polymer donor and a soluble C(60) derivative acceptor sandwiched between an ITO anode and a low-workfunction metal cathode (46). P3HT and [6,6]-phenyl-C-61-butyric acid methyl ester

(PCBM) are the most widely used donor and acceptor materials, respectively.

However, the low LUMO-energy level of PCBM limits the VOC of the P3HT-based polymer solar cells to ca. 0.6 V. A soluble C(60) derivative was synthesized, i.e., indene-C(60) bisadduct (ICBA), with a LUMO-energy level 0.17 eV higher than that of PCBM. The polymer solar cell based on P3HT with an ICBA as acceptor shows a higher VOC of 0.84 V and higher PCE of 5.44% under the illumination of AM1.5, 100 $mW\,cm^{-2}$, while the PSC based on P3HT/PCBM displays a VOC of 0.58 V and PCE of 3.88% under the same experimental conditions. The results indicate that the ICBA is an alternative high-performance acceptor and could be widely used in high-performance polymer solar cells (46).

4.2.13 *Spiro Derivatives*

Spiro-OMeTAD is also known as $N^2,N^2,N^{2\prime},N^{2\prime},N^7,N^7,N^{7\prime},N^{7\prime}$-octakis(4-methoxyphenyl)-9,9′-spirobi[9H-fluorene]-2,2′,7,7′-tetramine, cf. Figure 4.10.

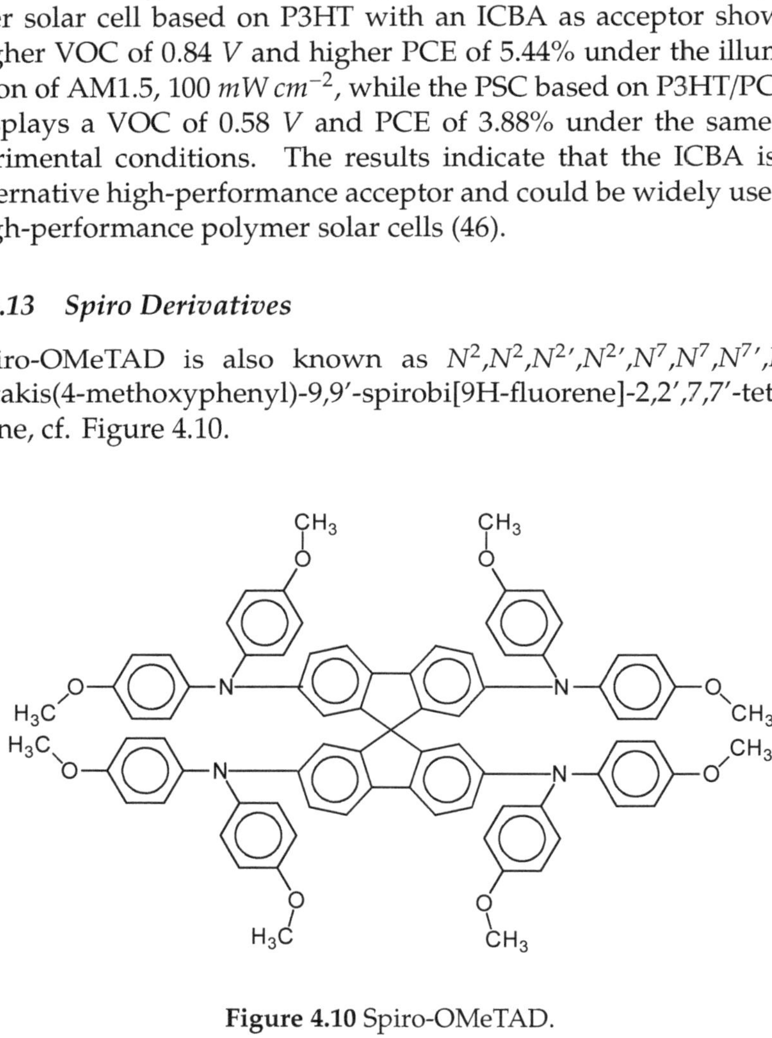

Figure 4.10 Spiro-OMeTAD.

Spiro-OMeTAD derivatives have been synthesized and characterized by 1H/13C nuclear magnetic resonance (NMR) spectroscopy and mass spectrometry (47). The optical and electronic properties of the derivatives were modified by changing the positions of the two methoxy substituents in each of the quadrants, as monitored by UV-Vis spectroscopy and cyclic voltammetry measurements.

These derivatives were employed as hole-transporting materials, and their performances were compared for the fabrication of mesoporous $TiO_2/CH_3NH_3PbI_3$/HTM/Au solar cells.

The cell performance was found to be dependent on the positions of the oxymethyl substituents. The derivative with *o*-oxymethyl substituents showed highly improved performance by exhibiting a J_{SC} of 21.2 $mAcm^{-2}$, a VOC of 1.02 V, and a fill factor of 77.6% under 1 sun illumination (100 $mW\,cm^{-2}$), which resulted in an overall PCE of 16.7%, in comparison to 15% for conventional *p*-oxymethyl substituents. The PCE of 16.7% is the highest value reported to date for perovskite-based solar cells with spiro-OMeTAD (47).

4.2.14 *Pyrene Derivatives*

A set of three *N,N*-di-*p*-methoxyphenylamine-substituted pyrene derivatives have successfully been synthesized and characterized by 1H/13C NMR spectroscopy, mass spectrometry, and elemental analysis. The basic structure is shown in Figure 4.11.

The optical and electronic structures of the pyrene derivatives were adjusted by controlling the ratio of *N,N*-di-*p*-methoxyphenylamine to pyrene, and investigated by UV/Vis spectroscopy and cyclic voltammetry. The pyrene derivatives were employed as hole-transporting materials in fabricating mesoporous $TiO_2/CH_3NH_3PbI_3$/HTMs/Au solar cells. The pyrene-based derivative Py-C exhibited a J_{SC} of 20.2 $mA\,cm^{-2}$, a VOC of 0.886 V, and a fill factor of 69.4% under an illumination of 1 sun (100 mW/cm2), resulting in an overall PCE of 12.4%. The performance is comparable to that of the well-studied spiro-OMeTAD, even though the VOC is slightly lower. Thus, this newly synthesized pyrene derivative holds promise as a hole-transporting material for highly efficient perovskite-based solar cells (48).

4.2.15 *Interfacial Materials for Organic Solar Cells*

Organic solar cells have shown great promise as low-cost photovoltaic devices for solar energy conversion over the past decade.

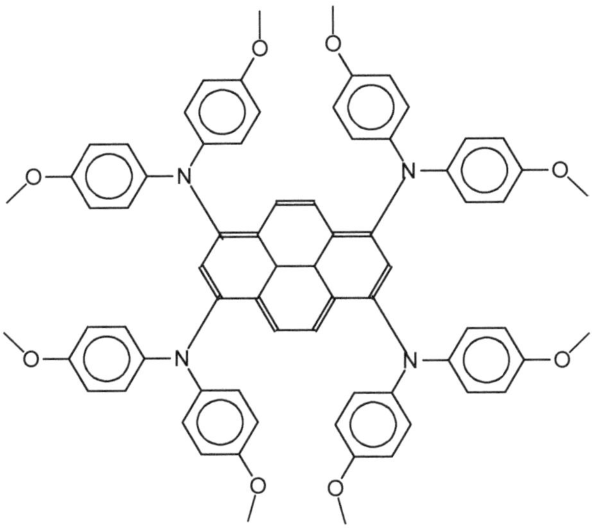

Figure 4.11 *N,N*-di-*p*-Methoxyphenylamine.

Interfacial engineering provides a powerful strategy to enhance the efficiency and stability of organic solar cells (49). With the rapid advances of interface layer materials and active layer materials, the power conversion efficiencies of both single-junction and tandem organic solar cells have exceeded a landmark value of 10%.

The recent advances in interfacial layers for single-junction and tandem organic solar cells have been reviewed. Electron or hole-transporting materials, including metal oxides, polymers/small molecules, metals and metal salts/complexes, carbon-based materials, organic-inorganic hybrids/composites, and other emerging materials, have been systemically presented as cathode and anode interface layers for high-performance organic solar cells.

The incorporation of these electron-transporting and hole-transporting layer materials as building blocks, and a variety of interconnecting layers for conventional or inverted tandem organic solar cells are discussed, along with their functions to bridge the difference between adjacent subcells.

By analyzing the structure-property relationships of some interfacial materials, the important design rules for such materials towards high efficiency and stable organic solar cells could be highlighted (49).

High power conversion efficiencies of 9–10% for single-junction organic solar cells are achieved by combining [6,6]-phenyl-C71-butyric acid methyl ester (PC71BM) as an acceptor with a low bandgap polymer, poly((4,8-bis[(2-ethylhexyl)oxy]benzo-[1,2-b:4,5-b′]dithiophene-2,6-diyl) (3-fluoro-2-[(2-ethylhexyl)carbonyl] thieno[3,4-b]thiophenediyl)) or its derivative (poly[4,8-bis-(5-(2-ethylhexyl)thiophen-2-yl)benzo[1,2-b:4,5-b′] dithiophene-co-3-fluorothieno[3,4-b]thiophene-2-carboxylate]) as a donor in the active layer (50–52).

When two photoactive materials with complementary absorption spectra are used to improve light harvesting of tandem organic solar cells, power conversion efficiencies of more than 11% for both polymer and small molecule solar cells have been achieved (53, 54).

4.2.16 *Improvement of Polymer Solar Cell Stability*

A polymer-based solar cell with improved operational lifetime has been reported (55). The employment of thermocleavable side groups allows the technique of solution processing and the subsequent formation of insoluble stable films by a thermal treatment. Efficiencies of up to around 0.2% were obtained with half-lives exceeding 3900 h of continuous illumination at 1000 $W m^{-2}$ at an accelerated testing at 72°C.

The side chains that are added to conjugated polymer materials convey desirable solubility and film-forming properties but they generally lead to a low glass transition temperature that is comparable or slightly higher than the operational temperature for the devices (56). The use of thermocleavable side chains allows for solution processing and film forming while a subsequent thermal treatment leads to efficient removal of the side chains, yielding a dense insoluble film which, in principle has a much higher glass transition temperature, making diffusion phenomena much slower.

The synthesis of regiorandom poly(2,5-thienyl-*co* -3′-(1″-valeryloxy-1″-ethyl)-2′,5′-thienyl), a poly(thiophene) based on a copolymer of thiophene and the valeric acid ester of 3-hydroxyethylthiophene, was demonstrated to thermocleave valeric acid efficiently at temperatures above 200°C, leaving vinyl groups on the poly(thiophene) backbone, thus giving regiorandom poly(2,5-thienyl-3′-vinyl-2′,5′-thienyl) materials (56).

4.3 Solar Cell Efficiency

Since January 1993, *Progress in Photovoltaics* has published 6 monthly listings of the highest confirmed efficiencies for a range of photovoltaic cell and module technologies (57). By providing guidelines for inclusion of results into these tables, this not only provides an authoritative summary of the current state-of-the-art but also encourages researchers to seek independent confirmation of results and to report results on a standardized basis.

In Tables 4.5 and 4.6, the most recent results are given. Still more information can be found in the special paper itself (57).

4.4 Fabrication Methods

Polymer solar cells are now considered one of the most promising low-cost alternatives for renewable energy production with devices that now reach power conversion efficiencies above 10% (77).

Enhanced performances could be achieved by developing new electron donor and electron acceptor materials, as well as finding the adequate morphologies in either bulk heterojunction or sequentially deposited active layers.

The introduction and development of active layers composed of P3HT and fullerene derivatives in the early 2000s has been a major achievement, as these layers resulted in a large increase in the PCE of more than 6% (78,79).

In particular, producing adequate vertical concentration gradients with higher concentrations of electron donor and electron acceptor close to the anode and cathode, respectively, results in an improved charge collection and consequently higher photovoltaic parameters such as the fill factor.

Theoretical results, as well as experimental results, have demonstrated that the vertical concentration gradients of electron donor and electron acceptor play a major role in the production of high-efficiency devices, especially when a layered structure is obtained

Table 4.5 Efficiencies of single-junction solar cells (57).

Cell Type	Efficiency/[%]	Reference
Crystalline cells		
Si crystalline cell	26.7	(58)
Si multicrystalline cell	21.9	(59)
Si thin transfer submodule	21.2	(60)
Si thin film minimodule	10.5	(61)
GaAs thin film cell	28.8	(62)
GaAs multicrystalline	18.4	(63)
InP crystalline cell	24.2	(64)
Thin film chalcogenide		
CIGS cell	21.7	
CdTe cell	21.0	
CZTS cell	10.0	(65)
Amorphous/microcrystalline		
Si amorphous cell	10.2	
Si microcrystalline cell	11.9	(66)
Perovskite		
Perovskite cell	19.7	(67)
Perovskite minimodule	16.0	
Dye		
Dye cell	11.9	(68)
Dye minimodule	10.7	(68)
Dye submodule	8.8	
Organic cell	11.2	(69)

Table 4.6 Efficiencies of direct beam solar cells (57).

Cell Type	Efficiency/[%]	Reference
Single cells		
GaAs	29.3	
Si	27.6	(70)
CIGS (thin-film)	23.3	(71)
Multijunction cells		
GaInP/GaAs; GaInAsP/GaInAs	46.0	(72)
GaInP/GaAs/GaInAs/GaInAs	45.7	
InGaP/GaAs/InGaAs	44.4	(73)
GaInP/GaInAs	35.1	(74)
Minimodule		
GaInP/GaAs; GaInAsP/GaInAs	43.4	(75)
Submodule		
GaInP/GaInAs/Ge; Si	40.6	(76)

composed of an electron donor-rich layer on the anode side, an electron acceptor-rich layer on the cathode side and an intermixed layer sandwiched between the two first layers (80, 81).

The processes to generate active layers with electron donor-electron acceptor vertical concentration gradients have been reviewed (77).

The sequential deposition of multilayered active layers can be an efficient approach to remarkably increase the fill factor and the PCE of polymer solar cells.

The effect of annealing at 130°C for 20 *min* in regular polymer solar cells was studied where the active layers with various thicknesses were annealed after deposition of the LiF/Al cathode (82). The results of these studies clearly emphasize that the active layer thickness and the annealing temperature are influence the formation of adequate vertical concentration gradients for regular polymer solar cells. In devices with 100 *nm* thick annealed active layers, an adequate P3HT vertical gradient is formed, leading to fill factors as high as 62%, along with a fill factor of 9.4 $mA\ cm^{-2}$ and a VOC of 0.6 V.

The fabrication of inverted architecture polymer solar cells has the potential to generate low-cost, high-efficiency and stable devices, which may revolutionize worldwide energy demand or help to develop next generation devices, such as semitransparent photovoltaic windows (77).

There are monographs concerning the issues of organic solar cells (83–86).

Polymeric solar cells have been reviewed with respect to the processing techniques (87).

There are several techniques, among which are film-forming techniques such as spin-coating, doctor-blading and casting. Other, more desirable film-forming techniques are slot-die coating, gravure coating, knife-over-edge coating, offset coating, and spray coating. Printing techniques include inkjet printing, pad printing and screen printing.

Subsequently, the various techniques are summarized (87).

Casting is the simplest film-forming technique. No equipment is needed apart from a very horizontal work surface. The technique consists of casting a solution onto a substrate followed by drying.

Spin-coating has been most important for the development of polymer solar cells. This technique allows for a highly reproducible formation of films and has several advantages over other coating techniques. Very homogeneous films over a large area can be formed.

Doctor-blading is a technique which has not been explored very much in the context of polymer solar cells. In contrast to spin-coating, the technique is economical. With some experience the loss of coating solution can be minimized. This technique works by placing a sharp blade at a fixed distance from the substrate surface to be coated.

Knife-over-edge coating and meniscus coating is similar to doctor-blading except that the knife in this case is stationary and the substrate is moving. The knife is suitably used in conjunction with an ink bath positioned in front of the knife.

Screen printing is a very versatile printing technique that allows a full two-dimensional patterning of the printed layer. There is essentially no loss of the coating solution during printing. Its main distinction from all other printing and coating techniques is a large wet film thickness and a requirement for a relatively high viscosity and a low volatility of the coating solution.

Inkjet printing is a comparatively new process. Technology has been driven forward by the typical low-cost inkjet printers for the home office.

Roll-to-roll printing needs a substrate in the form of a long sheet that is wound on a roll. During printing and coating the substrate is unwound from the roll and passed through the printing or coating machine. Then the material is again rewound on a roll.

Slot-die coating allows the coating of stripes for making a multi-layer solar cell with stripes of different materials layered on top of each other. The alignment of the pattern is easy since the coating head is translated along the direction perpendicular to the direction of the movement of the substrate. This technique belongs to the premetered coating techniques, where all the ink supplied to the coating head is coated with no loss. There, the ink is fed to the coating head with a pump.

Curtain, multilayer slot and slide coating have the potential to become the most important coating techniques in the context of polymer photovoltaics. However, these techniques are possibly also the most costly and complex coating techniques.

Slide and curtain coating allow the simultaneous coating of a multilayer film of up to 18 layers. These techniques have been developed in the photographic film industry where many layers have to be coated simultaneously on top of each other.

Spray coating forces the printing ink through a nozzle, whereby a fine aerosol is formed. A carrier gas and electrostatic charging may be used to direct the aerosol onto the surface that has to be coated.

Flexographic printing is similar to gravure printing except that the printed image stands up on the printing roller, the surface of which is typically made from rubber (87).

4.4.1 Slot-Die Coating

The method of slot-die coating has been described (88). This is a method of forming a coating layer on a base film. the schematics of a slot-die coating roller is shown in Figure 4.12

The development and the characterization of a lab-scale slot-die coater has been reported. The advantage of this coating equipment is the cost, which is comparable to that of spin-coating equipment, and its easy applicability for coating of different solubilized materials.

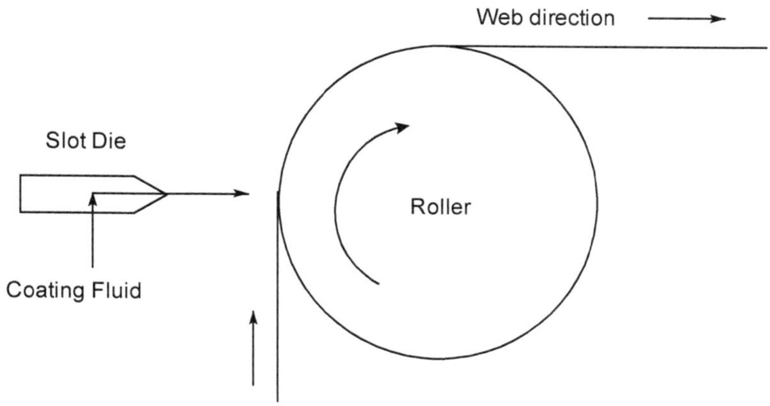

Figure 4.12 Slot-die coating roller.

Its use to fabricate air-stable, large-area, solar cell modules has been demonstrated (89). An entry level paint applicator has been adapted to a fully functional S2S slot-die coater. The layers with a photoactive ink were deposited on glass substrates.

The optimization of the process parameters results in homogeneous layers that have been extensively characterized by light beam induced current, micro-photoluminescence, and micro-Raman mapping of the whole modules.

The fabrication of polymer solar cell modules has been described with an active area above 35 cm^2 and a PCE exceeding 3%. Also, the behavior of the module characteristics at different annealing temperatures and its stability during operation under ambient conditions have been investigated (89). The results have been detailed elsewhere (90).

4.4.2 *Full Roll-to-Roll Processing*

4.4.2.1 *Processing in Ambient Atmosphere*

A complete polymer solar cell module could be prepared in ambient atmosphere using all-solution processing with no vacuum steps and full roll-to-roll processing (91).

The modules have layers that were prepared on a 175 μm flexible poly(ethylene terephthalate) (PET) substrate with an 80 nm layer of transparent conducting indium tin oxide. The indium tin oxide layer was first patterned by screen printing an etch resist followed by etching. The second layer was applied by either knife-over-edge coating or slot-die coating a solution of zinc oxide nanoparticles followed by curing. The second layer contains a mixture of the thermocleavable poly-(3-(2-methylhexan-2-yl)-oxy-carbonyldithiophene) and zinc oxide nanoparticles and was applied by a modified slot-die coating procedure, enabling slow coating speeds with low viscosity and low surface tension ink solutions. The third layer was patterned into stripes and juxtaposed with the indium tin oxide layer.

The fourth layer comprised a screen-printed or slot-die-coated poly(3,4-ethylenedioxythiophene) (PEDOT):PSS and the fifth and the final layer also comprised a screen-printed or slot-die-coated silver electrode. The final module dimensions were 28 $cm \times 32$ cm and presented four individual solar cell modules (91):

1. A single-stripe cell,
2. A two-stripe serially connected module,
3. A three-stripe serially connected module, and
4. An eight-stripe serially connected module.

The length of the individual stripes was 25 cm and the width was 0.9 cm. With overlaps of the individual layers this gave a width of the active layer of 0.6 cm and an active area for each stripe of 15 cm^2. The performance was increased tenfold compared to mass-produced modules employing screen printing for all five layers of the device.

The processing speeds employed for the roll-to-roll processed layers were in the range of 40–50 $m\,h^{-1}$ (91).

4.4.2.2 *Performance Improvement Through Miniaturization*

The improvement of the performance of roll-to-roll processed polymer solar cell modules through miniaturization of the device outline has been described.

The devices were prepared using full roll-to-roll processing comprising flexographic printing, slot-die coating and rotary screen printing to create 5 mm wide lines of ZnO, P3HT:[60/70]PCBM, PEDOT:PSS and silver on an ITO-PET substrate. The lines were spaced by 1 mm and the devices were completed by encapsulation using roll-to-roll lamination on both sides using a pressure-sensitive adhesive and a multilayered barrier material having a UV-filter with a cut-off at 390 *nm*, oxygen and water vapor transmission rates of 0.01 $cm^3m^{-2}bar^{-1}d^{-1}$ and 0.04 $gm^{-2}d{-}1$ respectively.

The final modules comprised 16 serially connected cells. The technical yield was 89% based on the criterion that the VOC had to be larger than 7.2 *V*.

A total of 1960 modules were prepared for each run and the best power conversion reached was 2.75% for devices based on P3HT and methanofullerene phenyl C_{61} butyric acid methyl ester. The solar cell modules were used to demonstrate the complete manufacture of a small lamp entirely using techniques of flexible electronics. The solar cell module was used to charge a polymer lithium-ion battery through a blocking diode. The entire process was fully automated and demonstrates the capacity of polymer solar cells in the context of flexible and printed electronics. Finally, a comparison was made between the learning curve for organic photovoltaics and crystalline silicon solar cells in terms of the cost per watt peak and the cumulative watt peak. Organic photovoltaics as a technology was found to have a significantly steeper learning curve.

4.4.2.3 *Upscaling*

The upscaling of the manufacture of polymer solar cells has been detailed with respect to costs and practical approach (92). The device modules were prepared using both slot-die coating and screen printing the active layers in the form of stripes that were serially connected. The stripe width was varied and the resultant performance analyzed.

Wider stripes give access to higher geometric fill factors and lower aperture loss while they also present larger sheet resistive losses. An optimum was found through preparation of serially connected stripes having widths of 9, 13 and 18 *mm* with nominal geometric fill factors (excluding bus bars) of 50, 67m and 75% respectively. In addition, modules with lengths of 6, 10, 20, 22.5 and 25 *cm* were explored. The devices were prepared by full roll-to-roll solution processing in a web width of 305 *mm* and roll lengths of up to 200 *m*. The devices were encapsulated with a barrier material in a full roll-to-roll process using standard adhesives, giving the devices excellent stability during storage and operation. The total area of processed polymer solar cell was around 60 m^2 per run.

The solar cells were characterized using a roll-to-roll system comprising a solar simulator and an IV-curve tracer. After characterization, the solar cell modules were cut into sheets using a sheeting machine and contacted using button contacts applied by crimping.

Based on this method, a detailed cost analysis was made showing that it is possible to prepare complete and contacted polymer solar cell modules on this scale at an area cost of 89 EURO per m^2 and an electricity cost of 8.1 EURO Wp^{-1}. The cost analysis was separated into the manufacturing cost, materials cost and also the capital investment required for setting up a complete production plant on this scale. Even though the cost in EURO Wp^{-1} is comparable to the cost for electricity using existing technologies the levelized cost of electricity is expected to be significantly higher than the existing technologies due to the inferior operational lifetime. The devices developed are thus competitive for consumer electronics but ill-suited for on-grid electricity production in their current form (92).

4.5 Silver Nanoplates and Core-Shell Nanoparticles

The localized surface plasmon resonance effect and the light-scattering effect of silver nanoplate and core-shell Ag–SiO_2 nanoparticles could enhance the photovoltaic performances of polymer solar cells (93).

To prevent the direct contact between silver nanoparticles and photoactive materials, which will cause electrons quenching, bare silver nanoplate was spin-coated on indium tin oxide and silica capsulated nanoparticles were incorporated into a PBDTTT-C-T:PC71BM active layer. PBDTTT-C-T is a polymer from 2,6-bis(trimethyltin)-4,8-bis(5-(2-ethylhexyl)thiophen-2-yl)benzo[1,2-b :4,5-b′]dithiophene and is shown in Figure 4.13.

As a result, the devices incorporated with silver nanoplate and Ag–SiO_2 nanoparticles showed great enhancements. With the dual effects of silver nanoplate and Ag–SiO_2 nanoparticles in devices, all wavelength sensitization in the visible range could be realized. Therefore, the PCE of these polymer solar cells showed a great

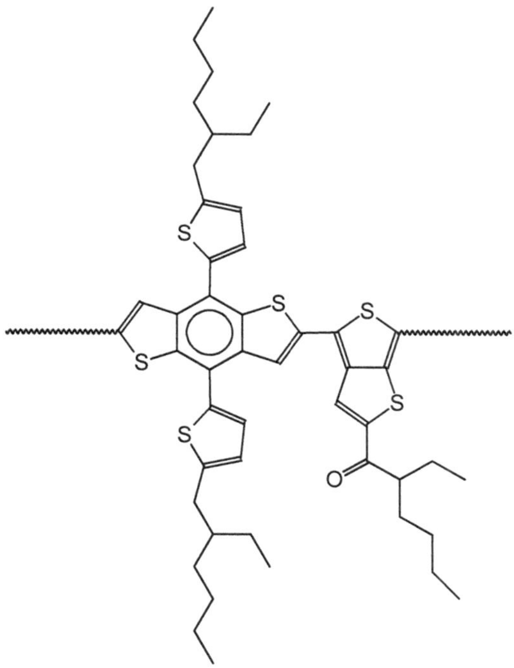

Figure 4.13 PBDTTT-C-T.

enhancement of 14.0–8.46%, with an increased J_{SC} of 17.23 $mA\,cm^{-2}$ (93).

The improved photovoltaic performance of the devices was attributed to the localized surface plasmon resonance effect and the light-scattering effect of metallic nanoparticles. Apart from optical effects, the charge collection efficiency of polymer solar cells was improved after the incorporation of a silver nanoplate (93).

4.6 Vanadium Oxide Hydrate as Hole-Transport Layer

A facile and green approach to prepare a vanadium oxide hydrate layer has been reported. This layer serves as the hole-transport layer in high-performance polymer solar cells (94).

The vanadium oxide hydrate layer was *in-situ* prepared by a combined H_2O_2 and ultraviolet-ozone processing on a vanadium oxide layer. The so-prepared a vanadium oxide hydrate layer featured a work function of $5.0 \pm 0.1\,eV$, high transmittance, and better interface properties compared to those of the generally prepared vanadium oxide (ultraviolet-ozone or thermal annealing) layers.

Polymer solar cells based on poly[(ethylhexyl-thiophenyl)-benzodithiophene-(ethylhexyl)-thienothiophene]/PC71BM using the vanadium oxide hydrate layer as the hole-transport layer yielded high power conversion efficiencies of up to 8.11%, thus outperforming the devices with vanadium oxide layers (94). Poly[(ethylhexyl-thiophenyl)-benzodithiophene-(ethylhexyl)-thienothiophene] is shown in Figure 4.14.

A PCE of 6.79% was observed for the ultraviolet-ozone-processed vanadium oxide layer and 6.10% for the thermally annealed vanadium oxide layer.

Conventional PEDOT-PSS layers have a PCE of 7.67%.

The improved PCE was attributed to the enhanced short-circuit current J_{SC} and/or fill factor, which mainly correlates with the improved interfacial contact between the photoactive layer and the indium tin oxide/hole-transport layer or the cathode when using a vanadium oxide hydrate layer as the hole-transport layer.

A similar improvement in the PCE was also observed for the polymer solar cells based on P3HT/[6,6]-phenyl C61 butyric acid methyl

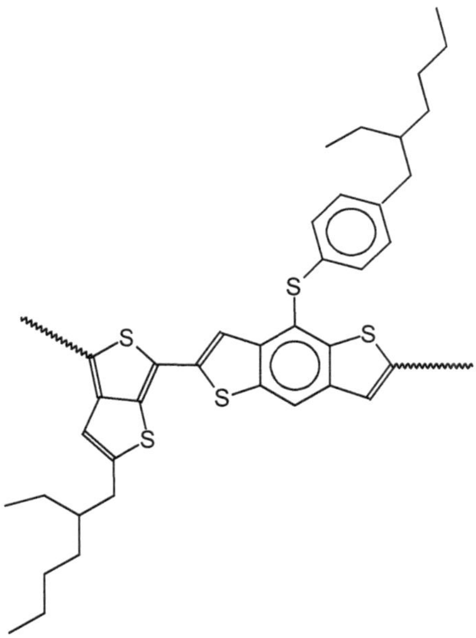

Figure 4.14 Poly[(ethylhexyl-thiophenyl)-benzodithiophene-(ethylhexyl)-thienothiophene].

ester. In addition, polymer solar cells with a vanadium oxide hydrate layer as the hole-transport layer showed a higher stability than that of those with a PEDOT:PSS layer. Hence, it would be possible to use this simply and *in-situ* prepared vanadium oxide hydrate layer as an inexpensive hole-transport layer for high-performance polymer solar cells (94).

4.7 Graphene Quantum Dot-Modified Electrodes

The graphene quantum dot is a new kind of anode/cathode interlayer material for polymer solar cells (95). The key requirement for a cathode interlayer is a low work function.

The application of a cathode interlayer for polymer solar cells, a general approach to tune the work function of graphene quantum dot-modified electrodes, has been demonstrated. Alkali metal cations are used, e.g., Li^+, Na^+, K^+, Rb^+ and Cs^+.

For ITO electrodes modified with these graphene quantum dots containing alkali metal cations, the work function can be finely tuned within the range of 4.0–4.5 eV. Owing to their low work function, graphene quantum dots containing K^+, Rb^+ and Cs^+ can be used as cathode interlayers for polymer solar cells.

Their device performance is fairly comparable to that of the state-of-the-art cathode interlayer material ZnO. This experiments provide a rational approach to tune the properties of a graphene quantum dot material and to design solution-processable electrode interlayer materials for organic electronic devices. A plot of the work function of the graphene quantum dot-modified electrodes with various metals is shown in Figure 4.15.

4.8 Enhancing Thermal Stability by Electron Beam Irradiation

Fullerene bulk heterojunction thin films show great promise for use as active layers in organic solar cells but their low thermal stability is a barrier. *In-situ* microscopy has been done and the effects of electron beam irradiation during transmission electron microscopy of polymer solar cell blends have been investigated (96).

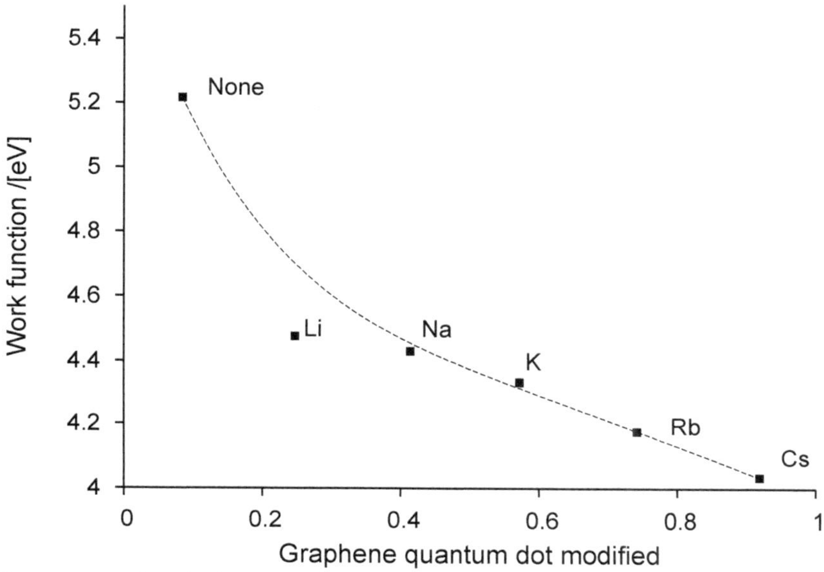

Figure 4.15 Work function of the graphene quantum dot-modified electrodes (95).

Irradiation can be used to lock the microstructural features and to enhance the structural thermal stability of a nanostructured polymer, i.e., a fullerene blend. A model bulk heterojunction film, based on a thiophene-quinoxaline copolymer and a fullerene derivative, was heat-treated *in-situ* in a transmission electron microscope. In the areas of the film that were exposed to the electron beam, the nanostructure of the film remained stable, while the nanostructure in areas not exposed to the electron beam underwent a large phase separation and nucleation of the fullerene crystals.

UV-Vis spectroscopy showed that the polymer fullerene films are stable for electron doses up to 2000 *kGy* (96).

4.9 Inverted Polymer Solar Cell

The use of annealed sol-gel derived ZnO nanoparticles acting as electron transport layer in inverted bulk heterojunction polymer solar cells has been investigated (97).

The photovoltaic performance of devices based on poly(2-methoxy-5-(2-ethylhexyloxy)-*p*-phenylene vinylene) (MEH-PPV): (6,6)-phenyl C61 butyric acid methyl ester (PC61BM) blend system has been examined, employing the ZnO nanoparticles as an electron transport layer with CuI as hole-transport layer. The performance was compared to a conventional hole-transport layer of PEDOT/PSS sulfonic acid. The effect of the presence of another layer of ZnO macrospheres attached to the ZnO nanoparticles has also been investigated.

The highest PCE value of 1.35% was achieved for a device of ITO/ZnO nanoparticles/MEH-PPV:PC61BM/CuI/Ag, which is 275% more than the value obtained when CuI was replaced by PEDOT:PSS.

The analysis of the structural and optical characteristics indicated that the use of the ZnO nanoparticles alone as electron transport layer, together with the CuI as hole-transport layer, could effectively reduce trap-assisted recombination and charge accumulation at the interface, which is beneficial for the enhanced performance of the devices (97).

4.10 Single-Junction Polymer Solar Cells

PEDOT:PSS is widely used as the hole-transporting layer for the fabrication of solar cells (98).

Water-containing methanol was used for the posttreatment of the PEDOT:PSS surface. Here, the insulating PSS component is partially washed out and the PEDOT-to-PSS weight ratio increases from 1:6.79 to 1:2.93.

As a result, the surface becomes more covered with the electrically conductive PEDOT nanodomains, and the mean current of the conductive nanodomains increases slightly from 6.68 pA to 7.28 pA, which could be demonstrated with conductive atomic force microscopy (AFM). The electrical conductivity of the bulk PEDOT:PSS layer increases from 5.51×10^{-4} to 5.51×10^{-4} $S\,cm^{-1}$.

The improvement in the surface conductivity allows for a more efficient collection of mobile holes with a bit higher value of the hole mobility from 5.56×10^{-4} $cm^2V^{-1}s^{-1}$ to 6.78×10^{-4} $cm^2V^{-1}s^{-1}$. The solution-processed single-junction polymer solar cell fabricated on the treated PEDOT:PSS surface shows a higher mean J_{SC} and, therefore, a higher mean PCE (8.23% vs. 9.28%) than that on the untreated surface, as calculated from over 200 cells (98).

4.11 Medium-Bandgap Polymer Donor

A medium bandgap copolymer based on benzodithiophene and benzoxadiazole, cf. Figure 4.16, was synthesized and used for polymer solar cells (99).

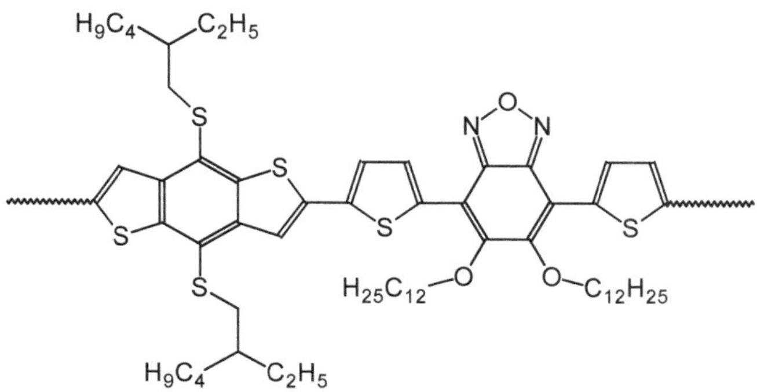

Figure 4.16 Bandgap copolymer (PBO) (99).

The introduction of two alkylthiol side chains onto the benzodithiophene unit can endow the resulting polymer with a good solubility in solutions and good crystallinity in the solid state (99).

The low highest occupied molecular orbital (HOMO) level of -5.52 *eV* and the broad absorption ranging from 350 to 700 *nm* make PBO a promising donor material for polymer solar cells. A PCE of higher than 7% has been achieved for devices using PBO as the donor material and [6,6]-phenyl C71 butyric acid methyl ester (PC71BM), a fullerene compound, or 3,9-bis(2-methylene-(3-(1,1-dicyanomethylene)-indanone))-5,5,11,11-tetrakis(4-hexylphenyl)-dithieno-[2,3-*d*:2′,3′-*d*′]-*s*-indaceno[1,2-*b*:5,6-*b*′]dithiophene (ITIC) as the acceptor material (99). ITIC is shown in Figure 4.17.

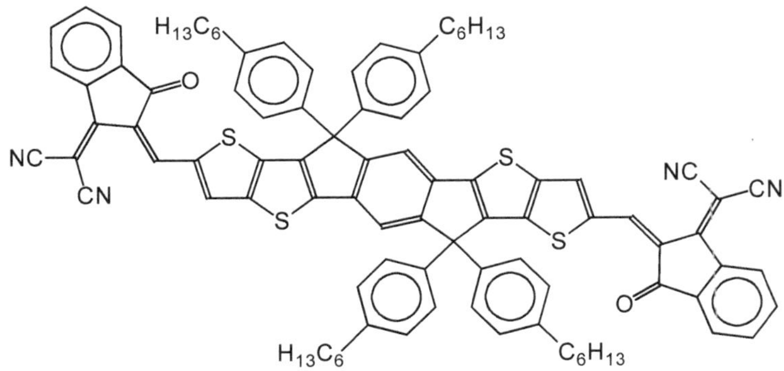

Figure 4.17 ITIC: 3,9-Bis(2-methylene-(3-(1,1-dicyanomethylene)-indanone))-5,5,11,11-tetrakis(4-hexylphenyl)-dithieno[2,3-*d*:2′,3′-*d*′]-*s*-indaceno[1,2-*b*:5,6-*b*′]dithiophene.

4.12 Flexible Polymer Solar Cells

Conventional organic solar cell architectures with a rigid transparent substrate, such as glass, a conductive electrode, e.g., indium tin oxide, as well with small working areas, are widely utilized in organic photovoltaic fields (100). However, such a structure as well as the conventional spin-coating method obviously restrict the industrial application of such devices.

The deposition of silver nanowires on the flexible substrate by slot-die printing has been investigated (100).

The thus-obtained silver nanowire films exhibited a high transmittance and a low resistance. The have been further used as the transparent conductive electrode for organic solar cells.

A typical conjugated polymer, poly[(2,5-bis(2-hexyldecyloxy)-phenylene)-*alt*-(5,6-difluoro-4,7-di(thiophen-2-yl)benzo[c] [1,2,5]-thiadiazole)] (PPDT2FBT), cf. Figure 4.18, was used as the active material to fabricate large-area solar cells of 7 cm^2 by a slot-die coating process.

The PCE initially reached 1.87% and could be further increased to 3.04% by thermal annealing. In comparison to the performance of a reference cell with an indium tin oxide substrate, these results indicated that the silver nanowires could be an alternative substitute

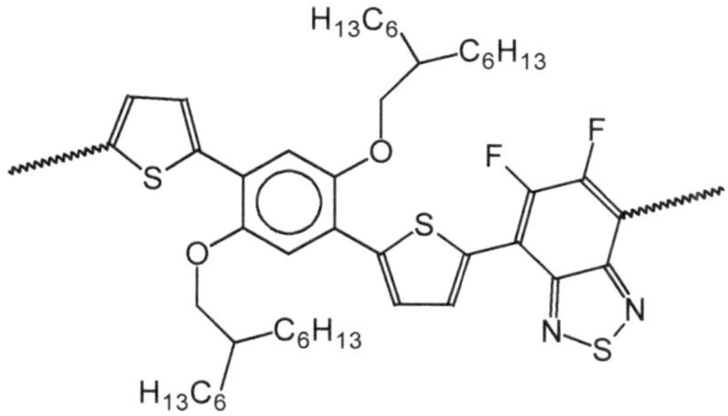

Figure 4.18 Poly[(2,5-bis(2-hexyldecyloxy)phenylene)-*alt*-(5,6-difluoro-4,7-di(thiophen-2-yl)benzo[c] [1,2,5]thiadiazole)].

for conductive electrodes for the fabrication of large-area flexible organic solar cells (100).

4.13 PCPDTBT

Donor-acceptor copolymers have been recognized as excellent materials for organic photovoltaic applications (101). Because of complex film formation properties, however, direct correlations between morphology and optical and electrical properties have been not investigated in detail.

The morphology control and the molecular doping of the polymer poly[2,6-(4,4-bis-(2-ethylhexyl)-4H-cyclopenta [2,1-b; 3,4-b′]dithiophene)-*alt*-4,7-(2,1,3-benzothiadiazole)] to control the optoelectronic properties have been highlighted (101).

This copolymer was first described in 2006 (102). This compound is also known as PCPDTBT and is shown in Figure 4.19.

PCPDTBT is based on alternating cyclopentadithiophene units that work as donor units and benzothiadiazole units that work as acceptor units.

There are also modified polymers, C-PCPDTBT and Si-PCPDTBT, which are shown in Figure 4.20.

The influence of processing conditions on polymorphism and the structure formation on the mesoscale for the family of PCPDTBT polymers with branched alkyl side chains have been detailed (104).

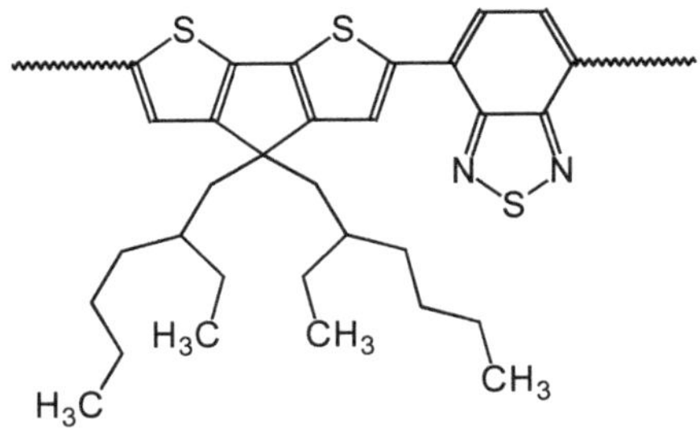

Figure 4.19 Poly[2,6-(4,4-bis-(2-ethylhexyl)-4H-cyclopenta[2,1-b;3,4-b′] dithiophene)-*alt*-4,7-(2,1,3-benzothiadiazole)].

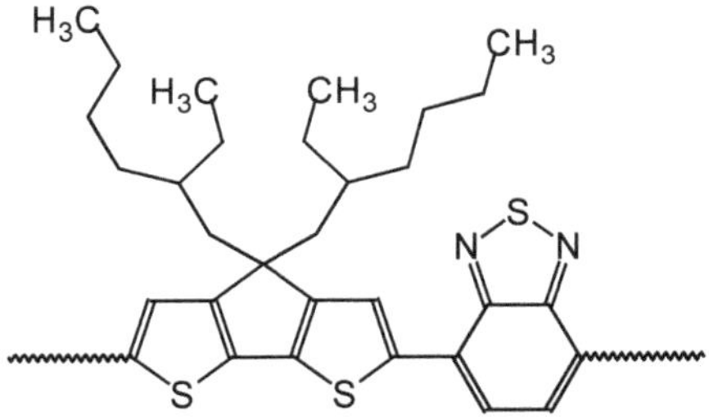

C-PCPDTBT

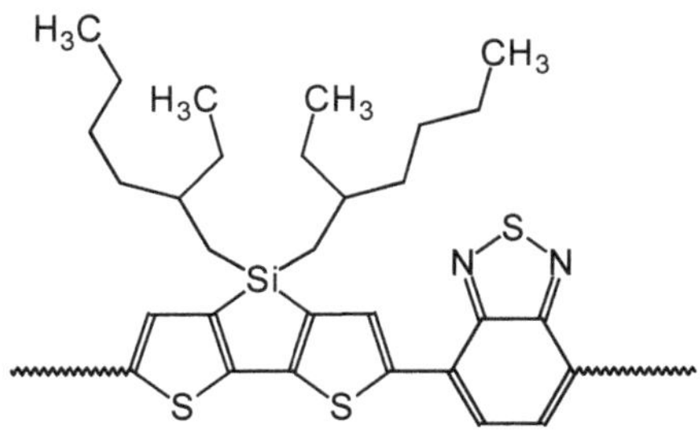

Si-PCPDTBT

Figure 4.20 C-PCPDTBT and Si-PCPDTBT (103).

Direct correlations of morphology with the chemical structure and transistor device performance could be established. Up to four different packing motifs could be realized depending on the polymer derivative and the processing conditions (104):

1. Amorphous,
2. *p*-Stacked,
3. Cross-hatched, and
4. Dimer-containing polymorphs.

While C-PCPDTBT and F-PCPDTBT display similar packing behavior, organizing in *p*-stacked and dimer-like structures, Si-PCPDTBT gives rise to cross-hatched structures upon simple deposition from solution.

The observed differences in chain packing for C-PCPDTBT and F-PCPDTBT versus Si-PCPDTBT have been attributed to the differences in backbone conformations and aggregation behavior in solution.

The effect of polymorphism on charge transport has been elucidated using field-effect transistors, in which both *p*-stacked and cross-hatched polymer chain arrangements yield the highest hole mobilities. Simulations of the mesoscopic morphology and mobility rationalize the experimental findings by relating mobility to distributions of electronic coupling elements between the chains (104).

4.13.1 *Direct Attachment and Growth of Gold or Silver Nanoparticles*

The direct attachment and growth of gold or silver nanoparticles on indium tin oxide surfaces could be demonstrated with a simple and inexpensive successive ionic layer adsorption and reaction method.

Here the chemical reduction of the precursor metal salts with dopamine aqueous solution occurs.

Ag nanoparticles on a indium tin oxide substrate were found to be approximately spherical with an average particle size of about 57 *nm*, but had a wide particle size distribution.

In comparison to Ag nanoparticles, under the same 10 successive ionic layer adsorption and reaction cycles, Au nanoparticles showed a higher density packing and a smaller average particle size of about 36 *nm*.

X-Ray diffraction (XRD) characterization and surface chemistry analysis confirmed the formation of Ag and Au nanoparticles on indium tin oxide substrate with small amounts of dopamine-quinone adsorbed on the surface of them. Although Au nanoparticles showed characteristic plasmon absorption, this did not result in performance enhancement in solar cell with the structure of indium tin oxide/ZnO/PCPDTBT:[6,6]-phenyl-C71/MoO_3/Ag, because of the energy level mismatch between ZnO and dopamine molecules adsorbed on the surface of metal nanoparticles.

4.13.2 *Photooxidation Behavior*

The photooxidation of a polymer blend film that is used in efficient solar cells has been investigated. The film is based on Si-PCPDTBT and PC71BM (105).

A set of experiments from complementary techniques was developed to monitor the modifications during aging that occur not only in the bulk but also at the surface.

Surface analysis has been performed by XPS and AFM. The bulk analysis was one using UV-visible spectroscopy and infrared (IR) spectroscopy. The results of these experiments revealed that the silicon bridge atom is the first target of degradation.

Also, the existence of a photooxidation profile within the 300 *nm* thick film could be identified. Such a heterogeneous degradation was confirmed by time-of-flight secondary ion mass spectrometry depth profiling (105).

4.13.3 *PCPDTBT:PC70BM Solar Cells*

The organic photovoltaic performance can be enhanced through processing additives that change the nanostructure. The critical structure-property relationships have been investigated in the organic photovoltaic system PCPDTBT:PC70BM by varying the amount of an additive (106). PC 70 BM is a fullerene-based compound and is shown in Figure 4.21.

Measuring structure, excited-state dynamics and device performance all on the same sample enables direct relationships to be measured. An appropriate balance of crystallinity, domain size and

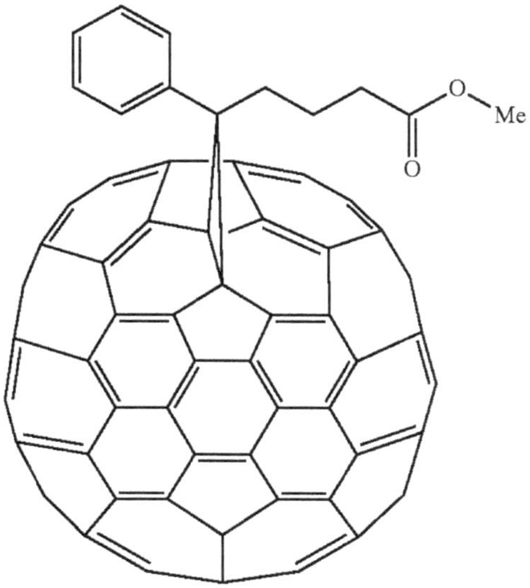

Figure 4.21 PC 70 BM (107).

domain purity are important for optimized excited-state dynamics and the performance of the device (106).

4.13.4 Ternary Blend of PCDTBT, PCPDTBT, and PC70BM

In order to improve the absorption range of binary blend devices, ternary blends with two push-pull polymer donor materials and one fullerene acceptor material have been developed (108). Push-pull polymers are a class of organic polymers with alternating electron-deficient and electron-rich units for easy transfer of charge carriers.

A ternary blend of two push-pull donor materials, PCPDTBT, PCDTBT ([Poly [*N*-9′-heptadecanyl-2,7-carbazole-alt-5,5-(4′,7′-di-2-thienyl-2′,1′,3′-benzothiadiazole)]), and one acceptor material, PC71BM, has been examined (108).

It has been found that the combination of these two donor materials showed better results in terms of efficiency and consistency than the individual donor materials. The reason for this increase is the extension of absorption spectrum from the visible to the IR region due to the addition of PCDTBT and PCPDTBT to the acceptor material.

Also, there is a cascading of energy levels between the highest occupied molecular orbital and the lowest unoccupied molecular orbital from the dominating donor material to the acceptor material to facilitate charge transport. Morphology studies, such as AFM and transmission electron microscopy (TEM), showed that the ternary blend exhibited a better nanomorphology than the binary blend. This is the primary reason for the improvement in the efficiency (108).

In addition, a ternary blend formed by adding a donor material to the already existing binary blend has been tested (109). The addition of P3HT (Polyhexylthiopene) to either donor-acceptor copolymer material PCPDTBT or PCDTBT with common acceptor PC60BM (phenyl C61 butyric acid) has been tested.

Donor-acceptor copolymers are materials with repeated units of electron donor and electron acceptor units connected by a *p*-conjugated small molecule. Interestingly, a decrease in the efficiency is observed when P3HT is added to the binary blend of PCDTBT:PCBM and an increase in efficiency is observed when P3HT is added to the binary blend of PCPDTBT:PCBM (109).

There is cascading of energy levels in both the ternary blends PCDTBT:P3HT:PCBM and PCPDTBT:P3HT:PCBM which helps in the movement of the free charge carriers. Also, the VOC decreased in both cases by the addition of P3HT. However, the J_{SC} increased in the PCPDTBT:P3HT:PCBM ternary blend due to the improvement in photon absorption (109).

4.13.5 PCPDTBT:PC71BM Devices with Gold Nanoparticles

In order to clarify the effect of Au nanoparticles on the device performance experimentally, PCPDTBT:PC71BM devices with and without Au nanoparticles were fabricated on the same electrode and compared (110).

The Au nanoparticles were deposited only on a partial area of indium tin oxide electrode, and the devices with and without Au nanoparticles were fabricated simultaneously by spin-coating of PEDOT:PSS and PCPDTBT:PC71BM.

This device fabrication enables the two cells to have the same device fabrication procedures, active layer thicknesses, and material components, meaning that the difference between the two devices is only the existence of Au nanoparticles. Consequently, the device with Au nanoparticles showed an increase in a short-circuit current of 7.2%. The incidence photon-to-current efficiency behavior of the device with Au nanoparticles was similar to the extinction spectrum of Au nanoparticles, implying that the near field effect rather than the scattering effect of Au nanoparticles is the dominant mechanism in the enhanced device performance (110).

4.13.6 P3HT and ICBA blends in C-PCPDTBT and Si-PCPDTBT

A systematic study on the morphology evolution of prototype ternary systems upon adding sensitizers featuring similar chemical structures but dramatically different crystallinity has been reported (111). The ingredients are namely P3HT and ICBA blends with poly-[(4,4′-bis(2-ethylhexyl)dithieno[3,2-b:2′,3′-d]silole)-2,6-diyl-*alt*-(4,7-bis(2-thienyl)-2,1,3-benzothiadi-azole)-5,5′-diyl] (Si-PCPDTBT) and poly[2,6-(4,4-bis(2-ethylhexyl)-4H-cyclopenta[2,1-b;3,4-b′]-dithiophene)-*alt*-4,7-(2,1,3-benzothiadiazole)] (C-PCPDTBT).

A combined density functional theory and artificial neuronal network computational approach has been utilized to calculate the solubility parameters and the Flory-Huggins intermolecular parameters to evaluate the influence of the miscibility on the final morphology.

The domain spacing and the purity of ICBA-rich domains are retained in Si-PCPDTBT-based systems, but are strongly reduced in C-PCPDTBT-based ternary systems. The P3HT fiber structure is retained at a low sensitizer content but dramatically reduced at a high sensitizer content. The theoretical calculations reveal a very similar miscibility and compatibility between the two sensitizers, ICBA as well as P3HT (111).

4.13.7 Influence of Environment Temperature

The influence of environment temperature on the performance of the organic bulk heterojunction organic solar cells has been investigated (112). The effect of ambient temperature on the efficiency of PCPDTBT and [6,6]-phenyl-C71-butyric-acid-methyl-ester (PC71BM)-based bulk heterojunction organic solar cells has been elucidated.

The current-voltage characteristics of ITO/PEDOT: PSS/PCPDTBT: PC71BM/Al solar cells have been recorded in the temperature range of 25–60°C at a solar irradiation of 100 $mW\,cm^{-2}$.

The short-circuit current of the solar cells increased from 4.28 $mA\,cm^{-2}$ to 9.23 $mA\,cm^{-2}$ when the temperature was elevated from 25°C to 55°C.

However, the VOC and fill factor of the cells remained almost unchanged over the whole investigated temperature range. The values of the VOC and fill factor were found to be 0.58 V and 0.60 V, respectively. These results clearly indicate that a maximum efficiency of the ITO/PEDOT:PSS/PCPDTBT:PC71BM/Al solar cells can be achieved in the range of 52–58°C (112).

4.14 Extended Storage Life

Most organic and polymeric semiconductor materials used in solar cell applications have a limited storage life, which makes their implementation difficult. For example, P3HT, the best known material in plastic solar cells, has a storage life of only about 1 y. Most organic solar active materials also require post-coating thermal or vacuum treatments, as well as additional buffer or blocking layers in their structure, to prevent leakage or facilitate photovoltaic effects. These factors make the fabrication process problematic.

A photovoltaic device has been reported that comprises an active layer, wherein the active layer comprises an electron acceptor and a poly(arylamine biscarbonate ester) (107). An example is shown in Figure 4.22.

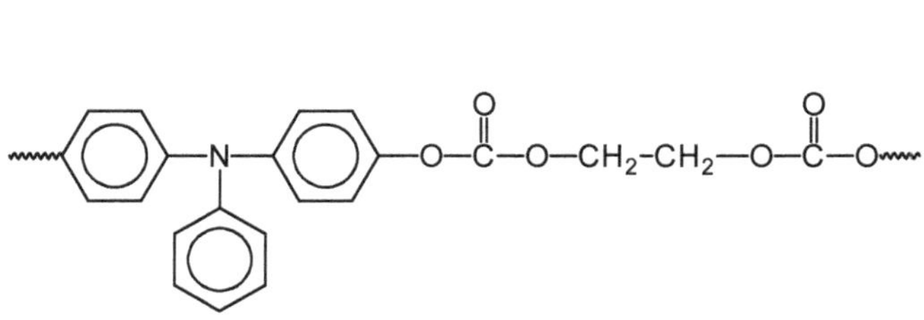

Figure 4.22 Poly(arylamine biscarbonate ester) (107).

The active layer between the first electrode and the second electrode contains PCBM and a poly(arylamine) biscarbonate ester. The active layer may have a thickness of 50–150 *nm*.

A major advantage of the poly(arylamine) biscarbonate esters is that they have a stable shelf life of over a decade as well as a long operating life. In contrast, the typical storage life of poly(thiophene)s is less than 18 *mon*. In addition, most photovoltaic materials are oxygen sensitive and fabrication must occur in an inert atmosphere. In contrast, the above-described semiconducting layer can be fabricated in an ambient environment. Also, no electron-blocking or hole-blocking layers are necessary to obtain a good performance (107).

4.15 Dye-Sensitized Solar Cells

4.15.1 Poly(ethylene oxide) Matrix

Gel polymer electrolytes modified with urea in a poly(ethylene oxide) (PEO) polymer matrix and iodine-iodide-based redox couple have been reported for the application of dye-sensitized solar cells (113).

The effect of urea on both molecular mobility and final morphology of gel polymer electrolytes has been characterized by Fourier transform infrared (FTIR) spectroscopy and scanning electron microscope technology.

Electrochemical impedance spectroscopy and linear sweep voltammetry showed that the addition of urea gives a general increment in both ionic conductivity and tri-iodide diffusion coefficient. In particular, gel polymer electrolytes containing 4% of urea have an ionic conductivity of $4.28 \times 10^{-4}\ S\,cm^{-1}$ and a tri-iodide diffusion coefficient of $2.06 \times 10^{-6}\ cm^2\,s^{-1}$. A maximum PCE of 6.82% in the photovoltaic performance could be achieved.

In addition, a variation of the charge transfer resistance and the chemical capacitance at the TiO_2 dye interfaces as a function of bias voltage was observed. This suggests an upward shift in the conduction band of TiO_2 in the case of gel electrolytes (113).

In a similar way, transparent gel polymer electrolytes have been prepared by adding thiourea coupled with PEO for the application of dye-sensitized solar cells (114).

The coupling of thiourea in the presence of iodine undergoes a dimerization reaction to produce formamidine disulfide. FTIR spectroscopy shows that the interactions of thiourea and formamidine disulfide with electronegative ether linkage of PEO results in conformational changes of gel polymer electrolytes.

Also, an increment in the ionic conductivity and tri-iodide diffusion coefficient, for thiourea modified gel polymer electrolytes has been found.

The prepared electrolytes can be used as a redox mediator in dye-sensitized solar cells. Apart from transparency, the gel polymer electrolytes with thiorurea show higher photovoltaic properties compared to a bare gel polymer electrolyte (114).

4.15.2 *Poly(methyl methacrylate) Matrix*

In order to improve the durability of dye-sensitized solar cells, a poly(methyl methacrylate) (PMMA)-based polymer gel electrolyte with different amounts of carbon black was studied to replace the conventional liquid electrolyte (115). Carbon black was used to improve the ionic conductivity of the polymer gel electrolyte.

Dye-sensitized solar cells fabricated with the prepared polymer gel electrolytes exhibit a very good long-term stability in comparison to a liquid electrolyte. The optimized dye-sensitized solar cell with 0.57% of carbon black in the PMMA polymer matrix exhibits the highest photo-conversion efficiency of 5.52 ± 0.03% with a J_{SC} value of 12.43 ± 0.04 $mA\,cm^{-2}$, a VOC value of 766.02 ± 0.52 mV and a fill factor value of 58.01 ± 0.02% (115).

A significant enhancement of VOC is observed with the employment of the polymer gel electrolyte. The impact of the polymer gel electrolyte in the enhancement of VOC was studied by analyzing the charge transfer kinetics data at the interface of the photoanode and the polymer gel electrolyte.

The long-term stability showed that after 1000 h of testing the optimized dye-sensitized solar cell (polymer gel electrolyte (0.57)) retains the short-circuit current value at 83% of the initial performance, thus exhibiting a very significant long-term stability in comparison to the dye-sensitized solar cell that is fabricated with a liquid electrolyte (115).

4.15.3 *Poly(propylene carbonate) Matrix*

Gel polymer electrolytes with incorporation of poly(propylene carbonate) and different weight percentages of sodium iodide salt have been prepared (116). Ethylene carbonate and propylene carbonate were used as plasticizers. The maximum ionic conductivity of 2.01 $mS\,cm^{-1}$ could be achieved at room temperature. Dye-sensitized solar cells have been fabricated and tested under one sun illumination. The highest energy conversion efficiency of 6.38% was achieved with the addition of 60% of sodium iodide.

Gel polymer electrolytes have been prepared by mixing poly-(propylene carbonate) with various weight percentages of 1-butyl-3-methyl imidazolium iodide as ionic liquid (117). The gel polymer electrolytes consist of poly(propylene carbonate) as the host polymer, sodium iodide salt, ethylene carbonate, propylene carbonate, 1-butyl-3-methyl imidazolium iodide ionic liquid, and iodine. 1-Butyl-3-methyl imidazolium iodide is shown in Figure 4.23.

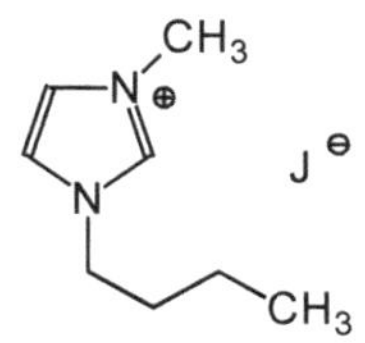

Figure 4.23 1-Butyl-3-methyl imidazolium iodide.

The optimum 1-butyl-3-methyl imidazolium iodide ionic liquid content was found to be 60% with respect to poly(propylene carbonate) with the highest ionic conductivity of $4.79 \times 10^{-3}\ S\,cm^{-1}$. Temperature-dependent ionic conductivity studies showed that the gel polymer electrolytes obey an Arrhenius model (117).

Dye-sensitized solar cells have been fabricated and gel polymer electrolytes were sandwiched between the working and counter electrodes and tested under one sun illumination. The highest energy conversion efficiency of 6.14% was achieved with the addition of 60% of 1-butyl-3-methyl imidazolium iodide (117).

4.15.4 Sulfobetaine-Based Polymer

An eco-friendly, efficient poly(sulfobetaine)-based gel electrolyte was synthesized as an alternative to liquid electrolyte in the fabrication of dye-sensitized solar cells (118).

This nitrogen-rich and highly conductive poly(sulfobetaine) was synthesized by an easy and facile method without the use of any catalyst and explored for its dye-sensitized solar cell application. The synthesized polymer gel electrolyte exhibited good ionic conductivity of about $6.8 \times 10^{-3}\ S\,cm^{-1}$ at ambient temperature.

Dye-sensitized solar cells were fabricated based on this poly-(sulfobetaine) gel electrolyte and studied for their performance based on photovoltaic parameters. The dye-sensitized solar cell photovoltaic results were appreciable and are VOC = 0.82 V, Jsc = 11.49 $mA\,cm^{-2}$, FF = 66%, and PCE = 6.26% at 1 sun intensity. These values are slightly lower than conventional liquid electrolyte-based dye-sensitized solar cells (118).

4.15.5 Titanium Dioxide-Based Cells

The performance of dye-sensitized nanocrystalline TiO_2 thin film-based photo-electrochemical solar cells that contain gel polymer electrolytes is largely governed by the nature of the cation in the electrolyte. The dependence of the photovoltaic performance in these quasi-solid-state photo-electrochemical solar cells on the alkaline cation size has already been investigated for single cation iodide salt-based electrolytes.

Here, the ionic conductivity dependence on the nature of alkaline cations as counterion in a gel polymer electrolyte based on binary iodides has been investigated (119). Several poly(acrylonitrile)-based gel polymer electrolytes containing binary iodide salts have been prepared using one of the alkaline iodides, i.e., LiI, NaI, KI, RbI, CsI, and and an organic compound, tetrapropylammonium iodide. All the electrolytes based on binary salts have shown a conductivity enhancement compared to their single cation counterparts.

When combined with tetrapropylammonium iodide, each of the Li^+, Na^+, K^+, Rb^+, and Cs^+ cations containing iodide salts incorporated into the gel electrolytes have shown a room-temperature conductivity enhancement of 85.59%, 12.03%, 12.71%, 20.77%, and

15.36%, respectively. The conductivities of gel electrolytes containing binary iodide systems with tetrapropylammonium iodide and KI/RbI/CsI are higher and have shown values of 3.28 $mS\,cm^{-1}$, 3.43 $mS\,cm^{-1}$, and 3.23 $mS\,cm^{-1}$, respectively, at room temperature (119).

The influence of the nature of counterions on the performance of quasi-solid-state dye-sensitized solar cells has been investigated by assembling two series of cells. All the binary cationic solar cells have shown more or less enhancements of the VOC, J_{SC}, fill factor, and efficiency in comparison to their single cation counterparts.

The importance of employing binary cations (a large and a small) in electrolytes intended for quasi-solid-state solar cells has been demonstrated. The percentage of energy conversion efficiency enhancement shown for the photo-electrochemical solar cells made with electrolytes containing tetrapropylammonium iodide along with Li^+, Na^+, K^+, Rb^+, and Cs^+ iodides is 260.27%, 133.65%, 65.27%, 25.32%, and 8.36%, respectively.

The highest efficiency of 4.93% has been shown from the solar cell containing KI and tetrapropylammonium iodide. However, the highest enhancements of ionic conductivity as well as the energy conversion efficiency were exhibited by the photo-electrochemical solar cell made with Li^+ containing binary cationic electrolyte (119).

4.15.6 *Quasi-Solid-State Gel Electrolytes*

A series of dual function quasi-solid-state gel electrolytes with high conductivity and good catalytic ability were prepared by integrating the carbon nanotubes and conducting polymers, including poly-(pyrrole) (PPy), poly(aniline) and PEDOT, into a poly(acrylic acid) gel (120).

A significant improvement in electrochemical and photoelectrochemistry capability was shown when used in dye-sensitized solar cells. These electrolytes provide three-dimensional network structures for transporting electrons, giving a similar conduction mechanism to that of I^-/I_3^- liquid electrolyte system.

The electrochemical performance of the CoS/Ag/Ti counter electrode was evaluated by electrochemical impedance spectroscopy, which revealed that the CoS/Ag/Ti counter electrode exhibited an excellent electrocatalytic ability for these electrolytes, as well as that of a I^-/I_3^- liquid system (120).

The quasi-solid-state flexible dye-sensitized solar cell fabricated with the CoS/Ag/Ti counter electrode and the gel electrolytes integrated poly(pyrrole), poly(aniline), and PEDOT achieved an enhanced PCE of 6.89%, 7.01% and 7.20% under the irradiation of 100 $mWcm^{-2}$, which has greatly approached that of the dye-sensitized solar cell (7.35%) based on a platinum electrode and an I^-/I_3^- liquid electrolyte (120).

4.15.7 Bio-based Electrolytes

4.15.7.1 Agar

Agar is a natural polymer and has been used to prepare quasi-solid-state polymer electrolytes. Two different iodide salts, i.e., sodium iodide and potassium iodide, were incorporated (121).

To enhance the ionic conductivity of the quasi-solid-state polymer electrolyte system, 1-methyl-3-propylimidazolium iodide (MPII) ionic liquid is added. The highest ionic conductivity of 1.48 ± 0.001 $S\,cm^{-1}$ was achieved after the addition of 50% of KI and 3.0 g of 1-methyl-3-propylimidazolium iodide ionic liquid. The quasi-solid-state polymer electrolytes have been studied for their temperature-dependent ionic conductivity behavior.

Structural studies revealed that the complexation between the agar polymer, iodide salts, and 1-methyl-3-propylimidazolium iodide ionic liquid has occurred. The quasi-solid-state polymer electrolytes are sandwiched between counter and working electrodes to fabricate dye-sensitized solar cells and are analyzed under a sun simulator. The highest efficiency of 2.16% is achieved with the incorporation of 3.0 g 1-methyl-3-propylimidazolium iodide ionic liquid (121). 1-Methyl-3-propylimidazolium iodide is shown in Figure 4.24.

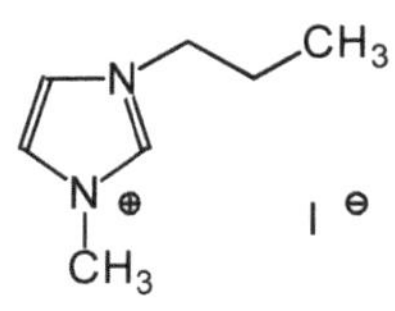

Figure 4.24 1-Methyl-3-propylimidazolium iodide.

4.15.7.2 Chitosan

Chitosan is a biopolymer which can be derived from crab shells. Chitosan is insoluble in common organic solvents. It could be converted to the organosoluble *N*-phthaloylchitosan by the reaction with phthalic anhydride in dimethylformamide (122). The formation is shown in Figure 4.25.

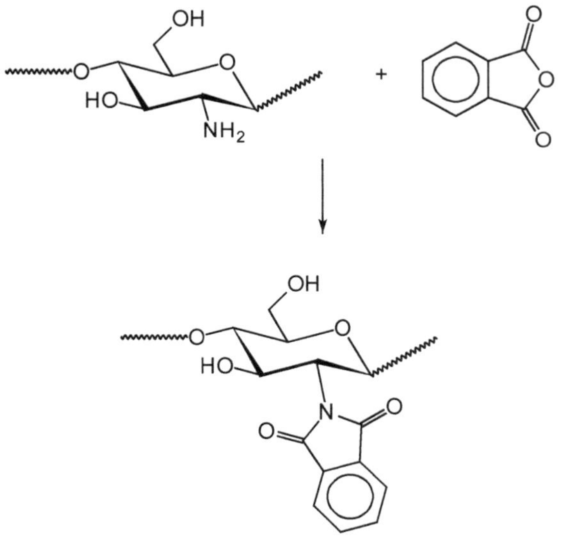

Figure 4.25 *N*-Phthaloylchitosan.

The formation and the structure of *N*-phthaloylchitosan was confirmed by the characteristic peaks of phthalimido and aromatic groups observed at 719, 1708 and 1772 cm^{-1} and two sets of peaks centered at 3.0 and 7.5 *ppm* obtained from FTIR and 1H NMR analyses, respectively. Gel polymer electrolytes consisting of *N*-phthaloylchitosan, ethylene carbonate, and dimethylformamide with various amounts of tetrapropylammonium iodide and iodine were prepared (122).

The interaction behavior between polymer-plasticizer-salt was thoroughly investigated using FTIR spectroscopy. The gel polymer electrolyte consisting of *N*-phthaloylchitosan : ethylene carbonate : dimethylformamide : tetrapropylammonium iodide : iodine in a weight ratio (g) of 0.1 : 0.3 : 0.3 : 0.12 : 0.012 showed the highest conductivity of $5.46\times10^{-3}\ S\,cm^{-1}$ at room temperature and exhibited the best performance in dye-sensitized solar cells with efficiency of 5.0%, with JSC of 12.72 $mA\,cm^{-2}$, VOC of 0.60 V and a fill factor of 0.66 (122).

4.16 Direct Arylation Polymerization

Direct arylation polymerization is a simple, cost-effective and efficient method for synthesizing conjugated polymers.

The synthesis of a narrow bandgap conjugated polymer, PCPDT-TBT, consisting of alternating cyclopentadithiophene (CPDT) and 4,7-di(thiophen-2-yl)benzo[c][1,2,5] thiadiazole (TBT) units, was optimized by a direct arylation polycondensation (123). The synthesis method is shown in Figure 4.26.

The synthesized polymer had a number average molecular weight of 36.3 $kg\,mol^{-1}$ with a low polydispersity index of 1.25, as measured by gel permeation chromatography against poly(styrene) standards. PCPDTTBT exhibits an absorption maximum at 617 nm in tetrahydrofuran solution, whereas in thin film, the absorption spectrum was broader and a maximum was observed at 650 nm. The HOMO, LUMO and bandgap calculations were estimated using cyclic voltammetry and were found to be -5.20 eV, -3.57 eV, and 1.63 eV, respectively (123).

Bulk heterojunction polymer solar cells were fabricated by blending PCPDTTBT and PC71BM in three different ratios with six cells for each ratio to optimize the efficiency. The device structure of the fabricated device with PCPDTTBT: PC71BM polymer-acceptor blends is shown in Figure 4.27.

It was found that the blend ratio of 1:2 exhibited a high short-circuit current of 10.03 $mAcm^{-2}$, VOC of 0.567 V and a PCE of 1.86%. The morphology of the active layer was investigated by employing AFM in tapping mode and the film of active layer with 1:2 ratio of PCPDTTBT: PC71BM showed the most favorable morphology with less phase separation (123).

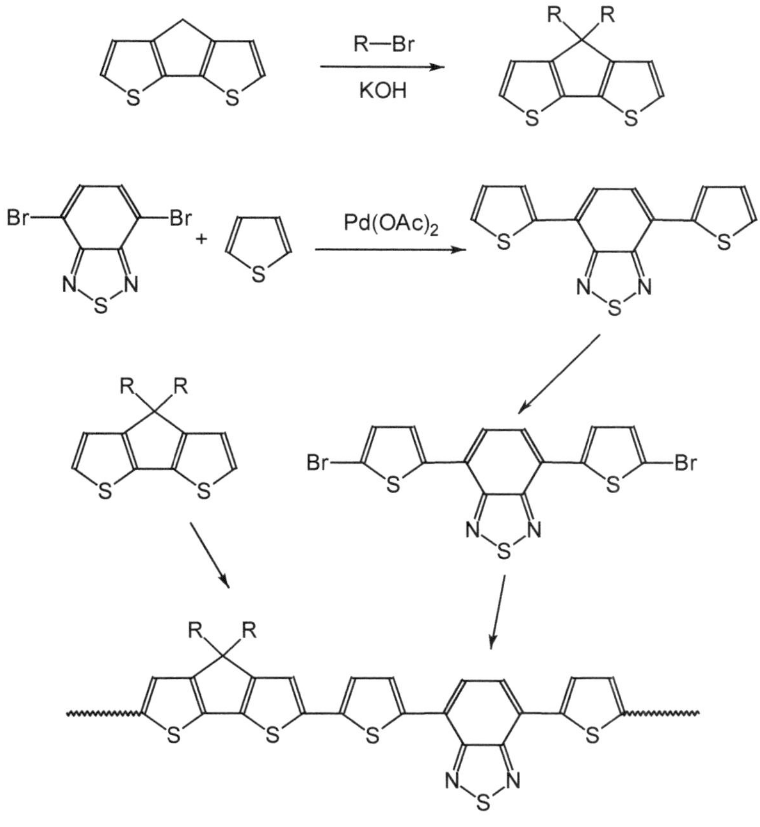

Figure 4.26 Direct arylation polymerization to prepare the polymer PCPDTTBT (123).

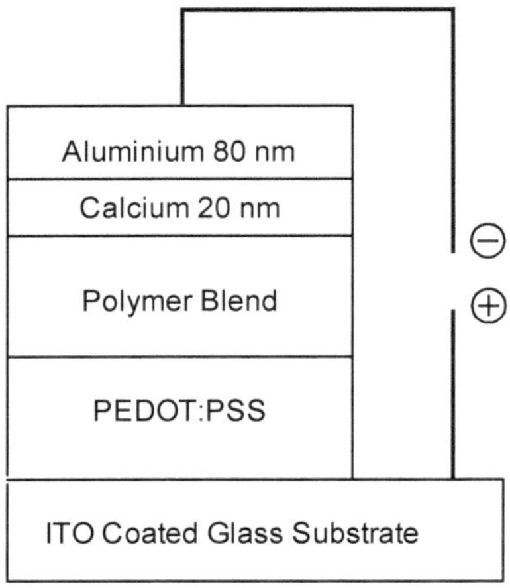

Figure 4.27 Device structure using PCPDTTBT: PC71BM (123).

4.17 Polymer-Fullerene Solar Cells

Polymer-fullerene solar cells have been detailed (124).

Polymer-fullerene solar cells are a type of organic solar cells made with conductive polymers and electron-accepting fullerene derivatives.

Compared to conventional solar cells, such as silicon-based solar cells, polymer-fullerene solar cells are lightweight, potentially disposable, and flexible. The main advantage of polymer-fullerene solar cells is that they are customizable at a molecular level (124).

Fullerenes have become the ubiquitous acceptors because of their high electron affinity and ability to transport charge effectively (125). The most effective solar cells have been made from bicontinuous polymer-fullerene composites, i.e., bulk heterojunctions.

Fullerenes exhibit an energetically deep-lying LUMO, which endows the molecule with a very high electron affinity relative to the numerous potential organic donors. The triply degenerate LUMO of C60 also allows the molecule to be reversibly reduced with up to six electrons, thus illustrating its ability to stabilize negative charge.

A number of conjugated polymer-fullerene blends exhibit an ultrafast photoinduced charge transfer of ca. 45 fs, with a back transfer that is orders of magnitude slower. A C60-based fullerene has been shown to have a very high electron mobility of up to 1 $cm^2V^{-1}s^{-1}$ in field-effect transistors.

Basically, the optimization of polymer-fullerene solar cells is done by fine-tuning the electronic properties and the interactions of the donor and the acceptor components so as (125):

- To absorb the most light,
- Generate the greatest number of free charges with minimal concomitant loss of energy, and
- Transport the charges to the respective electrodes at a maximum rate and with a minimum of recombination.

However, such an approach that focuses solely on the electronic characteristics of the individual components, such as absorption coefficient and charge carrier mobility, ignores the morphological issues, which are also of critical importance in such devices.

The two components required in solar cell devices for electronic optimization are a soluble fullerene-based acceptor, generally a C60 derivative, and a polymeric donor that can be processed in solution. Fullerenes have been considered to be the ideal acceptors for organic solar cells (125).

The use of a C70 derivative shows an increase in performance. The main reason for this increase in performance is the much greater absorption of C70 in the visible region relative to that of C60. The high symmetry of C60 renders low-energy transitions formally dipole forbidden, thereby resulting in a very weak absorption of light in the visible region, despite the bandgap of 1.8 eV (125).

The measured extinction coefficient of a PCBM is nearly five times that of [60]PCBM at 600 nm and nearly 20 times higher at 475 nm (126).

4.18 Functionalized Poly(thiophene)

Poly[1,5-naphthyridine-(3-hexylthiophene)] has been synthesized by both a conventional and a microwave-assisted Suzuki-Miyaura cross-coupling reaction using 3-hexylthiophene-2,5-diboronic ester and 2,6-dibromo-1,5-naphthyridine (127). In this way a semiconducting polymer was formed. 2,6-Dibromo-1,5-naphthyridine is shown in Figure 4.28.

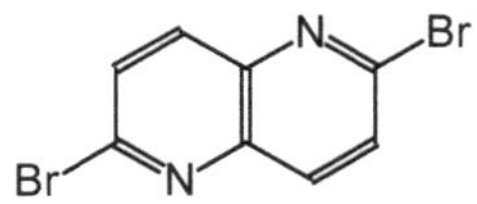

Figure 4.28 2,6-Dibromo-1,5-naphthyridine.

The electrochemical and transport properties of the polymer were investigated both in the bulk as well as in thin-film form (127). Cyclic voltammetry results of the polymer in bulk form and in H_2SO_4 solution indicated that the concentration of the polymer in the solution is not well defined because of the poor solubility of the polymer in aqueous solutions.

On the other hand, the sulfur group, which works as electron-donating, makes the system more electron-rich. This can be explained by the absence of the reduction peak. For the thin film, two single oxidation peaks were obtained at around 0 *V* and 0.3 *V* for both cases.

Different solvents can tune the transport properties of the polymer, as can be seen from the two cyclic voltammetry measurements, where BF_3 exhibited enhanced transport properties over ACN. This polymer was also employed in dye-sensitized solar cells as a photosensitizer (127).

4.19 Fullerene

There are monographs concerning the issues of fullerene (128, 129).

Fullerenes are an allotrope of carbon in which the carbon atoms are present in even numbers and are arranged at the vertices of a closed cagelike structure composed of 12 pentagons and at least 20 hexagons (130). Fullerene types are C_60, C_70, C_84. Here, the number refers to the number of carbon atoms in the molecule. C60 Fullerene is shown in Figure 4.29.

Initially, for the synthesis of fullerene, graphite has been vaporized by laser irradiation (131). Then, fullerenes have been synthesized at a temperature of formation of 2700°C at a helium pressure of 150 *kPa*. Here, cylindrical carbon bodies are inductively heated

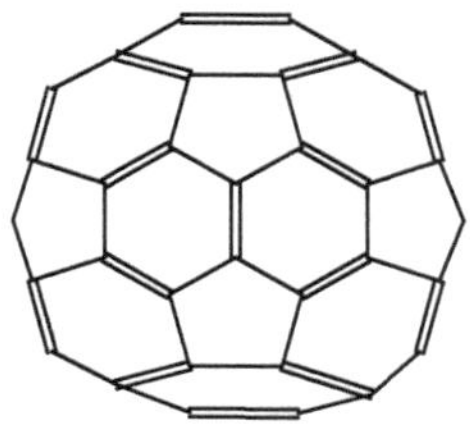

Figure 4.29 C60 Fullerene.

and evaporated and the resulting fullerenes are extracted from the soot formed (132).

Nowadays, three methods are known for the synthesis of fullerenes (133). The Krätschmer-Huffmann method (134) uses the arc discharge between graphite rods in helium atmosphere. Another method is the combustion of benzene in a deficiency of oxygen. Also, the condensation of polycyclic aromatic compounds by dehydrogenation or dehydrohalogenation results in fullerenes. An example is shown in Figure 4.30.

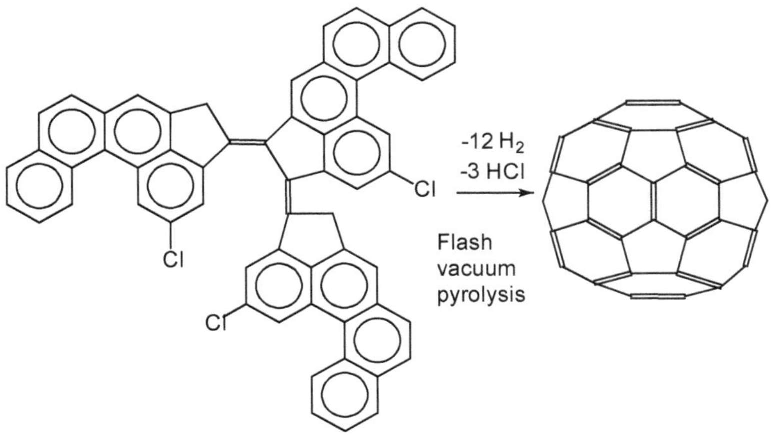

Figure 4.30 Synthesis of C60 Fullerene by dehydrohalogenation (133).

Fullerenes are sparingly soluble in most solvents. However, the chemical functionalization of fullerenes allows the preparation of soluble fullerene compounds. The basic principles of the chemical reactivity of fullerenes have been detailed (135).

The cycloaddition reaction plays an important role in the functionalization of fullerenes. Cyclopropanated fullerenes can be synthesized by three methods (135):

1. Thermal addition of diazo compounds followed by thermolysis or photolysis,
2. Addition of free carbenes, and
3. Bingel reaction, an addition-elimination reaction (136, 137).

4.20 Transparent Window Materials

Zinc oxide thin films have been deposited onto PET and poly(imide) (PI) substrates using the chemical spray pyrolysis technique in order to explore their potential use as transparent window materials for solar cells (138).

The substrate temperature along deposition of the material was maintained at 250°C. The effects of substrate types on the structural and optical characteristics of the formed films were studied. XRD patterns confirmed the proper phase formation of crystalline ZnO films.

Films deposited on PI exhibited a larger roughness compared to those deposited onto PET substrates because of the large particles adsorbed on the former. Optical transmittance values exceeding 80% in the visible and IR region on both substrates were found.

Surface reflectance measurements showed that ZnO on PI has a higher surface reflectance of ca. 2% throughout the spectral region compared to ZnO films on PET substrates, while both showed a parasitic absorbance below 10% within the region of interest (138).

4.21 Solar Cell Encapsulants

Solar cell encapsulants are required to achieve a weather resistance because use over a long period of time is required.

An ethylene-vinyl acetate copolymer is usually synthesized by radically polymerizing ethylene with vinyl acetate under high-temperature and high-pressure conditions.

An ethylene-vinyl acetate copolymer prepared by this method has a structure that has many branches or two or more continuous repeating units derived from vinyl acetate.

A coupling agent has been added. Examples of silane coupling agents are collected in Table 4.7. Some of these compounds are shown in Figure 4.31.

Table 4.7 Silane coupling agents (139).

Compound
3-Chloropropyltrimethoxysilane
Vinyltrichlorosilane
Vinyltriethoxysilane
Vinyl-tris(2-methoxyethoxy)silane
γ-Methacryloxypropyltrimethoxysilane
β-(3,4-Ethoxycyclohexyl)ethyl-trimethoxysilane
γ-Glycidoxypropyltrimethoxysilane
Vinyltriacetoxysilane
γ-Mercaptopropyltrimethoxysilane
γ-Aminopropyltrimethoxysilane
N-β-(Aminoethyl)-γ-aminopropyltrimethoxysilane

In order to obtain an encapsulant having more stable adhesive force and high volume resistivity, the addition proportion of the silane coupling agent per 100 parts by mass of the polymer is preferably 0.01 parts by mass to 0.6 parts by mass. The preparation of a crosslinked sheet runs as (139):

Preparation 4–1: One hundred parts by weight of a polymer made from cyclooctene and 5-methoxycarbonyl-1-cyclooctene was impregnated with 1.0 or 2.0 part by weight of *tert*-butylperoxy-2-ethylhexyl carbonate and 0.5 parts by mass of γ-methacryloxypropyltrimethoxysilane. The polymer impregnated with the organic peroxide and the auxiliary crosslinking agent was pressed with a pressure of 10 *MPa* for 5 *min* with a hot presser at 90°C, then pressed with a pressure of 10 *MPa* for 20 *min* with a hot presser at 150°C, and then cooled for 5 *min* with a cooling presser at 30°C, thereby preparing a crosslinked sheet of about 500 μm in thickness.

4.22 Anti-reflection Coating

A polymer thin film, PSS, has been employed in interdigitated back contact solar cells as an anti-reflection coating and front surface

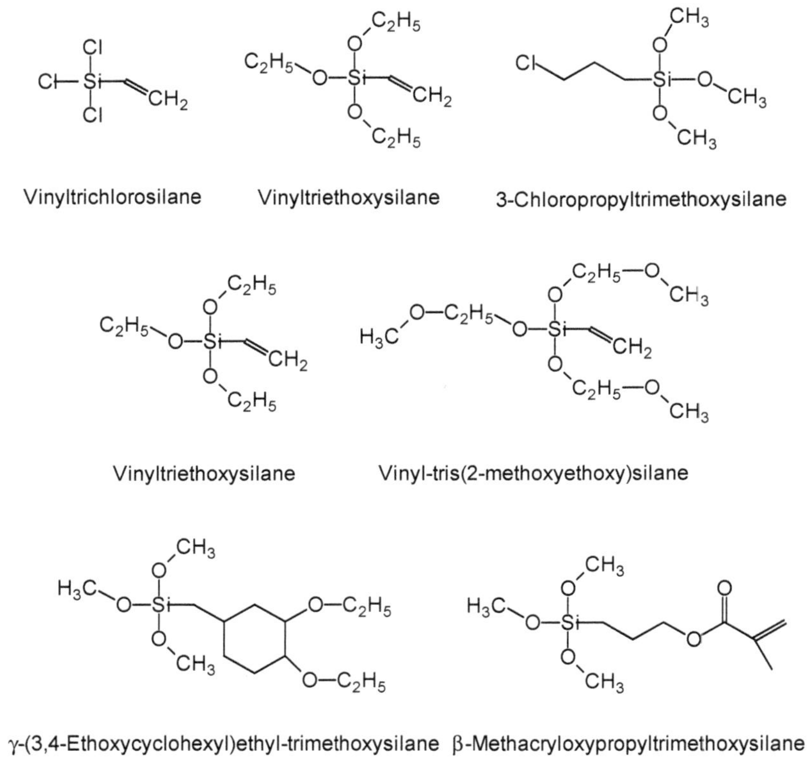

Figure 4.31 Silane coupling agents (139).

passivation layer (140). It has been found that the PSS thin film is highly transparent and possesses a refraction index of about 1.5, and thus functions well as anti-reflection coating for Si wafer-based solar cells.

An effective minority carrier lifetime of 2.3 *ms* could be obtained on 1–5 Ωcm *n*-type crystalline Si wafer with both sides symmetrically coated by the PSS thin film, proving a good Si surface passivation by this polymer.

An increase in PCE is obtained when 150 *nm* thick PSS thin film is coated on the front surface of interdigitated back contact solar cells without any anti-reflection/surface passivation layers, resulted from the increased J_{SC} and VOC.

Thus, a new approach has been found using an organic polymer thin film deposited with low-temperature and vacuum-free technique as anti-reflection/surface passivation multifunctional layer in Si solar cells (140).

4.23 Fullerene-Free Polymer Solar Cells

Fullerene derivatives, especially for PC71BM, have been predominately used in highly efficient polymer solar cells (141). However, nonfullerene-based acceptors have attracted much attention because of their easily tunable molecular energy levels, excellent optical absorption properties, and potential for low-cost production processes (142, 143).

However, the PCE of the fullerene-free polymer solar cells has still been lower than the state-of-art PCEs of the polymer:PC71BM-based polymer solar cells (144, 145).

The PCE has now surpassed 10% for single-junction organic solar cells (146). This occurred mainly through the design and the synthesis of novel donor materials, the optimization of film morphology and the evolution of the devices. However, the development of novel acceptor materials is relatively sluggish compared with the donor compounds.

Nowadays, fullerene derivatives, such as PC61BM and PC71BM, are still the dominant acceptors due to their superior charge transporting properties (146). Unfortunately, these two acceptors suffer from some intrinsic shortcomings such as limited absorption, difficult functionalization, and high production cost.

Therefore, the development of novel nonfullerene acceptors that can overcome the above-mentioned disadvantages is desirable. For these reasons, research on nonfullerene acceptors has made considerable progress in the last two years and in this field a highest PCE of around 12% could be achieved (146).

The progress of recent research in nonfullerene small molecule acceptors has been summarized. Also, the performance of these molecules in organic solar cells has been detailed where the same donor materials are used. Moreover, the acceptors with excellent photovoltaic performance have been highlighted and the reasons for this behavior have been explained (146).

4.23.1 *PBDB-T Fullerene-Free Solar Cells*

A nonfullerene-based polymer solar cell that significantly outperforms fullerene-based polymer solar cells with respect to the power conversion efficiency has been demonstrated. An efficiency of greater than 11%, which is among the top values in the field, and excellent thermal stability could be obtained using poly[(2,6-(4,8-bis(5-(2-ethylhexyl)thiophen-2-yl)-benzo[1,2-b:4,5-*b*′]dithiophene))-*alt*-(5,5-(1′,3′-di-2-thienyl-5′,7′-bis(2-ethylhexyl)benzo[1′,2′-*c*:4′,5′-*c*′]dithiophene-4,8-dione))] (PBDB-T), cf. Figure 4.32, 3,9-bis(2-methylene-(3-(1,1-dicyanomethylene)-indanone))-5,5,11,11-tetrakis(4-hexylphenyl)-dithieno[2,3-*d*:2′,3′-*d*′]-*s*-indaceno-[1,2-*b*:5,6-*b*′]dithiophene, cf., Figure 4.17, as donor and acceptor, respectively (141).

4.23.2 *P3HT-Based Fullerene-Free Solar Cells*

A nonfullerene acceptor has been presented that has been specifically designed to give an improved performance alongside the wide bandgap donor P3HT, a polymer with significantly better prospects for commercial organic photovoltaics due to its relative scalability and stability (147).

Due to the well-matched optoelectronic and morphological properties of these materials, efficiencies of 6.4% could be achieved,

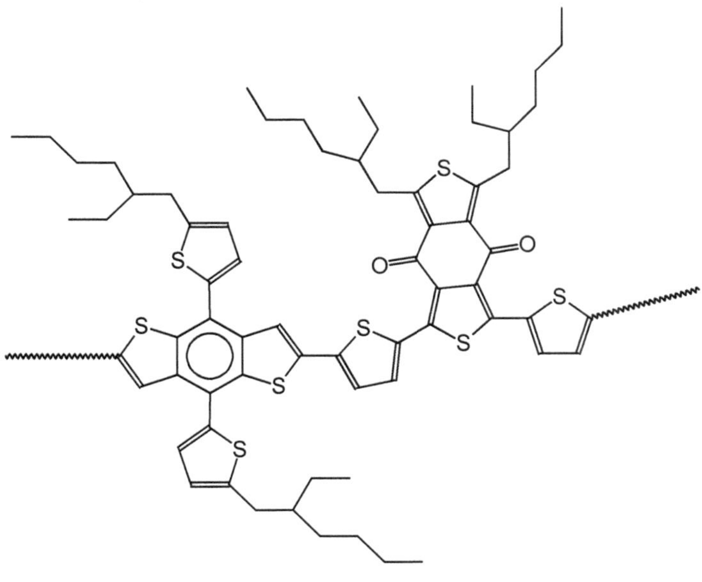

Figure 4.32 Poly[(2,6-(4,8-bis(5-(2-ethylhexyl)thiophen-2-yl)-benzo-[1,2-b:4,5-*b*′]dithiophene))-*alt*-(5,5-(1′,3′-di-2-thienyl-5′,7′-bis(2-ethylhex-yl)benzo[1′,2′-*c*:4′,5′-*c*′]dithiophene-4,8-dione))].

which is the highest hitherto reported for fullerene-free P3HT devices. In addition, dramatically improved air stability is demonstrated relative to other high-efficiency organic photovoltaics, showing the excellent potential of this new material combination for future technological applications (147).

4.23.3 Poly(thiophene)-Based Fullerene-Free Solar Cells

A highly efficient fullerene-free polymer solar cell based on polymeric 3,3′-dichloro-2,2′-bithiophene (PDCBT), a poly(thiophene) derivative substituted with alkoxycarbonyl, achieves an impressive PCE of 10.16%, which is the best result in polymer solar cells based on polythiophene derivatives to date (148). PDCBT is shown in Figure 4.33.

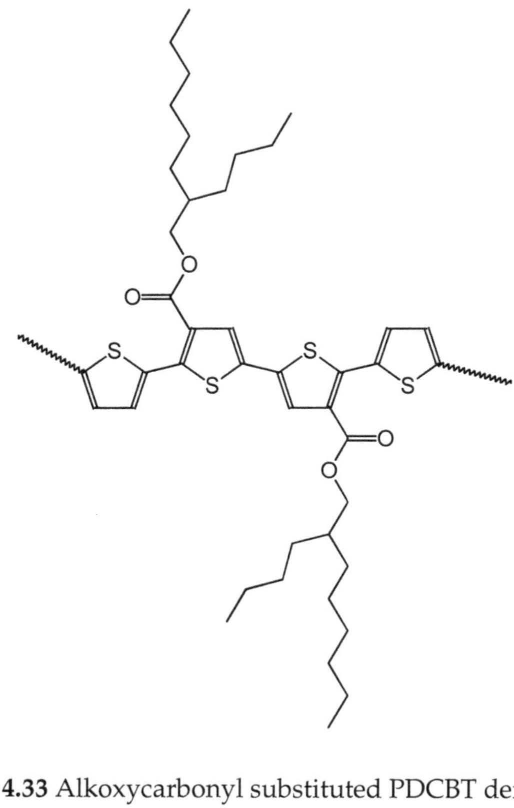

Figure 4.33 Alkoxycarbonyl substituted PDCBT derivative.

In comparison to a P3HT:ITIC-based device, the photovoltaic and morphological properties of the PDCBT:ITIC-based device have been investigated and interpreted. In comparison to a P3HT:ITIC-based device, the PDCBT:ITIC device after thermal annealing shows (148):

1. Higher crystalline and well-distributed nanofibrillar structures (with face-on stacking) in the blend film,
2. A comparable hole mobility but a higher electron mobility, and
3. Efficient charge generation and extraction with little geminate and nongeminate charge recombinations.

In contrast, the as-casted P3HT:ITIC device shows an almost amorphous morphology and the crystalline interchain ordering in P3HT decreased substantially even with thermal annealing by blending with ITIC (148).

Also, a fluorinated PDCBT derivative has been used as donor, and a methyl-end-capped ITIC derivative was used as acceptor (149). ITIC is shown in Figure 4.17. Here, at both of the endings, benzene moieties methyl groups are pending.

The methyl-end-capped ITIC derivative, with elevated HOMO and LUMO levels, was selected as the acceptor in the pursuit of a higher VOC. A best PCE of 6.6% with an extremely high VOC of 1.13 *V* could be obtained after a careful optimization of the morphology (149).

4.23.4 *Trialkylsilyl Substituted 2D-Conjugated Polymer*

A trialkylsilyl substituted 2D-conjugated polymer has been developed with the highest occupied molecular orbital level downshifted by a Si–C bond interaction (150). The synthesis is shown in Figure 4.34.

Polymer solar cells obtained by pairing this polymer with a nonfullerene acceptor demonstrated a high PCE of 11.41% with both high VOC of 0.94 *V* and high J_{SC} of 17.32 $mA\ cm^{-2}$.

This benefits from the complementary absorption of the donor and acceptor, and the high hole transfer efficiency from acceptor to donor, although the highest occupied molecular orbital level difference between the donor and acceptor is only 0.11 eV. The results

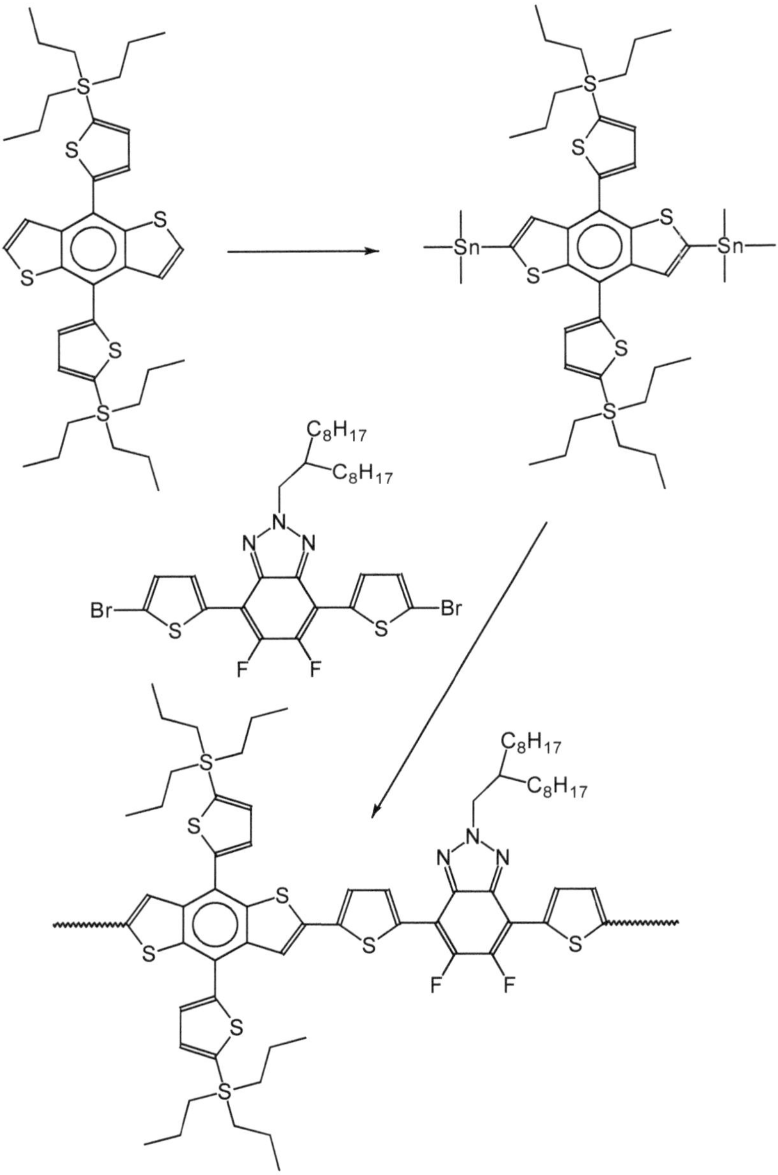

Figure 4.34 Trialkylsilyl substituted 2D-conjugated polymer (150).

indicate that the alkylsilyl substitution is an effective way to design high-performance conjugated polymer photovoltaic materials (150).

4.23.5 *Electron Acceptor Dimer*

A nonfullerene electron acceptor dimer, i.e., 2,5-bis(8-(17-phenyl)-7,9,16,18-tetraazabenzodifluoranthene-3,4,12,13-tetracarboxylic acid diimide)-3,4-ethylenedioxythiophene (DBFI-EDOT), has been described (151). DBFI-EDOT is shown in Figure 4.35.

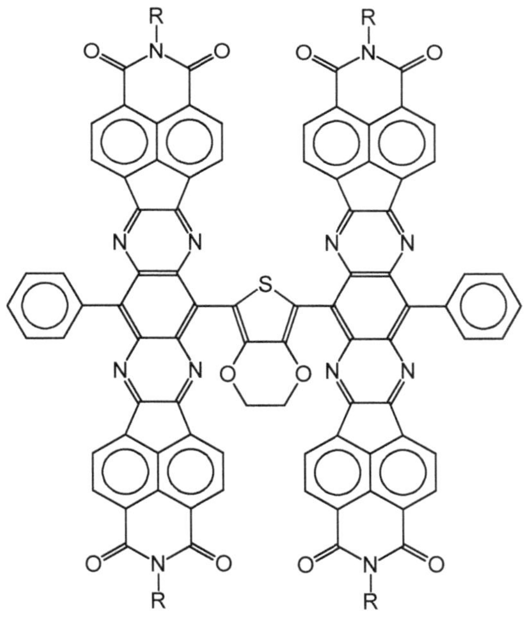

Figure 4.35 2,5-Bis(8-(17-phenyl)-7,9,16,18-tetraazabenzodifluoranthene-3,4,12,13-tetracarboxylic acid diimide)-3,4-ethylenedioxythiophene (R=2-decyltetrdecyl).

The material has a highly twisted, nonplanar 3D conformation. Polymer solar cells that have incorporated DBFI-EDOT and a thiazolothiazole-dithienylsilole copolymer donor, without using a processing additive, exhibit 8.1% PCE with a high VOC of 0.93 *V*.

Furthermore, 6.7% efficient polymer solar cells with a VOC of 0.95 *V* could be achieved when DBFI-EDOT acceptor is paired with the smaller bandgap poly(4,8-bis(5-(2-ethylhexyl)thiophen-2-yl)-benzo[1,2-b;4,5-b′]dithiophene-2,6-diyl-*alt*-(4-(2-ethylhexyl)-3-fluorothieno[3,4-b]thiophene-)-2-carboxylate-2-6-diyl)) (PBDTT-FTTE) donor polymer (151). PBDTT-FTTE is shown in Figure 4.36.

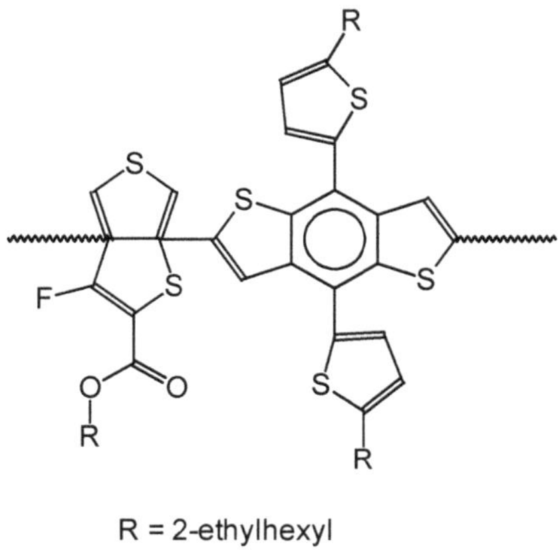

Figure 4.36 PBDTT-FTTE.

Combining DBFI-EDOT acceptor with these two different donor polymers (PSEHTT and PBDTT-FTTE) in a ternary blend active layer produced polymer solar cells with a PCE of 8.5%, a maximum photocurrent of 15.67 $mA\,cm^{-2}$, and a maximum external quantum efficiency of 83% (151). PSEHTT is shown in Figure 4.37.

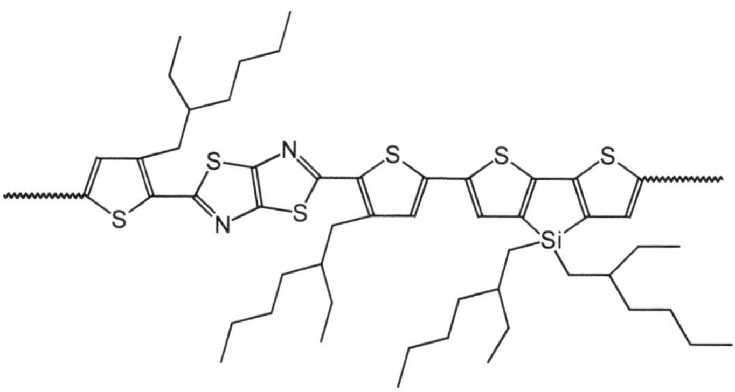

Figure 4.37 PSEHTT: Thiazolothiazole-dithienylsilole donor polymer.

These DBFI-EDOT BHJ devices combine maximum external quantum efficiency values of 78–83% with high VOC of 0.91–0.95 *V*, and thus have rather low optical bandgap energy losses of 0.62–0.77 *eV* (151).

4.23.6 *Wide Bandgap Polymer Donor*

A wide bandgap polymer donor PBDTS-DTBTO has been designed and synthesized (152). The alkoxyl modified 4,7-bis-thienyl-benzo-thiadiazole (DTBT) moiety acts as a strong electron-withdrawing unit.

The synthesis of PBDTS-DTBTO by Stille coupling is shown in Figure 4.38.

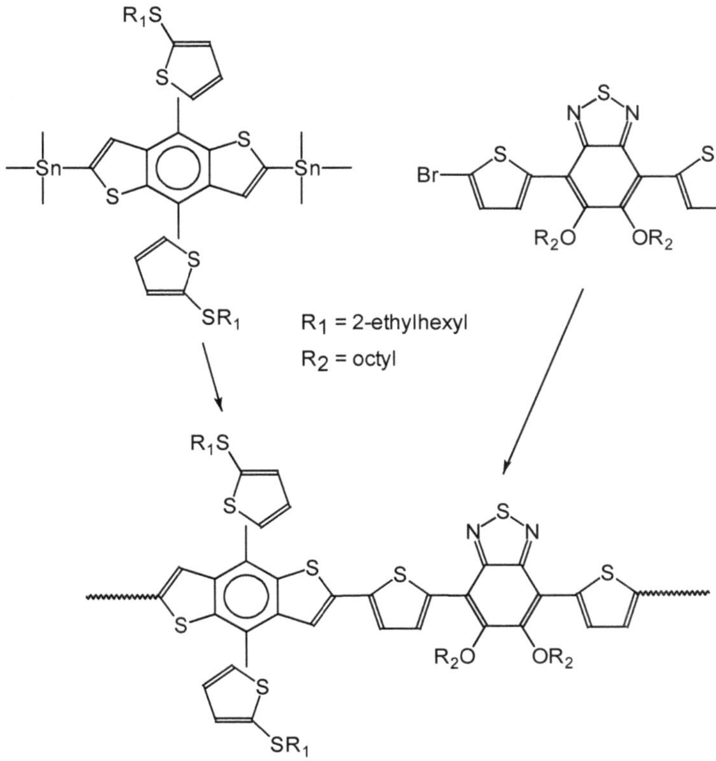

Figure 4.38 Synthesis of PBDTS-DTBTO by Stille coupling.

The material shows an optical bandgap of 1.76 *eV* and strong p-p interaction (152). By using a low bandgap acceptor ITIC, PCE over 9% could be achieved in a fullerene-free polymer solar cell device. Furthermore, the PSC devices fabricated by PBDTS-DTBTO:ITIC show a relatively small sensitivity to variations of the active layer thickness (152).

4.23.7 *Spirobifluorene- and Diketopyrrolopyrrole-Based Non-fullerene Acceptor*

A nonfullerene electron acceptor, SF(DPPB)4, in which a spirobifluorene (SF) core is installed with four benzene end-capped diketopyrrolopyrrole (DPP) arms has been presented (153). The compound is shown in Figure 4.39.

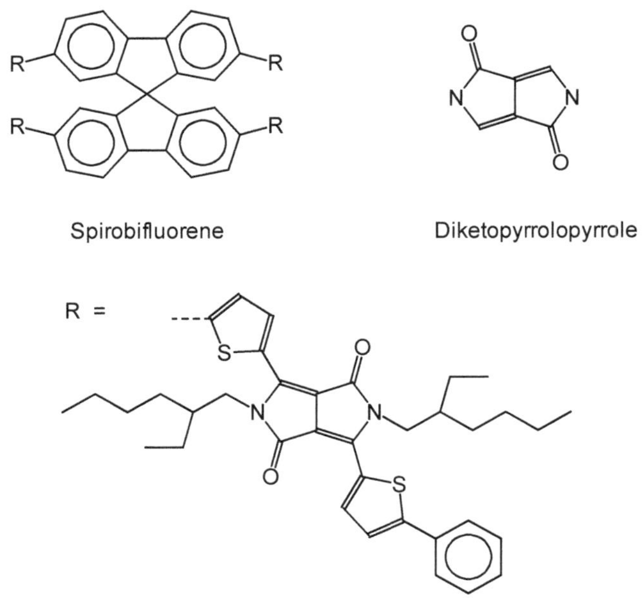

Figure 4.39 Spirobifluorene compound.

SF(DPPB)4 was synthesized via a one-step palladium-catalyzed Suzuki coupling between a tetra-boric ester functionalized spirobifluorene and four brominated benzene end-capped diketopyrrolo-pyrrole units in a good yield of 80%.

This compound exhibits energy levels that match perfectly with those of the commonly used P3HT donor in polymer solar cells. In addition, a designed cross-shaped molecular geometry helps to suppress a strong intermolecular aggregation in the P3HT:SF(DPPB)4 blend, leading to efficient nonfullerene polymer solar cells (153).

The resultant devices have a maximum PCE of 5.16% with an extremely high VOC of 1.14 V. In contrast, the devices based on P3HT:PC61BM blends provide a PCE of 3.18% with a VOC of 0.62 V. Finally, it was observed that the P3HT: SF(DPPB)4 devices exhibit significantly improved thermal stability from that of the P3HT:PC61BM devices; upon thermal treatment at 150°C for 3 h, the PCEs of P3HT: SF(DPPB)4 devices remain unchanged, whereas those of the P3HT: PC61BM devices drop drastically to below 1%. These results demonstrate that the design strategy of employing a high-performance nonfullerene acceptor, SF(DPPB)4, is promising for a practical application of polymer solar cells (153).

4.23.8 Selenophene-Containing Fused-Ring Acceptor

A nonfullerene electron acceptor with a fused five-heterocyclic ring containing selenium atoms has been developed, denoted as IDSe-T-IC. IDSe-T-IC is shown in Figure 4.40.

This compound is used for fullerene-free polymer solar cell (PSC) (154). This molecule exhibits a low bandgap of 1.52 eV, a strong absorption in the region of 600–850 nm and a high LUMO level of -3.79 eV.

When a large bandgap polymer was used as the donor, a complementary absorption of the polymer donor and the acceptor was obtained in the wavelength range of 350–850 nm. A solar cell based on J51:IDSe-T-IC gives a maximum PCE of 8.6%, with a high VOC of 0.91 V, a J_{SC} of 15.20 $mA\,cm^{-2}$ and a fill factor of 62.0%.

This performance is much higher than that of J51:PC71BM-based PSCs under similar device fabrication conditions with a PCE of 6.0%.

The trade-off features of the J_{SC} and VOC existing in PSCs with fullerene acceptors have been minimized in the fullerene-free PSCs based on IDSe-T-IC and J51.

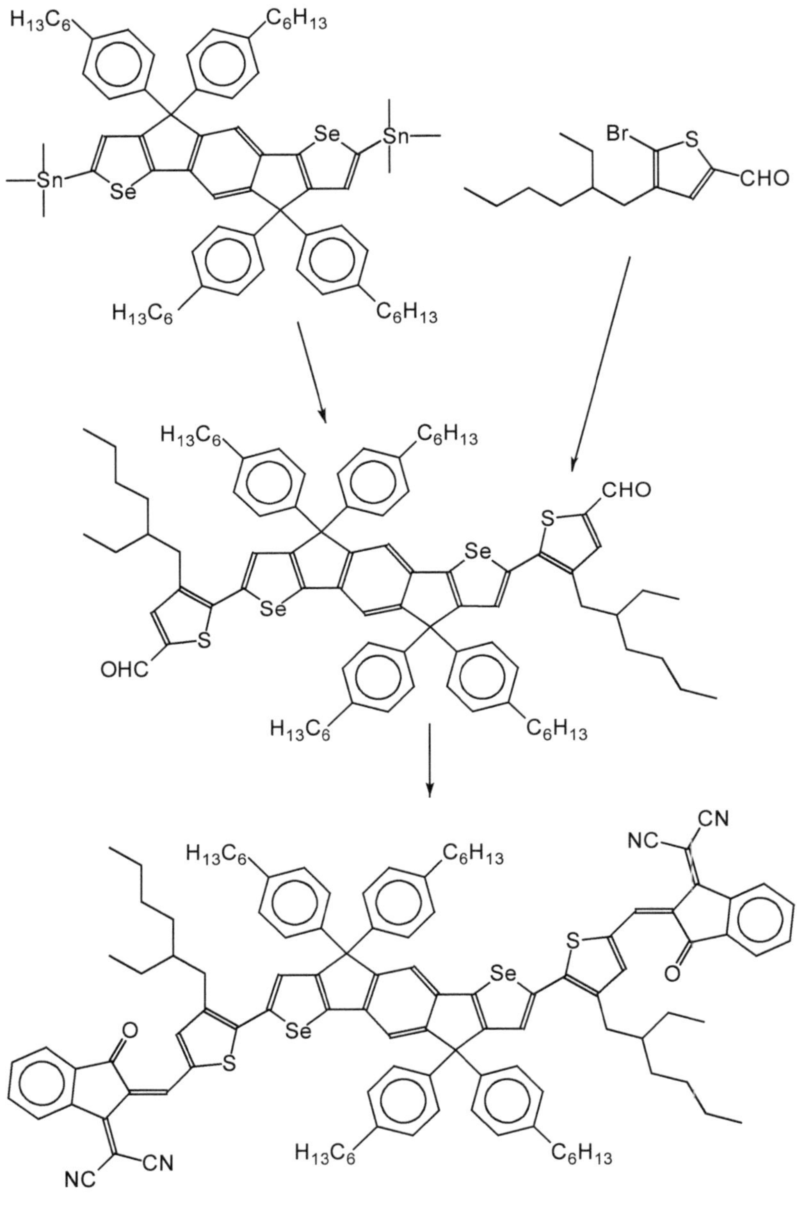

Figure 4.40 Synthesis of IDSe-T-IC (154).

These results demonstrate that a fine-tuning of the absorption and electronic energy levels of nonfullerene acceptors, and a proper selection of a polymer donor to achieve complementary absorption, is a promising way to further improve the performance of PSCs (154).

4.23.9 *Rhodanine Flanked Nonfullerene Acceptor*

A small molecule bearing 3-ethylrhodanine flanking groups was synthesized as a nonfullerene electron acceptor for a solution-processed bulk heterojunction organic photovoltaic cell (155). The compound is shown in Figure 4.41.

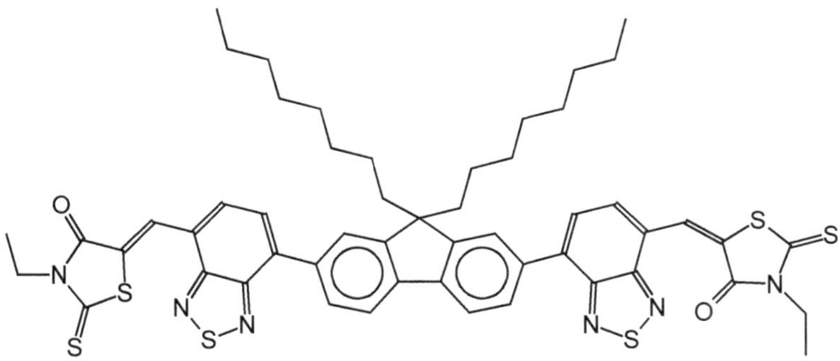

Figure 4.41 FBR.

Inverted organic photovoltaic cell devices employing P3HT as the donor polymer and FBR as the acceptor have a PCE up to 4.1%.

Optical spectroscopy investigations indicated an efficient, ultrafast charge generation and an efficient photocurrent generation from both donor and acceptor. Ultrafast transient absorption spectroscopy was used to investigate polaron generation efficiency as well as recombination dynamics. It was found that a P3HT:FBR blend is highly intermixed, leading to an increased charge generation relative to comparative devices with P3HT:PC60BM, but also faster recombination due to a nonideal morphology in which, in contrast to P3HT:PC60BM devices, the acceptor does not aggregate enough to create appropriate percolation pathways that prevent fast nongeminate recombination.

Despite this nonoptimal morphology, the P3HT:FBR devices exhibit a better performance than the P3HT:PC60BM devices (155).

4.23.10 *Indacenodithiopheno-indacenodithiophene*

A nonfullerene electron acceptor with a fused 10-heterocyclic ring, indacenodithiopheno-indacenodithiophene with a narrow bandgap of around 1.5 *eV* was synthesized (156). This molecule is shown in Figure 4.42.

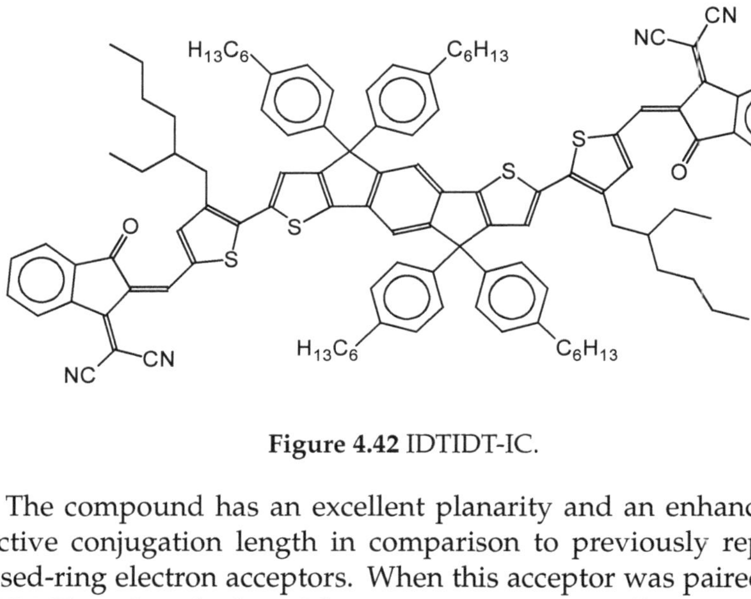

Figure 4.42 IDTIDT-IC.

The compound has an excellent planarity and an enhanced effective conjugation length in comparison to previously reported fused-ring electron acceptors. When this acceptor was paired with PTB7-Th and applied in PSCs, a power conversion efficiency of 6.5% was achieved with a high open-circuit voltage of 0.94 *V*. More significantly, an energy loss as low as 0.59 *eV* and an external quantum efficiency of as high as 63% could be simultaneously obtained (156).

Similarly, a nonfullerene electron acceptor with a backbone of a fused 10-heterocyclic ring (indacenodithiopheno-indacenodiselenophene), denoted by IDTIDSe-IC, has been developed for nonfullerene solar cells (157).

This molecule exhibits a low bandgap (E_g =1.52 *eV*), and a strong absorption in the 600–850 *nm* region. When using a large bandgap polymer J51 (E_g=1.91 *eV*) as donor, complementary absorption of the polymer donor and acceptor was obtained (157).

4.23.11 DTBTF with Thiobarbituric Acid

The synthesis of FTTB has been as described in another paper (158). A new small molecule named DTBTF with thiobarbituric acid as a terminal group was designed and synthesized as an acceptor for organic photovoltaic applications. The molecular structure is shown in Figure 4.43.

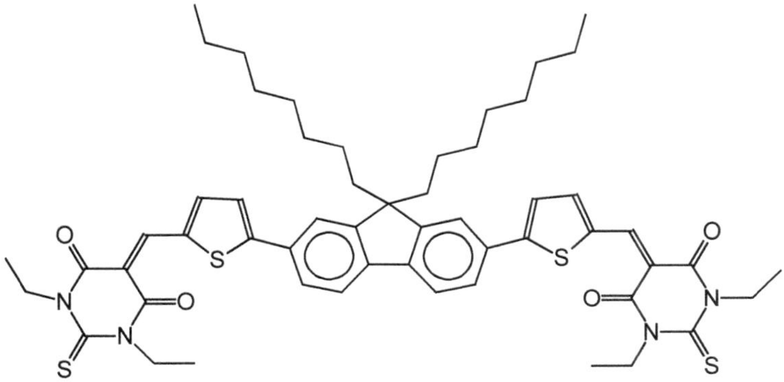

Figure 4.43 DTBTF (158).

DTBTF exhibits a strong absorption in the visible region, and a relatively high-lying LUMO-energy level of -3.62 *eV*. All-small-molecule organic solar cells based on DR3TSBDT:DTBTF blend films show a considerable PCE of 3.84% with a high VOC of 1.15 *V* (158).

4.23.12 2-Vinyl-4,5-dicyanoimidazole

A small molecule electron acceptor has been described that is based on 2-vinyl-4,5-dicyanoimidazole (Vinazene™) for use in solution-processed organic solar cells (159). The electron acceptor is shown in Figure 4.44.

This material has a favorably located LUMO level of -3.6 *eV* and absorbs strongly in the visible spectrum up to 520 *nm*. These are attractive properties in comparison to the widely used acceptor 6,6-phenyl C60 butyric acid methyl ester (PCBM). The Vinazene derivative was blended with a poly(2,7-carbazole) donor, chosen for its complementary absorption range and comparatively high-lying

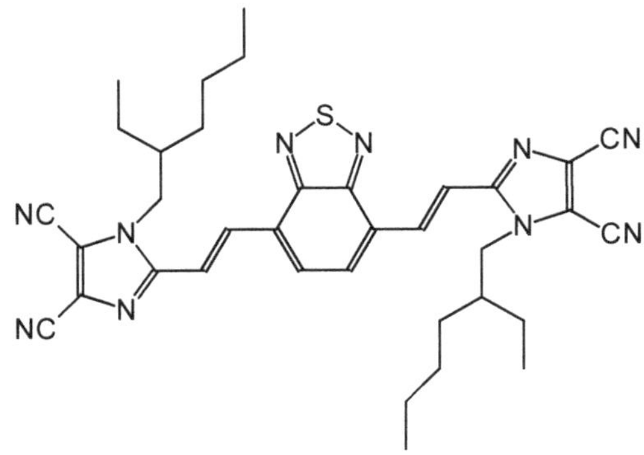

Figure 4.44 Electron acceptor based on 2-Vinyl-4,5-dicyanoimidazole.

HOMO level of -5.6 *eV* and incorporated into bulk heterojunction devices.

The influence of the donor-acceptor composition and the annealing temperature on device performance were investigated. The best performing devices exhibited power conversion efficiencies of 0.75% and open-circuit voltages of more than 1.3 *V*, which are substantially higher than former developed devices with small molecule acceptors (159).

4.23.13 *Thiophene-Based Polymers*

4.23.13.1 *Quarterly Thiophene-Containing Polymers*

The optimization of the energy levels at the donor-acceptor interface of organic solar cells has driven their efficiencies to above 10% (160). However, further improvements towards efficiencies comparable with inorganic solar cells remain challenging because of high recombination losses, which empirically limit the VOC to typically less than 1 *V*. It could be shown that this empirical limit can be overcome using nonfullerene acceptors blended with the low bandgap polymer PffBT4T-2DT, leading to efficiencies now approaching nearly 10%. A VOC of up to 1.12 *V* can be achieved, which corresponds to a loss of only VOC = 0.5 ± 0.01 *V* between the optical bandgap of the polymer and VOC. PffBT4T-2DT is poly[(5,6-difluoro-2,1,3-benzothiadiazol-4,7-diyl)-*alt*-(3,3‴-di(2-

decyltetradecyl)-2,2′;5′,2″;5″,2‴-quaterthiophen-5,5‴-diyl)]. The structure of PffBT4T-2DT is shown in Figure 4.45.

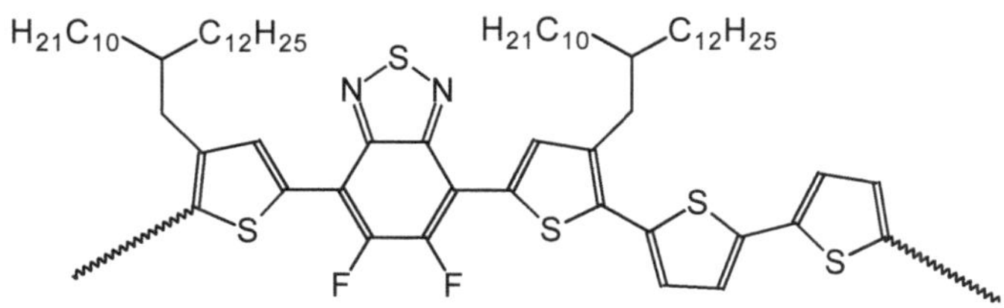

Figure 4.45 Poly[(5,6-difluoro-2,1,3-benzothiadiazol-4,7-diyl)-*alt*-(3,3‴-di-(2-decyltetradecyl)-2,2′;5′,2″;5″,2‴-quaterthiophen-5,5‴-diyl)] (PffBT4T-2DT) (160).

This high VOC could be shown to be associated with the achievement of remarkably low nongeminate and non-radiative recombination losses in these devices. The suppression of non-radiative recombination implies high external electroluminescence quantum efficiencies which are some magnitude higher than those of equivalent devices employing fullerene acceptors.

Using the balance between reduced recombination losses and good photocurrent generation efficiencies achieved experimentally as a baseline for simulations of the efficiency potential of organic solar cells, it has been estimated that efficiencies of up to 20% are achievable if bandgaps and fill factors are further optimized (160).

The PffBT4T-2DT polymer that was supplied from the He Yan group was synthesized according to procedures reported elsewhere (161). The FBR acceptor was synthesized as previously described (155).

The PTFB polymers are poly(bithiophene fluorenebenzothiadiazole)-based polymers (162). The structures of a PTFB-P polymer and a PTFB-O polymer are shown in Figure 4.46.

When the difluorinated monomer unit has two isomers with the two fluorine atoms at para or ortho positions the orientation of the thiophene rings are opposite to each other. When the isomer with two fluorine atoms are on ortho positions, the two thiophene units point to the same side where the two fluorine atoms are located. Thus, the positions of the fluorine atoms dictate the relative orientation of the thiophene units (163).

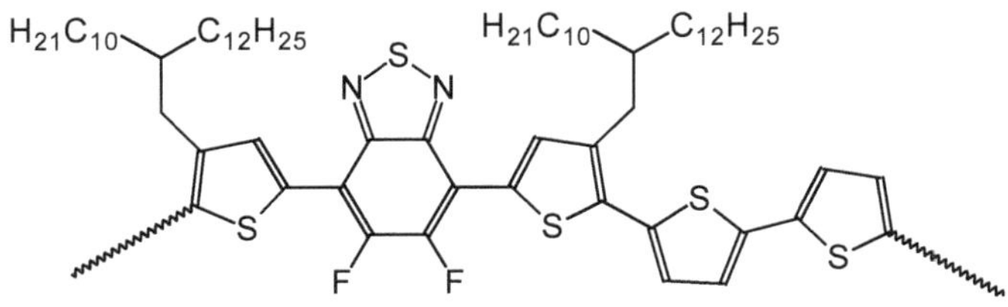

Figure 4.46 PTFB-O polymer and PTFB-P polymer (163).

This subtle difference of the fluorine position in the structures causes a dramatic difference in the performance of the respective organic solar cells. This affects the polymer crystallinity (163).

4.23.13.2 Fluorinated Poly(thiophene) Derivatives

A poly(thiophene) derivative (PBDD4T) was used as a starting polymer (164). This polymer is shown in Figure 4.47.

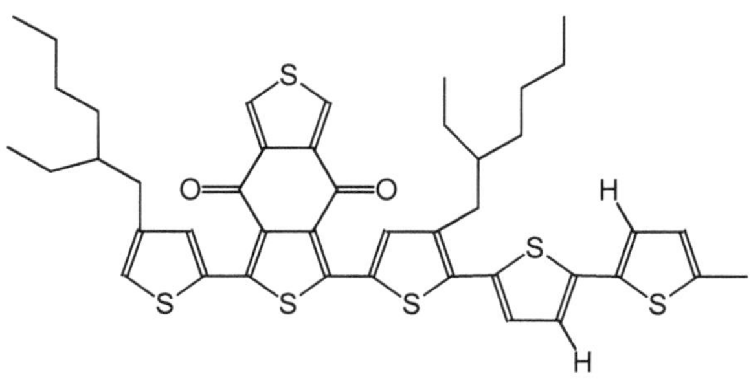

Figure 4.47 PBDD4T (164).

An attempt was made increase the rotation barrier and hence to stabilize its backbone conformation by introducing fluorine into the β- and β'-position of the linked bithiophene segments. Here, a new polymer named PBDD4T-2F was synthesized. It could be demonstrated that the rotation barrier between the α-linked bithiophene significantly increases after the fluorination, so PBDD4T-2F has a more stable backbone conformation than PBDD4T.

Compared to PBDD4T, PBDD4T-2F shows a stronger aggregation

effect in the solution state and also a more compact p-p stacking in a solid thin film and it possesses a deeper HOMO level.

These properties make PBDD4T-2F an ideal donor material in PSCs (164).

When blended with PC71BM, a fullerene acceptor, the PBDD4T-2F-based device showed a PCE of 9.04%, which is 38% higher than that of the PBDD4T-based device. When blended with ITIC, a non-fullerene acceptor, the PBDD4T-2F-based device showed a PCE of 8.69%, which is almost 20 times higher than that of the PBDD4T-based device.

A tandem cell, in which the blend of PBDD4T-2F:PC61BM was used for making the front subcell, exhibited a high PCE of 10.12%. The photovoltaic results indicate that the fluorination is an effective method to enhance interchain p-p interaction for the poly(thiophene) and hence to tune its photovoltaic properties in PSCs, especially for the fullerene-free device based on ITIC (164).

4.23.13.3 Thiophene-Thiazolothiazole-Based Solar Cells

Two wide bandgap polymers based on thiophene-thiazolothiazole (TTz) units, PBT-TTz and PBT-S-TTz, cf. Figure 4.48, have been synthesized (165).

Both polymers showed absorption onsets at 635 *nm* in solid films. Although PBT-TTz and PBT-S-TTz are wide bandgap materials with relatively narrow absorption spectra, they have a great potential for constructing high-performance PSCs.

By replacing the alkyl side chain of PBT-TTz with an alkylthiol side chain, the HOMO level of PBT-S-TTz was lowered to -5.45 *eV* (165).

A PCE of 7.92% was then obtained in a single-junction PSC device based on a PBT-S-TTz:PC71BM active layer.

Also, high-performance fullerene-free PSCs could be fabricated using these polymers and a high PCE of 8.22% was achieved.

Thus, TTz-based polymers PBT-TTz and PBT-S-TTz are promising candidates as efficient wide bandgap polymers for constructing high-performance PSC devices (165).

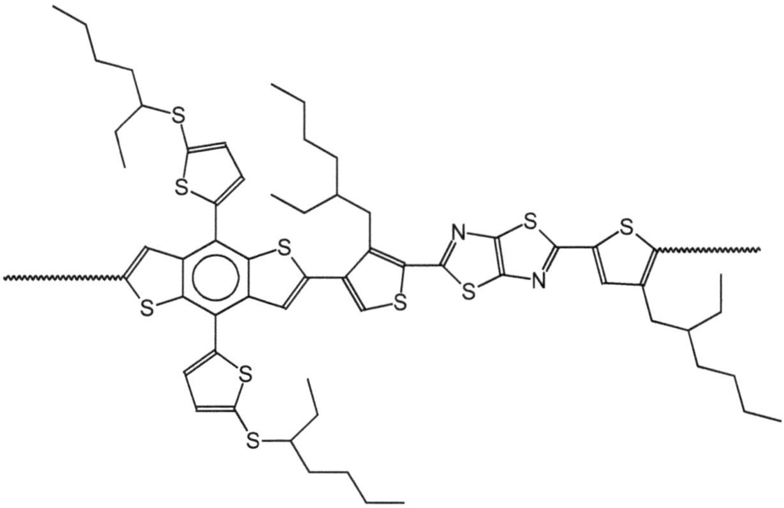

PBT-TTz

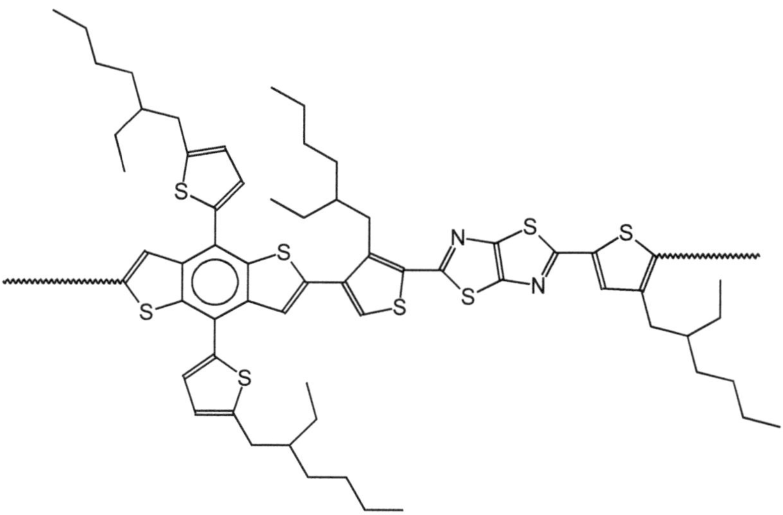

PBT-S-TTz

Figure 4.48 PBT-TTz and PBT-S-TTz (165).

4.23.13.4 Tetrafluoroquinoxaline-Based Polymers

In order to increase the PCE of nonfullerene PSCs, the absorption spectra of donor and acceptor should be complementary for efficient light harvesting (166). This polymer is shown in Figure 4.49.

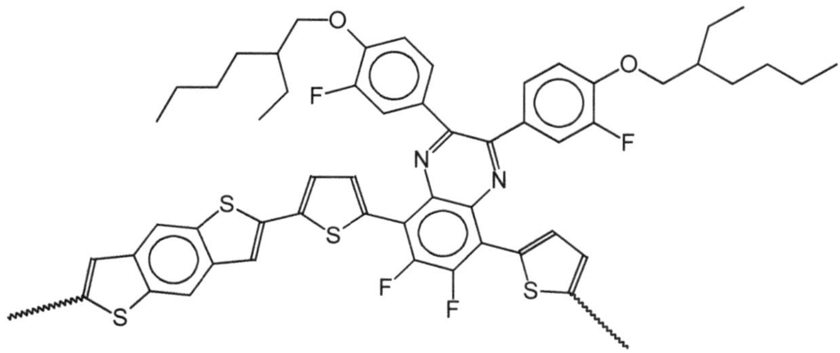

Figure 4.49 Tetrafluoroquinoxaline-based polymer (166).

Two types of medium bandgap polymers were designed and synthesized, in which two-dimension-conjugated benzodithiophene (B-DT) (BDTT and BDTPS) were used as the electron-donating units and tetrafluoroquinoxaline (ffQx) was used as electron-accepting unit, namely PffQx-T and PffQx-PS, for the application as donor in the PSCs with a popular nonfullerene small molecule ITIC as acceptor.

The optical, electrochemical and photovoltaic properties were investigated. Under AM 1.5G, 100 $mW\,cm^{-2}$, all the PSCs with the ffQx-based polymers as donor exhibited a PCE of more than 8%, i.e., 8.47% for PffQx-T and 9.12% for PffQx-PS. The PCE of 9.12% is the highest reported value for BDT-Qx fullerene-free PSCs, which is even higher than that of fullerene-based devices (166).

References

1. P. Würfel and U. Würfel, *Physics of Solar Cells: From Basic Principles to Advanced Concepts*, Wiley-VCH, Weinheim, 2nd edition, 2009.
2. J.G. Conibeer and A. Willoughby, eds., *Solar Cell Materials: Developing Tecnologies*, Wiley Series in Materials for Electronic & Optoelectronic

Applications), isbn = 9781118695814,, Wiley, Chichester, West Sussex, United Kingdom, 2014.
3. M.P. Paranthaman, W. Wong-Ng, and R.N. Bhattacharya, eds., *Semiconductor Materials for Solar Photovoltaic Cells*, Vol. 218 of Springer Series in Material Science, Springer, Cham, 2015.
4. W.C.H. Choy, ed., *Organic Solar Cells: Materials and Device Physics*, Springer, London New York, 2013.
5. Q. Qiao, ed., *Organic Solar Cells: Materials, Devices, Interfaces, and Modeling*, Vol. 38, CRC Press, Florida, USA, 2015.
6. L. Schmidt-Mende and J. Weickert, *Organic and Hybrid Solar Cells: An Introduction*, De Gruyter, Berlin Boston, 2016.
7. M. Boxwell, *The Solar Electricity Handbook - 2016 Edition: A simple, practical guide to solar energy: how to design and install photovoltaic solar electric systems*, Greenstream Publishing, 2016.
8. N.-G. Park, M. Grätzel, and T. Miyasaka, eds., *Organic-Inorganic Halide Perovskite Photovoltaics. From Fundamentals to Device Architectures*, Springer International Publishing, Switzerland, 2016.
9. J. Luo, M.T. Mayer, M. Grätzel, and N.-G. Park, Perovskite solar cells for the generation of fuels from sunlight in M. Grätzel and T. Miyasaka, eds., *Organic-Inorganic Halide Perovskite Photovoltaics: From Fundamentals to Device Architectures*, pp. 285–305. Springer International Publishing, Cham, 2016.
10. M. Helgesen, R. Sondergaard, and F.C. Krebs, *Journal of Materials Chemistry*, Vol. 20, p. 36, 2010.
11. A. Baker, A history of solar cells: How technology has evolved, electronic: https://www.solarpowerauthority.com/a-history-of-solar-cells/, 2016.
12. Wikipedia, Edmond Becquerel — wikipedia, the free encyclopedia, 2017. [Online; accessed 25-July-2017].
13. A.E. Becquerel, *Comptes Rendus*, Vol. 9, p. 561, 1839.
14. W. Smith, *Journal of the Society of Telegraph Engineers*, Vol. 2, p. 31, 1873.
15. W.G. Adams and R.E. Day, *Proceedings of the Royal Society of London*, Vol. 25, p. 113, 1876.
16. J.H. Heo, S.H. Im, J.H. Noh, T.N. Mandal, C.-S. Lim, J.A. Chang, Y.H. Lee, H.-j. Kim, A. Sarkar, M.K. Nazeeruddin, et al., *Nature Photonics*, Vol. 7, p. 486, 2013.
17. O. Malinkiewicz, A. Yella, Y.H. Lee, G.M. Espallargas, M. Graetzel, M.K. Nazeeruddin, and H.J. Bolink, *Nature Photonics*, Vol. 8, p. 128, 2014.
18. N.J. Jeon, J.H. Noh, Y.C. Kim, W.S. Yang, S. Ryu, and S.I. Seok, *Nature Materials*, Vol. 13, p. 897, September 2014.
19. F. Hao, C.C. Stoumpos, D.H. Cao, R.P.H. Chang, and M.G. Kanatzidis, *Nature Photonics*, Vol. 8, p. 489, 2014.

20. M. Kaltenbrunner, N.S. Sariciftci, and S. Bauer, Solar & alternative energy ultrathin, air-stable perovskite solar cells for powering unmanned aircraft, in *Solar & Alternative Energy*, San Diego, California, 2016. SPIE Optics + Photonics.
21. F.D. Sisler, Biochemical fuel cell, US Patent 3 477 879, November 11, 1969.
22. T.A. Beck, Solar powered biological fuel cell, US Patent 4 117 202, September 26, 1978.
23. S. Günes, H. Neugebauer, and N.S. Sariciftci, *Chemical Reviews*, Vol. 107, p. 1324, 2007.
24. T.B. Singh and N.S. Sariciftci, *Annual Review of Materials Research*, Vol. 36, p. 199, 2006.
25. Y.-H. So, P. Garrou, J.-H. Im, and D.M. Scheck, *Chemical Innovation*, Vol. 31, p. 40, 2001.
26. Wikipedia, Pullulan — wikipedia, the free encyclopedia, 2016. [Online; accessed 21-August-2017].
27. Y. Onda, H. Muto, and H. Suzuki, Cyanoethylpullulan, US Patent 4 322 524, assigned to Shin-Etsu Chemical Co. Ltd. (Tokyo, JP), March 30, 1982.
28. I. Fukui, K. Hayakawa, S. Tanioka, M. Ohgata, and M. Kajitani, Method for producing 2-cyanoethyl group-containing organic compound, US Patent 8 729 185, assigned to Shin-Etsu Chemical Co., Ltd. (JP) Matsugaki Chemical Industries Co., Ltd. (JP), May 20, 2014.
29. H.-H. Liao, L.-M. Chen, Z. Xu, G. Li, and Y. Yang, *Applied Physics Letters*, Vol. 92, p. 156, 2008.
30. M. Bajpai, R. Srivastava, and R. Dhar, Effect of plasmonic enhancement of light absorption on the efficiency of polymer solar cell in V.K. Jain, S. Rattan, and A. Verma, eds., *Recent Trends in Materials and Devices: Proceedings ICRTMD 2015*, pp. 315–317. Springer International Publishing, Cham, 2017.
31. Wikipedia, Poly-3,4-ethylendioxythiophen — wikipedia, die freie enzyklopädie, 2017. [Online; accessed Aug. 62017].
32. A. Tada, Y. Geng, Q. Wei, K. Hashimoto, and K. Tajima, *Nature Materials*, Vol. 10, p. 450, 2011.
33. W. Xu, F. Tan, X. Liu, W. Zhang, S. Qu, Z. Wang, and Z. Wang, *Nanoscale Research Letters*, Vol. 12, p. 11, 2017.
34. W.Y. Lynn Ko, H.G. Bagaria, S. Asokan, K.-J. Lin, and M.S. Wong, *Journal of Materials Chemistry*, Vol. 20, p. 2474, 2010.
35. C.-C. Chen, W.-H. Chang, K. Yoshimura, K. Ohya, J. You, J. Gao, Z. Hong, and Y. Yang, *Advanced Materials*, Vol. 26, p. 5670, 2014.
36. H. Tan, A. Furlan, W. Li, K. Arapov, R. Santbergen, M.M. Wienk, M. Zeman, A.H.M. Smets, and R.A.J. Janssen, *Advanced Materials*, Vol. 28, p. 2170, 2016.

37. C. Duan, A. Furlan, J.J. van Franeker, R.E.M. Willems, M.M. Wienk, and R.A.J. Janssen, *Advanced Materials*, Vol. 27, p. 4461, 2015.
38. Y. Cai, L. Huo, and Y. Sun, *Advanced Materials*, Vol. 29, p. 1605437, 2017.
39. J. You, L. Dou, K. Yoshimura, T. Kato, K. Ohya, T. Moriarty, K. Emery, C.-C. Chen, J. Gao, G. Li, et al., *Nature Communications*, Vol. 4, p. 1446, 2013.
40. G. Li, C.-W. Chu, V. Shrotriya, J. Huang, and Y. Yang, *Applied Physics Letters*, Vol. 88, p. 253503, 2006.
41. M.S. White, D.C. Olson, S.E. Shaheen, N. Kopidakis, and D.S. Ginley, *Applied Physics Letters*, Vol. 89, p. 143517, 2006.
42. S.K. Hau, H.-L. Yip, N.S. Baek, J. Zou, K. O'Malley, and A.K.-Y. Jen, *Applied Physics Letters*, Vol. 92, p. 253301, 2008.
43. M.-H. Park, J.-H. Li, A. Kumar, G. Li, and Y. Yang, *Advanced Functional Materials*, Vol. 19, p. 1241, 2009.
44. Y. Sun, J.H. Seo, C.J. Takacs, J. Seifter, and A.J. Heeger, *Advanced Materials*, Vol. 23, p. 1679, 2011.
45. H. Zhou, L. Yang, A.C. Stuart, S.C. Price, S. Liu, and W. You, *Angewandte Chemie*, Vol. 123, p. 3051, 2011.
46. Y. He, H.-Y. Chen, J. Hou, and Y. Li, *Journal of the American Chemical Society*, Vol. 132, p. 1377, 2010.
47. N.J. Jeon, H.G. Lee, Y.C. Kim, J. Seo, J.H. Noh, J. Lee, and S.I. Seok, *Journal of the American Chemical Society*, Vol. 136, p. 7837, 2014.
48. N.J. Jeon, J. Lee, J.H. Noh, M.K. Nazeeruddin, M. Grätzel, and S.I. Seok, *Journal of the American Chemical Society*, Vol. 135, p. 19087, 2013.
49. Z. Yin, J. Wei, and Q. Zheng, *Advanced Science*, Vol. 3, p. 1500362, 2016.
50. Y. Liang, Z. Xu, J. Xia, S.-T. Tsai, Y. Wu, G. Li, C. Ray, and L. Yu, *Advanced Materials*, Vol. 22, p. E135, 2010.
51. S.-H. Liao, H.-J. Jhuo, Y.-S. Cheng, and S.-A. Chen, *Advanced Materials*, Vol. 25, p. 4766, 2013.
52. A. Dantas, R. Consani, J. Sardi, M. Mesquita, M. da Silva, and M. Sinhoreti, *Journal of Research and Practice in Dentistry*, pp. 1–9, February 2014.
53. X. Che, X. Xiao, J.D. Zimmerman, D. Fan, and S.R. Forrest, *Advanced Energy Materials*, Vol. 4, p. 1400568, 2014.
54. H. Zhou, Y. Zhang, C.-K. Mai, S.D. Collins, G.C. Bazan, T.-Q. Nguyen, and A.J. Heeger, *Advanced Materials*, Vol. 27, p. 1767, 2015.
55. F.C. Krebs and H. Spanggaard, *Chemistry of Materials*, Vol. 17, p. 5235, 2005.

56. F.C. Krebs, Design and applications of polymer solar cells with lifetimes longer than 10000 hours, in Z.H. Kafafi and P.A. Lane, eds., *Organic Photovoltaics Proc. SPIE*, Vol. 5938, pp. 59380Y–59380Y–11, San Diego, California, 2005.
57. M.A. Green, Y. Hishikawa, W. Warta, E.D. Dunlop, D.H. Levi, J. Hohl-Ebinger, and A.W. Ho-Baillie, *Progress in Photovoltaics: Research and Applications*, Vol. 25, p. 668, 2017.
58. K. Yoshikawa, H. Kawasaki, W. Yoshida, T. Irie, K. Konishi, K. Nakano, T. Uto, D. Adachi, M. Kanematsu, H. Uzu, and K. Yamamoto, *Nature Energy*, Vol. 2, p. 17032, March 2017.
59. J. Benick, A. Richter, R. Müller, H. Hauser, F. Feldmann, P. Krenckel, S. Riepe, F. Schindler, M.C. Schubert, M. Hermle, A.W. Bett, and S.W. Glunz, *IEEE Journal of Photovoltaics*, Vol. PP, p. 1, 2017.
60. M. Moslehi, P. Kapur, J. Kramer, V. Rana, S. Seutter, A. Deshpande, T. Stalcup, S. Kommera, J. Ashjaee, A. Calcaterra, et al., World-record 20.6% efficiency 156 mm x 156 mm full-square solar cells using low-cost kerfless ultrathin epitaxial silicon & porous silicon lift-off technology for industry-leading high-performance smart PV modules, in *PV Asia Pacific Conference (APVIA/PVAP)*, Vol. 24, 2012.
61. M.J. Keevers, T.L. Young, U. Schubert, and M.A. Green, 10% efficient CSG minimodules, in *22nd European Photovoltaic Solar Energy Conference*, pp. 1783–1790, 2007.
62. B.M. Kayes, H. Nie, R. Twist, S.G. Spruytte, F. Reinhardt, I.C. Kizilyalli, and G.S. Higashi, 27.6% conversion efficiency, a new record for single-junction solar cells under 1 sun illumination, in *2011 37th IEEE Photovoltaic Specialists Conference*, pp. 000004–000008, June 2011.
63. R. Venkatasubramanian, B.C. O'Quinn, J.S. Hills, P.R. Sharps, M.L. Timmons, J.A. Hutchby, H. Field, R. Ahrenkiel, and B. Keyes, 18.2% (am1.5) efficient GaAs solar cell on optical-grade polycrystalline Ge substrate, in *Conference Record of the Twenty Fifth IEEE Photovoltaic Specialists Conference - 1996*, pp. 31–36, May 1996.
64. M. Wanlass, Systems and methods for advanced ultra-high-performance InP solar cells, US Patent 9 590 131, assigned to Alliance for Sustainable Energy, LLC (Golden, CO), March 7, 2017.
65. K. Sun, C. Yan, F. Liu, J. Huang, F. Zhou, J.A. Stride, M. Green, and X. Hao, *Advanced Energy Materials*, Vol. 6, p. 1600046, 2016.
66. H. Sai, K. Maejima, T. Matsui, T. Koida, K. Matsubara, M. Kondo, Y. Takeuchi, S. Sugiyama, H. Katayama, and I. Yoshida, *IEEE Journal of Photovoltaics*, Vol. 5, p. 1528, November 2015.
67. W.S. Yang, J.H. Noh, N.J. Jeon, Y.C. Kim, S. Ryu, J. Seo, and S.I. Seok, *Science*, Vol. 348, p. 1234, 2015.
68. R. Komiya, A. Fukui, N. Murofushi, N. Koide, R. Yamanaka, and H. Katayama, Improvement of the conversion efficiency of a monolithic type dye-sensitized solar cell module, in *Technical Digest, 21st*

International Photovoltaic Science and Engineering Conference, pp. 2C–5O, 2011.
69. S. Mori, H. Oh-oka, H. Nakao, T. Gotanda, Y. Nakano, H. Jung, A. Iida, R. Hayase, N. Shida, and M. Saito, *MRS Proceedings*, Vol. 1737, 2015.
70. A. Slade and V. Garboushian, 27.6% efficient silicon concentrator solar cells for mass production, in *Technical Digest, 15th International Photovoltaic Science and Engineering Conference, Beijing*, 2005.
71. J. Ward, K. Ramanathan, F. Hasoon, T.J. Coutts, J. Keane, M. Contreras, T. Moriarty, and R. Noufi, *Progress in Photovoltaics: Research and Applications*, Vol. 10, p. 41, 2002.
72. F. Dimroth, New world record for solar cell efficiency at 46% - French-German cooperation confirms competitive advantage of european photovoltaic industry, electronic: https://www.ise.fraunhofer.de/en/press-media/press-releases/2014/new-world-record-for-solar-cell-efficiency-at-46-percent.html, 2014.
73. Sharp, Sharp develops concentrator solar cell with world's highest conversion efficiency of 43.5% achieved with concentrator triple-junction compound solar cell, electronic: http://www.sharp-world.com/corporate/news/120531.html, 2012.
74. J. Ohlmann, D. Lackner, J.F. Sanchez, M. Zedda, A. Wekkeli, M. Steiner, A. Fallisch, and F. Dimroth, 35.1% efficient GaInP/GaInAs dual-junction solar cells optimized for direct hydrogen generation, in *44th IEEE Photovoltaic Specialists Conference*, Washington, DC, 2017.
75. M. Steiner, G. Siefer, T. Schmidt, M. Wiesenfarth, F. Dimroth, and A.W. Bett, *IEEE Journal of Photovoltaics*, Vol. 6, p. 1020, July 2016.
76. M.A. Green, M.J. Keevers, I. Thomas, J.B. Lasich, K. Emery, and R.R. King, *Progress in Photovoltaics: Research and Applications*, Vol. 23, p. 685, 2015.
77. S. Inaba and V. Vohra, *Materials*, Vol. 10, 2017.
78. F. Padinger, R.S. Rittberger, and N.S. Sariciftci, *Advanced Functional Materials*, Vol. 13, p. 85, 2003.
79. G. Zhao, Y. He, and Y. Li, *Advanced Materials*, Vol. 22, p. 4355, 2010.
80. B. Gao, *High Performance Polymers*, Vol. 26, p. 197, 2014.
81. V. Vohra, K. Higashimine, S. Tsuzaki, K. Ohdaira, and H. Murata, *Thin Solid Films*, Vol. 554, p. 41, 2014. 10th International Conference on Nano-Molecular Electronics (ICNME2012).
82. S. van Bavel, E. Sourty, G. de With, K. Frolic, and J. Loos, *Macromolecules*, Vol. 42, p. 7396, 2009.
83. S. Sun and N. Sariciftci, eds., *Organic Photovoltaics: Mechanisms, Materials and Devices*, CRC Press, Florida, USA, 2005.
84. F.C. Krebs, ed., *Polymer Photovoltaics: A Practical Approach*, SPIE Press, Bellingham, 2008.

85. C.J. Brabec, U. Scherf, and V. Dyakonov, eds., *Organic Photovoltaics: Materials, Device Physics and Manufacturing Technologies*, Wiley-VCH, Weinheim, 2008.
86. C.J. Brabec, V. Dyakonov, J. Parisi, and N.S. Sariciftci, eds., *Organic Photovoltaics: Concepts and Realization*, Vol. 60 of Springer Series in Material Science, Springer Science & Business Media, New York, 2013.
87. F.C. Krebs, *Solar Energy Materials and Solar Cells*, Vol. 93, p. 394, 2009.
88. W.C. Park, J.H. Yeo, and Y.H. Im, Slot die coating apparatus, US Patent 9 682 395, assigned to LG CHEM, LTD. (Seoul, KR), June 20, 2017.
89. D.I. Kutsarov, E. New, F. Bausi, A. Zoladek-Lemanczyk, F.A. Castro, and S.R.P. Silva, *Solar Energy Materials and Solar Cells*, Vol. 161, p. 388, 2017.
90. D.I. Kutsarov, E. New, F. Bausi, A. Zoladek-Lemanczyk, F.A. Castro, and S.R.P. Silva, *Data in Brief*, Vol. 11, p. 44, 2017.
91. F.C. Krebs, *Solar Energy Materials and Solar Cells*, Vol. 93, p. 465, 2009.
92. F.C. Krebs, T. Tromholt, and M. Jørgensen, *Nanoscale*, Vol. 2, p. 873, 2010.
93. W. Shen, J. Tang, Y. Wang, J. Liu, L. Huang, W. Chen, L. Yang, W. Wang, Y. Wang, R. Yang, J. Yun, and L.A. Belfiore, *ACS Applied Materials & Interfaces*, Vol. 9, p. 5358, 2017.
94. H. Cong, D. Han, B. Sun, D. Zhou, C. Wang, P. Liu, and L. Feng, *ACS Applied Materials & Interfaces*, Vol. 9, p. 18087, 2017.
95. L. Zhang, Z.C. Ding, T. Tong, and J. Liu, *Nanoscale*, Vol. 9, p. 3524, 2017.
96. O. Bäcke, C. Lindqvist, A.D. de Zerio Mendaza, S. Gustafsson, E. Wang, M.R. Andersson, C. Müller, P.M. Kristiansen, and E. Olsson, *Ultramicroscopy*, Vol. 176, p. 23 , 2017. 70th Birthday of Robert Sinclair and 65th Birthday of Nestor J. Zaluzec PICO 2017 – Fourth Conference on Frontiers of Aberration Corrected Electron Microscopy.
97. A.M.S. Salem, S.M. El-Sheikh, F.A. Harraz, S. Ebrahim, M. Soliman, H.S. Hafez, I.A. Ibrahim, and M.S.A. Abdel-Mottaleb, *Applied Surface Science*, Vol. 425, p. 156, 2017.
98. W. Li, X. Zhang, X. Zhang, J. Yao, and C. Zhan, *ACS Applied Materials & Interfaces*, Vol. 9, p. 1446, 2017.
99. X. Gong, S. Feng, G. Li, R. Hou, Y. Liu, Z. Zhang, C. Li, and Z. Bo, *Dyes and Pigments*, Vol. 141, p. 342, 2017.
100. Y.-F. Zhao, W.-J. Zou, H. Li, K. Lu, W. Yan, and Z.-X. Wei, *Chinese Journal of Polymer Science*, Vol. 35, p. 261, February 2017.
101. E. von Hauff, E. da Como, and S. Ludwigs, Optoelectronic properties of PCPDTBT for photovoltaics: Morphology control and molecular doping in K. Leo, ed., *Elementary Processes in Organic Photovoltaics*, pp. 109–138. Springer International Publishing, Cham, 2017.

102. D. Mühlbacher, M. Scharber, M. Morana, Z. Zhu, D. Waller, R. Gaudiana, and C. Brabec, *Advanced Materials*, Vol. 18, p. 2884, 2006.
103. X. Wang, H.-J. Egelhaaf, H.-G. Mack, H. Azimi, C.J. Brabec, A.J. Meixner, and D. Zhang, *Advanced Energy Materials*, Vol. 4, p. 1400497, 2014. 1400497.
104. G.L. Schulz, F.S.U. Fischer, D. Trefz, A. Melnyk, A. Hamidi-Sakr, M. Brinkmann, D. Andrienko, and S. Ludwigs, *Macromolecules*, Vol. 50, p. 1402, 2017.
105. A. Tournebize, M. Seck, A. Vincze, A. Distler, H.-J. Egelhaaf, C.J. Brabec, A. Rivaton, H. Peisert, and T. Chassé, *Solar Energy Materials and Solar Cells*, Vol. 155, p. 323, 2016.
106. M. Pope, M. Waldrip, T. Ferron, and B. Collins, Using resonant X-ray scattering to determine how structure controls the charge generation process in PCPDTBT:PC70BM solar cells, in C. Wang, ed., *APS March Meeting 2017*, Vol. 62, New Orleans, Louisiana, 2017. APS.
107. L.-B. Lin, G.C. Cardoso, A.E. Preske, and K. Balantrapu, Photovoltaic device, US Patent 8 975 511, assigned to Xerox Corporation (Norwalk, CT), March 10, 2015.
108. T. Pratyusha, G. Sivakumar, A. Yella, and D. Gupta, *Materials Today: Proceedings*, Vol. 4, p. 5067, 2017. 9th International Symposium on Flexible Organic Electronics (ISFOE16), July (4-7) 2016, Thessaloniki, Greece.
109. G. Sivakumar, T. Pratyusha, W. Shen, and D. Gupta, *Materials Today: Proceedings*, Vol. 4, p. 5060 , 2017. 9th International Symposium on Flexible Organic Electronics (ISFOE16), July (4-7) 2016, Thessaloniki, Greece.
110. W. Kubo, *Physica Status Solidi A*, p. 1700110, 2017.
111. X. Du, X. Jiao, S. Rechberger, J.D. Perea, M. Meyer, N. Kazerouni, E. Spiecker, H. Ade, C.J. Brabec, R.H. Fink, and T. Ameri, *Macromolecules*, Vol. 50, p. 2415, 2017.
112. Z. Ahmad, F. Touati, F.F. Muhammad, M.A. Najeeb, and R.A. Shakoor, *Applied Physics A*, Vol. 123, p. 486, June 2017.
113. N. Pavithra, D. Velayutham, A. Sorrentino, and S. Anandan, *Synthetic Metals*, Vol. 226, p. 62, 2017.
114. N. Pavithra, D. Velayutham, A. Sorrentino, and S. Anandan, *Journal of Power Sources*, Vol. 353, p. 245, 2017.
115. K. Mohan, S. Dolui, B.C. Nath, A. Bora, S. Sharma, and S.K. Dolui, *Electrochimica Acta*, Vol. 247, p. 216, 2017.
116. N.K. Farhana, M.H. Khanmirzaei, S. Ramesh, and K. Ramesh, *Journal of Applied Polymer Science*, Vol. 134, p. 45091, 2017.
117. N.K. Farhana, M.H. Khanmirzaei, F.S. Omar, S. Ramesh, and K. Ramesh, *Ionics*, Vol. 23, p. 1601, June 2017.
118. N. Tarannum and M.M. Varishetty, *Polymers for Advanced Technologies*, 2017.

119. T.M.W.J. Bandara, H.D.N.S. Fernando, M. Furlani, I. Albinsson, M.A.K.L. Dissanayake, J.L. Ratnasekera, and B.-E. Mellander, *Journal of Solid State Electrochemistry*, Vol. 21, p. 1571, June 2017.
120. X. Liu, Y. Liang, G. Yue, Y. Tu, and H. Zheng, *Solar Energy*, Vol. 148, p. 63, 2017.
121. S.R. Nadia, M.H. Khanmirzaei, S. Ramesh, and K. Ramesh, *Ionics*, Vol. 23, p. 1585, June 2017.
122. S.N.F. Yusuf, A.D. Azzahari, R. Yahya, S.R. Majid, M.A. Careem, and A.K. Arof, *RSC Advances*, Vol. 6, p. 27714, 2016.
123. B. Sharma, A. Singh, M.A. Afroz, P.K. Iyer, and J. Jacob, *Synthetic Metals*, Vol. 226, p. 56, 2017.
124. I. Jeon and Y. Matsuo, Polymer-fullerene solar cells in *Encyclopedia of Polymer Science and Technology*. John Wiley & Sons, Inc., 2002.
125. B.C. Thompson and J.M.J. Fréchet, *Angewandte Chemie International Edition*, Vol. 47, p. 58, 2008.
126. F.B. Kooistra, V.D. Mihailetchi, L.M. Popescu, D. Kronholm, P.W.M. Blom, and J.C. Hummelen, *Chemistry of Materials*, Vol. 18, p. 3068, 2006.
127. M.N. Siddiqui, M. Mansha, U. Mehmood, N. Ullah, A.F. Al-Betar, and A.A. Al-Saadi, *Dyes and Pigments*, Vol. 141, p. 406, 2017.
128. C. Kramer, ed., *Fullerene Research Advances*, Nova Science Publishers, New York, 2007.
129. F. Langa and J.-F. Nierengarten, eds., *Fullerenes: Principles and Applications*, Royal Society of Chemistry, Cambridge, 2007.
130. J.M. McConnachie and E.I. Stiefel, Fullerene compositions and preparation, US Patent 5 372 798, assigned to Exxon Research and Engineering Company (Florham Park, NJ), December 13, 1994.
131. H.W. Kroto, J.R. Heath, S.C. O'Brien, R.F. Curl, and R.E. Smalley, *Nature*, Vol. 318, p. 162, 1985.
132. G. Peters and M. Jansen, *Angewandte Chemie International Edition in English*, Vol. 31, p. 223, 1992.
133. R. Taylor and G.L. Burley, Production. isolation and purification of fullerenes in F. Langa and J.-F. Nierengarten, eds., *Fullerenes: Principles and Applications*, chapter 1, pp. 1–14. Royal Society of Chemistry, Cambridge, 2007.
134. W. Krätschmer, L.D. Lamb, K. Fostiropoulos, and D.R. Huffman, *Nature*, Vol. 347, p. 354, 1990.
135. F. Langa and P. de la Cruz, Basic principles of the chemical reactivity of fullerenes in F. Langa and J.-F. Nierengarten, eds., *Fullerenes: Principles and Applications*, chapter 2, pp. 16–50. Royal Society of Chemistry, Cambridge, 2007.
136. C. Bingel, *Chemische Berichte*, Vol. 126, p. 1957, 1993.
137. Wikipedia, Bingel reaction — wikipedia, the free encyclopedia, 2017. [Online; accessed 25-July-2017].

138. M.G. Faraj and P. Taboada, *Journal of Inorganic and Organometallic Polymers and Materials*, June 2017.
139. H. Yoda, Polymer and solar cell encapsulant using the polymer, US Patent 9 570 641, assigned to Sumitomo Chemical Company, Limited (Tokyo, JP), February 14, 2017.
140. J. Chen, Y. Shen, B. Chen, K. Ge, J. Guo, Z. Wang, F. Li, Y. Xu, and Y. Mai, *Solar RRL*, Vol. 1, p. 1700079, 2017.
141. W. Zhao, D. Qian, S. Zhang, S. Li, O. Inganäs, F. Gao, and J. Hou, *Advanced Materials*, Vol. 28, p. 4734, 2016.
142. A. Facchetti, *Materials Today*, Vol. 16, p. 123, 2013.
143. Y. Lin and X. Zhan, *Materials Horizons*, Vol. 1, p. 470, 2014.
144. J.-D. Chen, C. Cui, Y.-Q. Li, L. Zhou, Q.-D. Ou, C. Li, Y. Li, and J.-X. Tang, *Advanced Materials*, Vol. 27, p. 1035, 2015.
145. W. Zhao, L. Ye, S. Zhang, M. Sun, and J. Hou, *Journal of Materials Chemistry A*, Vol. 3, p. 12723, 2015.
146. W. Chen and Q. Zhang, *Journal of Materials Chemistry C*, Vol. 5, p. 1275, 2017.
147. S. Holliday, R.S. Ashraf, A. Wadsworth, D. Baran, S.A. Yousaf, C.B. Nielsen, C.-H. Tan, S.D. Dimitrov, Z. Shang, N. Gasparini, M. Alamoudi, F. Laquai, C.J. Brabec, A. Salleo, J.R. Durrant, and I. McCulloch, *Nature Communications*, Vol. 7, p. 11585, 2016.
148. Y. Qin, M.A. Uddin, Y. Chen, B. Jang, K. Zhao, Z. Zheng, R. Yu, T.J. Shin, H.Y. Woo, and J. Hou, *Advanced Materials*, Vol. 28, p. 9416, 2016.
149. H. Zhang, S. Li, B. Xu, H. Yao, B. Yang, and J. Hou, *Journal of Materials Chemistry A*, Vol. 4, p. 18043, 2016.
150. H. Bin, L. Gao, Z.-G. Zhang, Y. Yang, Y. Zhang, C. Zhang, S. Chen, L. Xue, C. Yang, M. Xiao, and Y. Li, *Nature Communications*, Vol. 7, p. 13651, December 2016.
151. Y.-J. Hwang, H. Li, B.A.E. Courtright, S. Subramaniyan, and S.A. Jenekhe, *Advanced Materials*, Vol. 28, p. 124, 2016.
152. H. Yao, R. Yu, T.J. Shin, H. Zhang, S. Zhang, B. Jang, M.A. Uddin, H.Y. Woo, and J. Hou, *Advanced Energy Materials*, Vol. 6, p. 1600742, 2016.
153. S. Li, W. Liu, M. Shi, J. Mai, T.-K. Lau, J. Wan, X. Lu, C.-Z. Li, and H. Chen, *Energy & Environmental Science*, Vol. 9, p. 604, 2016.
154. Y. Li, L. Zhong, F.-P. Wu, Y. Yuan, H.-J. Bin, Z.-Q. Jiang, Z. Zhang, Z.-G. Zhang, Y. Li, and L.-S. Liao, *Energy & Environmental Science*, Vol. 9, p. 3429, 2016.
155. S. Holliday, R.S. Ashraf, C.B. Nielsen, M. Kirkus, J.A. Röhr, C.-H. Tan, E. Collado-Fregoso, A.-C. Knall, J.R. Durrant, J. Nelson, and I. McCulloch, *Journal of the American Chemical Society*, Vol. 137, p. 898, 2015.

156. Y. Li, X. Liu, F.-P. Wu, Y. Zhou, Z.-Q. Jiang, B. Song, Y. Xia, Z.-G. Zhang, F. Gao, O. Inganas, Y. Li, and L.-S. Liao, *Journal of Materials Chemistry A*, Vol. 4, p. 5890, 2016.
157. Y. Li, D. Qian, L. Zhong, J.-D. Lin, Z.-Q. Jiang, Z.-G. Zhang, Z. Zhang, Y. Li, L.-S. Liao, and F. Zhang, *Nano Energy*, Vol. 27, p. 430, 2016.
158. W. Ni, M. Li, B. Kan, F. Liu, X. Wan, Q. Zhang, H. Zhang, T.P. Russell, and Y. Chen, *Chemical Communications*, Vol. 52, p. 465, 2016.
159. Z.E. Ooi, T.L. Tam, R.Y.C. Shin, Z.K. Chen, T. Kietzke, A. Sellinger, M. Baumgarten, K. Mullen, and J.C. deMello, *Journal of Materials Chemistry*, Vol. 18, p. 4619, 2008.
160. D. Baran, T. Kirchartz, S. Wheeler, S. Dimitrov, M. Abdelsamie, J. Gorman, R.S. Ashraf, S. Holliday, A. Wadsworth, N. Gasparini, P. Kaienburg, H. Yan, A. Amassian, C.J. Brabec, J.R. Durrant, and I. McCulloch, *Energy & Environmental Science*, Vol. 9, p. 3783, 2016.
161. Y. Liu, J. Zhao, Z. Li, C. Mu, W. Ma, H. Hu, K. Jiang, H. Lin, H. Ade, and H. Yan, *Nature Communications*, Vol. 5, 2014.
162. W.Z.N. Yahya, *Synthesis and Characterisation of Nanostructured π-conjugated Oligomers and Polymers for Organic Photovoltaic*. Ph.D thesis, University of Joseph Fourier, Grenoble, 2012.
163. Z. Li, K. Jiang, G. Yang, J. Yuk Lin Lai, T. Ma, J. Zhao, W. Ma, and H. Yan, *Nature Communications*, Vol. 7, p. 13094, 2016.
164. S. Zhang, Y. Qin, M.A. Uddin, B. Jang, W. Zhao, D. Liu, H.Y. Woo, and J. Hou, *Macromolecules*, Vol. 49, p. 2993, 2016.
165. K. Zhao, Q. Wang, B. Xu, W. Zhao, X. Liu, B. Yang, M. Sun, and J. Hou, *Journal of Materials Chemistry A*, Vol. 4, p. 9511, 2016.
166. J. Yuan, L. Qiu, Z.-G. Zhang, Y. Li, Y. Chen, and Y. Zou, *Nano Energy*, Vol. 30, p. 312, 2016.

5

Rechargeable Batteries

5.1 Aluminium Batteries

Aluminum and its many versatile alloys are routinely used as surface coatings for the corrosion protection of many metals, offering both barrier and sacrificial protection (1). Among the various methods for aluminum coating, electrodeposition is the most attractive one because it leads to thin, economical coatings that usually are adherent and do not affect the structural and mechanical properties of the substrate. Unfortunately, neither aluminum nor its alloys can be electrodeposited from aqueous solutions because hydrogen is evolved before the aluminum is plated. Thus, it is necessary to employ nonaqueous solvents for this purpose, both molecular and ionic.

Low-temperature molten salts as ionic liquids have a unique set of physical properties such as nonflammability, negligible vapor pressure, high ionic conductivity, and high thermal, chemical and electrochemical stability (1).

Most research about the use of ionic liquids for electrodeposition of aluminum and its alloys has focused on chloroaluminate anions, which can be obtained by mixing anhydrous $AlCl_3$ with an organic chloride salt such as 1-ethyl-3-methyl imidazolium chloride or 1-butylpyridinium chloride, cf. Figure 5.1.

Because of the hygroscopic nature of $AlCl_3$ the electroplating process must be performed in an inert-gas atmosphere. The moisture sensitivity of chloroaluminate-based ionic liquids can be reduced by polymer gel electrolytes, either by impregnating liquid electro-

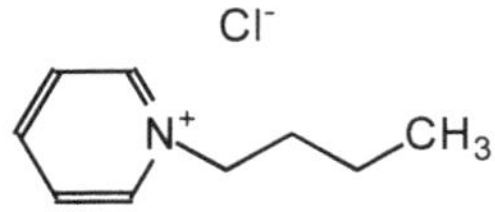

Figure 5.1 1-Butylpyridinium chloride.

lytes into preformed membranes, to co-cast polymer and liquid electrolytes, or by the copolymerization of monomers in the presence of plasticizers.

Polymer gel membranes have been synthesized using the copolymerization of monomers in the presence of plasticizers (1). The gel membranes are transparent with good mechanical properties. These materials can be used for aluminium batteries.

There, reversible aluminum deposition and stripping has been demonstrated. The current densities increase with increasing the scan cycles, indicating an activation process, probably due to the residual surface oxide on the aluminium plate (1).

A polymer gel electrolyte using $AlCl_3$ complexed acrylamide as a functional monomer and acidic ionic liquid-based on a mixture of 1-ethyl-3-methyl imidazolium chloride, cf. Figure 5.2, and $AlCl_3$ in molar ratio of 1:1.5 as a plasticizer has been successfully prepared via free-radical polymerization (2).

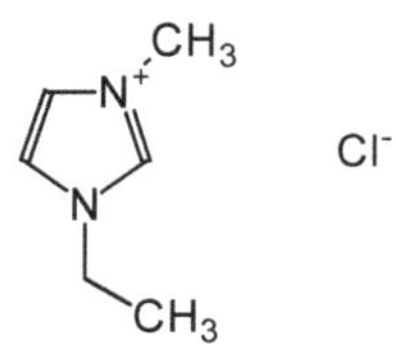

Figure 5.2 1-Ethyl-3-methyl imidazolium chloride.

The deposition of aluminum can be successfully achieved using a polymer gel electrolyte containing 80% of the ionic liquid. The polymer gel electrolytes are good candidates for rechargeable aluminum ion batteries (2).

5.2 Zinc Batteries

5.2.1 *Zinc-Poly(aniline) Batteries*

Poly(aniline) (PANI) is a promising electrode active material for secondary batteries because of its high conductivity, light weight, good redox reversibility and high environmental stability (3).

A nonaqueous zinc-PANI secondary battery could be fabricated using a PANI emeraldine base as cathode and zinc metal as anode in an electrolyte consisting of 0.3 *M* zinc-bis(trifluoromethyl-sulfonyl)imide which was dissolved in propylene carbonate (4).

The formation of the battery required a prerequisite condition to stabilize the interfaces in order to maintain a stable capacity. The battery suffered from Zn dissolution, which induces a competition between concurrent Zn dissolution and plating when the battery is in charge mode, and thus inefficient cycles are obtained. The capacity and coulombic efficiency of the battery depends on the charge-discharge rates (4).

Cycling protocols have been proposed at different rates in order to determine the steady-state rates of competing reactions. When the cell is cycled at 1C rate, the coulombic efficiency improves. The maximum capacity and energy densities of the battery are 148 $mAhg^{-1}$ and 127 $mWhg^{-1}$, respectively, for discharge at 0.5 C.

The battery was successively charged/discharged at constant current densities at a 1C rate. A high cycling stability was obtained for more than 1700 cycles at 99.8% efficiency. The dissolution of zinc and the self-discharge of the battery were investigated after 24 *h* of standby. This investigation showed that the battery experiences a severe self-discharge of 48% per day (4).

The low attainable specific capacity of PANI limits its applicability in commercial battery systems (3). A copolymer, poly(aniline-*co*-*N*-methylthionine), was prepared by incorporating a redox-active *N*-methylthionine unit into a PANI chain via electrochemical copolymerization. The copolymer is shown in Figure 5.3.

The resultant polymeric film exhibited greatly enhanced electrochemical properties and cycling stability when used as a cathode active material in an aqueous Zn-polymer secondary battery. It delivers a high specific capacity of 146.3 $Ahkg^{-1}$ at a current den-

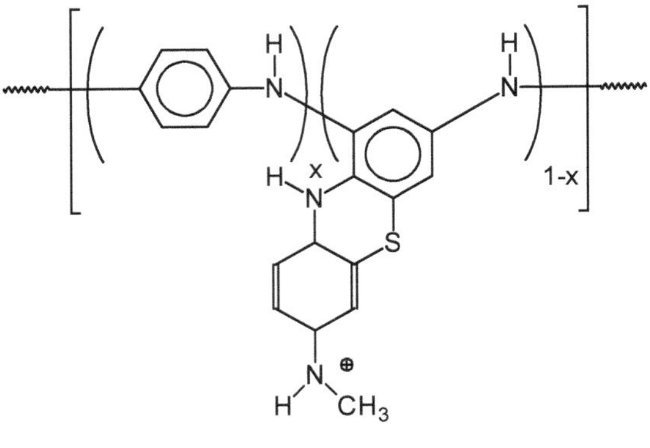

Figure 5.3 Poly(aniline-*co*-*N*-methylthionine).

sity of 1 $mA\,cm^{-2}$ and retains about 99.4% of the capacity over 150 consecutive cycles at a current density of 2 $mAcm^{-2}$ (3).

5.2.2 *Zinc Deposition and Stripping*

The zinc deposition and stripping in an ionic liquid polymer gel electrolyte on gold and copper substrates has been investigated (5).

The ionic liquid-based polymer gel electrolyte is prepared by combining the ionic liquid 1-butyl-1-methylpyrrolidinium trifluoromethylsulfonate, cf. Figure 5.4, with zinc trifluoromethylsulfonate and poly(vinylidene fluoride-*co*-hexafluoropropylene).

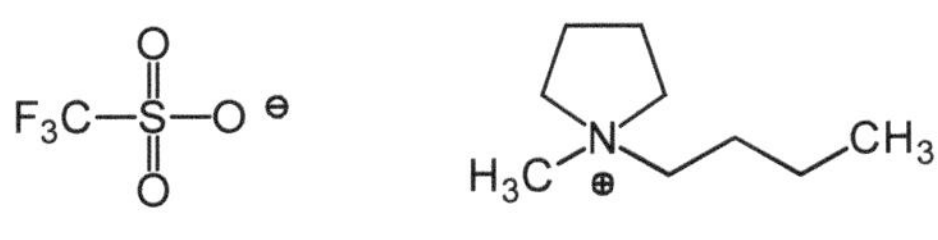

Figure 5.4 1-Butyl-1-methylpyrrolidinium trifluoromethylsulfonate.

The ionic liquid polymer gel electrolyte exhibits a good conductivity of 2.2 $mS\,cm^{-1}$ and a good mechanical stability. The zinc deposition and the stripping in the ionic liquid polymer gel electrolyte were studied by cyclic voltammetry, potentiostatic and galvanostatic cycling (charging/discharging) experiments.

The gel electrolyte exhibits a promising electrochemical stability and allows a quasi-reversible zinc deposition and stripping. The morphology of the zinc deposits after 10 cycles of zinc deposition and stripping is compact and dense, and deposits without any dendrite formation can be obtained. The quasi-reversibility of the electrochemical deposition and stripping of zinc in this ionic liquid polymer gel electrolyte is of interest for rechargeable zinc-based batteries (5).

5.2.3 *Zinc-Air Batteries*

In recent years, the increasing need for portable electronic devices and electric vehicles have significantly stimulated the development of energy storage systems with high efficiency, low cost, and long life circle (6). Compared to conventional lithium-ion rechargeable batteries, zinc-air batteries have a very high theoretical energy density, low cost, less safety risk, and thus have attracted attention. One of the key challenges for zinc-air batteries is the bifunctional air electrode, on which the oxygen reduction and oxygen evolution reactions occur during discharge and charge processes with very sluggish kinetics.

Cobalt-based spinel oxides, such as Co_3O_4, $NiCo_2O_4$, and $MnCo_2O_4$, have been intensively studied as the electrode materials for rechargeable zinc-air batteries and supercapacitors due to their high electrocatalytic activities.

Since the electrical conductivity of these oxides is poor, they are usually supported on carbon or porous metals to act as electrocatalysts. Pristine multiwall carbon nanotubes were used as the support material because of the following advantages (6):

- They have excellent chemical stability and resistance to electrooxidation even at high anodic potentials.
- They are easily dispersed in some organic solvents, which allows multiwall carbon nanotubes to easily form a freestanding film with sufficient gas diffusion path.

Such a porous electrode structure will significantly support the practical oxygen reduction and evolution on the electrode. However, it is difficult to decorate pristine multiwall carbon nanotubes with metal oxides because multiwall have rare binding sites on the highly crystallized graphitic surface. The conventional way to create binding sites for multiwall carbon nanotubes is to oxidize them in a strong acid. As a result, the surface of multiwall carbon nanotubes will be damaged, leading to a decrease in the electrical conductivity and stability.

A novel strategy has been proposed for decorating polymer-wrapped pristine multiwall carbon nanotubes with metal oxides, including NiO, Co_3O_4, and $NiCo_2O_4$. Uniform $NiCo_2O_4$ nanoparticles were homogeneously dispersed on the surface of pyridine-based poly(benzimidazole)-wrapped pristine multiwall carbon nanotubes via a solvothermal synthesis method. The resultant catalysts exhibited promising activity and durability as the bifunctional catalysts for zinc-air batteries.

The pyridine-based poly(benzimidazole)-wrapped multiwall carbon nanotubes were obtained by a sonication method (6). Then, nickel, manganese, and cobalt acetylacetonates with corresponding molar ratios were dissolved together with the wrapped nanotubes in a mixed solution of ethanol, water, and ammonia water. The suspension was refluxed at 80°C for 20 *h*, and subsequently transferred into a Teflon autoclave and solvothermally treated at 150°C for 3 *h*. The products were collected by filtration and vacuum drying.

The electrocatalytic properties of the samples were investigated in 0.1 *M* KOH solution by using a rotating ring disk electrode. The pyridine-based poly(benzimidazole)-wrapped multiwall carbon nanotube supported spinel oxides showed a promising activity for both the oxygen reduction and oxygen evolution reaction. A durability test was carried out on the samples which exhibited the best activity. A cathodic current of -1.0 $mA\,cm^{-2}$ was loaded for 30 *min* and then an anodic current of 1.0 $mA\,cm^{-2}$ was loaded for another 30 *min*.

The galvanic square-wave cycle was repeated for 60 cycles and the potential of the materials was monitored against time. It was confirmed that even after 60 cycles the oxygen evolution reaction potential did not increase at all while the oxygen reduction potential decreased for ca. 80 *mV*, demonstrating the excellent durability of the devices (6).

A thin-film, flexible, and rechargeable zinc-air battery having high energy density has been reported for portable and wearable electronic applications (7,8).

This freeform battery design has created by sandwiching a porous-gelled polymer electrolyte with a freestanding zinc film and a bifunctional catalytic electrode film.

The flexibility of both the electrode films and polymer electrolyte membrane gives great freedom in tailoring the battery geometry and performance (8).

5.3 Sodium Batteries

Rechargeable lithium batteries accelerated the wireless revolution over the last two decades. These batteries are now a mature technology for transportation applications in electric vehicles. However, several studies have concluded that the proven lithium reserves can hardly absorb the growth in demand (9).

For these reasons, sustainable sodium batteries have been considered to overcome the lithium resource shortages that may arise from large-scale application in electric vehicles and stationary energy storage. On the other hand, it is difficult to find a suitable host material for the reversible Na ion storage due to the size of the Na^+ ion of 0.102 *nm* compared to the Li^+ ion with a size of 0.076 *nm* (9).

A low-cost and simple sodium technology has been presented that is based on a metal-free cathode material. Sodium metal is used as the anode with a conducting polymer cathode using PANI emeraldine base as cathode. The construction has been electrochemically tested in a liquid electrolyte. With this technology, a host material for Na intercalation is not required, and because a polymer conductor is used, the size of the Na ion is not an issue (9).

5.3.1 *Organosodium Polymer Batteries*

An electrochemical cell may incorporate two types of conducting polymers each located at an electrode, a cation, a polycyclic aromatic hydrocarbon radical anion that contacts one of the conducting polymers, and an electrolyte (10). The polycyclic aromatic hydrocarbon radical anion may be a covalent substituent of one of the conducting polymers or may be in noncovalent contact with one of the conducting polymers.

The polycyclic aromatic hydrocarbon radical anion may permit the use of cations other than lithium, e.g., an alkali metal cation such as sodium or alkali earth metal cation such as calcium.

Such an electrochemical cell may provide alternative batteries to existing lithium-ion batteries, permitting the use of cations that may be more abundant, more easily extracted, or more sustainable in comparison to the known lithium devices (10).

The first conductive polymer may be: A poly(fluorene), a poly-(pyrene), a poly(azepine), and a poly(phenylene ethynylene), or a combination of these polymers. This conductive polymer is substituted by a fused polycyclic aromatic hydrocarbon radical anion. The fused polycyclic aromatic hydrocarbon radical anion includes an naphthalene or an anthracene radical anion.

For example, sodium naphthalene, the sodium salt of naphthalene radical anion, may be prepared by stirring an anhydrous tetrahydrofuran (THF) solution of naphthalene with metallic sodium. Likewise, the potassium salt of anthracene radical anion may be prepared by stirring an anhydrous THF solution of anthracene with metallic potassium.

The second conductive polymer includes: A poly(arylene ethynylene), a poly(phenylene ethynylene), and a poly(carbazole), or a combination thereof.

The preparation of an electrochemical cell with a noncovalently attached polycyclic aromatic hydrocarbon may be done as follows (10):

Preparation 5–1: A solution of PANI may be formed by the dissolution in anhydrous THF at a concentration of 0.005 *mol* of aniline repeat units in 100 *ml* of THF. The PANI-THF solution may be combined with an anhydrous THF solution containing about 0.005 *mol* or more of sodium naphthalene. The combined mixture of PANI-sodium naphthalene-THF solution may be sonicated for about 20 *min* to assist mixing. The sonicated PANI-sodium naphthalene-THF solution may be formed into a thin layer by spin-coating on the first electrode, e.g., a metal foil at about 30°C and anhydrous, atmospheric pressure. The thin layer may be baked 1 *min* at about 150°C to evaporate the THF to produce the sodium naphthalene-doped PANI as a thin film of the first conducting polymer. Separately, a solution of poly(*p*-phenylene vinylene) as second conducting polymer may be prepared, formed into a thin layer by spin-coating on second electrode, e.g., a metal foil at about 30°C and anhydrous, atmospheric pressure, and baked to evaporate the THF to produce the second conducting polymer as a thin film. The first and second conducting polymers may be prepared as thin films at the first and second electrodes. Next, the first electrode and the first conducting polymer may be contacted to the second electrode and the second polymer. Then, electrolyte components may be added, e.g., poly-(ethylene oxide) (PEO) and sodium perchlorate, and allowed to permeate the conducting polymer layers.

5.3.2 *Sodium Nickel Batteries*

Sodium metal halide batteries have been seriously considered as a low-cost alternative energy storage device for stationary energy storage systems (11). However, there are a number of challenges to be solved in order for there to be successful market penetration, such as high operating temperature and hermetic sealing of batteries that trigger an expensive manufacturing process.

Simple, economical and practical sealing technologies for $Na-NiCl_2$ batteries operated at an intermediate temperature of 190°C have been developed (11).

Conventional polymers have been implemented in planar $Na-NiCl_2$ batteries after a prescreening test, and their excellent compatibilities and durability could be demonstrated by a stable performance of the $Na-NiCl_2$-based battery for more than 300 cycles. The polymers used are listed in Table 5.1.

Table 5.1 Conventional polymers used (11).

Polymer
Ultrahigh molecular weight poly(ethylene)
Poly(vinylidene fluoride)
Poly(tetrafluoroethylene)
Fluorinated ethylene propylene copolymer
Perfluoroalkoxy alkane polymer
Poly(ether ether ketone)
Poly(imide) (Kapton®)
Ultra-temperature poly(etherimide) (Ultem PEI)

The developed sealing methods are highly beneficial and feasible for prolonging the battery cycle life and reducing the manufacturing cost for sodium-based batteries at elevated temperatures of less than 200°C (11).

5.4 Magnesium Batteries

Magnesium batteries are a promising battery technology that could lead to safer and significantly less expensive nonaqueous batteries with energy densities comparable or even better than common Li-ion batteries. The first prototype of a Mg battery using stable Mo_6S_8 as cathode was introduced more than fifteen years ago (12).

5.4.1 *Coordination Polymer Cathode*

A rechargeable magnesium battery with high volumetric capacity has been developed (13). A distinct amorphous molybdenum sulfide, which is a coordination polymer of disulfide-bridged Mo_3S_{11} clusters, has a great potential for a rechargeable magnesium battery cathode.

This material shows a good reversible capacity. This property has been attributed to its unique structure with high flexibility and capability of deformation upon Mg insertion. The free-terminal disulfide moiety may act as the active site for the reversible insertion and extraction of magnesium (13).

5.4.2 *Nanocomposite Polymer Electrolyte*

Nanocomposite polymer electrolytes present new opportunities for rechargeable magnesium batteries (14). However, only a few polymer electrolytes have demonstrated the reversible Mg deposition and dissolution. These polymer electrolytes also contain volatile liquids such as THF.

A nanocomposite polymer electrolyte for rechargeable Mg batteries has been described that is based on PEO, $Mg(BH_4)_2$ and MgO nanoparticles (14). Cells with this electrolyte have a high coulombic efficiency of 98% for Mg plating and stripping and a high cycling stability.

A correlation between the improved solvation of the salt and the solvent chain length, chelation and oxygen denticity could be established. The nanocomposite polymer electrolyte is inferred to enhance the dissociation of the salt $Mg(BH_4)_2$ and thus the electrochemical performance is improved (14).

5.4.3 *Solid Polymer Electrolytes*

5.4.3.1 *Magnesium Triflate*

Solid polymer electrolytes based on PEO complexed with magnesium triflate $Mg(CF_3SO_3)_2$ and incorporation of the ionic liquid 1-butyl-1-methylpyrrolidinium bis(trifluoromethanesulfonyl)imide were prepared by a solution cast technique (15). Triflate has the systematic name trifluoromethanesulfonate, $CF_3SO_3^-$.

The electrolyte was optimized and characterized using electrical conductivity, cationic transport number measurements, and cyclic voltammetry. The highest conductivity of the PEO/$Mg(CF_3SO_3)_2$ electrolyte in a molar ratio of 15:1 at room temperature was 1.19×10^{-2} $S\,cm^{-1}$. The conductivity could be increased to 3.66×10^{-4} $S\,cm^{-1}$ with the addition of 10% ionic liquid.

A significant increase in the Mg^{2+} ion transport number was observed with increasing content of the ionic liquid in the PEO/$Mg(CF_3SO_3)_2$ electrolyte.

The maximum Mg^{2+} ion transport number obtained was 0.40 at the optimized electrolyte composition. A battery with the optimized composition was assembled. The discharge capacity of the battery was 45 $mA\,h\,g^{-1}$ (15).

5.4.3.2 *Cardanol-Based Polymers*

A series of self-crosslinkable polymers composed of different amounts of ionic conducting units, i.e., poly(ethylene glycol) methyl ether methacrylate and crosslinkable units (2-hydroxy-3-cardanylpropyl methacrylate) obtained from a renewable resource, cardanol, were prepared for their application to solid polymer electrolytes (16). 2-Hydroxy-3-cardanylpropyl methacrylate is shown in Figure 5.5.

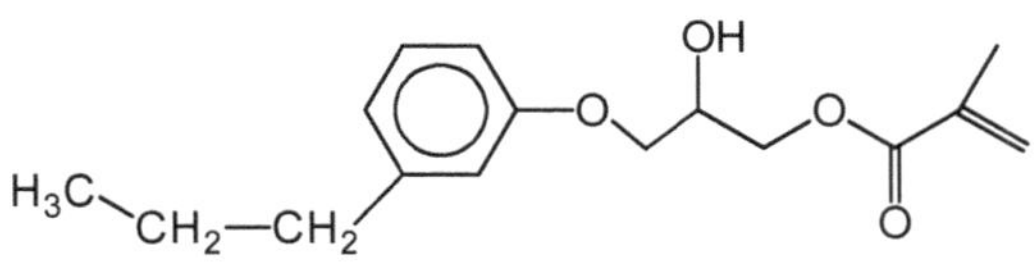

Figure 5.5 2-Hydroxy-3-cardanylpropyl methacrylate.

The electrolytes were prepared by mixing the polymers with lithium bis(trifluoromethanesulfonyl)imide followed by UV irradiation to induce the reaction of the double bonds in the cardanol moiety, thus forming the crosslinked structures.

The ionic conductivity of the solid crosslinked polymer electrolyte prepared from the polymers containing 8 mol-% of the crosslinkable cardanol monomeric units was $1.9 \times 10^{-4}\ S\,cm^{-1}$ at 60°C, which is close to that of poly(poly(ethylene glycol) methyl ether methacrylate) in the waxy state. The all-solid-state lithium battery prepared from this solid polymer electrolyte without a separator exhibited stable cell operation, showing 81.4% of capacity retention after 100 charge-discharge cycles, and demonstrating that the self-crosslinkable polymer from the renewable resource is suitable for high-temperature and high-voltage lithium secondary battery applications (16).

5.4.4 *Anthraquinone-Based Polymer as Cathode*

The design of high-energy cathode materials and the development of noncorrosive electrolytes with high oxidative stability are still issues in the field of magnesium batteries (12).

A robust approach towards achieving a stable cycling of Mg batteries has been presented. The use of a stable polymer cathode and a Mg powder anode coupled with non-nucleophilic electrolytes has been tested. These systems exhibit an excellent rate capability and a significant improvement in the electrochemical stability (12).

Also, two anthraquinone-based polymers have been synthesized (17). An excellent battery cycling performance could be demonstrated with an electrolyte consisting of magnesium bis(hexamethyldisilazide) and magnesium chloride. Magnesium bis(hexamethyldisilazide) is shown in Figure 5.6.

The factors that affect the battery performance of anthraquinone-based organic cathode materials have been elucidated (18).

Two organic cathode materials based on the poly(anthraquinonyl sulfide) structure with different substitution positions were synthesized and their electrochemical behavior and the battery performance were investigated. It has been found that the substitution positions on the anthraquinone structure, the type of binders for

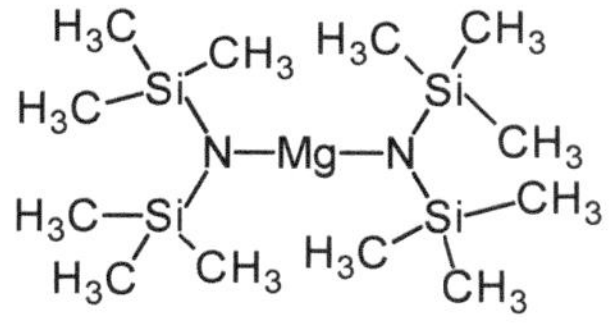

Figure 5.6 Magnesium bis(hexamethyldisilazide).

electrode preparation, and the electrolyte formulations exhibit significant effects on the performance of batteries that contain these organic cathode materials.

A polymer with less steric hindrance at the substitution positions shows a higher capacity, longer cycle life and a better high-rate capability (18).

5.5 Lithium Batteries

A historical review of the development of lithium-based rechargeable batteries has been presented (19).

A rechargeable lithium polymer electrolyte battery for oilfield use has been described (20). Many of the tools, sensors, and other equipment used in downhole applications use electrical power in order to operate or actuate the device. Tools located on the drill string may be powered by a turbine or other motor through which the drilling fluid is circulated.

However, when there is a lack of fluid circulation, or when the tool is located on a wireline, an auxiliary power may be required. This auxiliary power may be in the form of a battery that is attached to the downhole tool. Some tools may be entirely powered by the battery (20).

5.5.1 *Polymeric Binders*

Polymeric binders are important for the electrochemical performance of high capacity silicon anodes that usually suffer from severe capacity fading due to the unparalleled volume change of silicon in the courses of cycling (21).

5.5.1.1 *β-Cyclodextrin*

A hyperbranched *β*-cyclodextrin polymer was shown to be an effective multidimensional binder for silicon anodes in lithium rechargeable batteries (21). *β*-Cyclodextrin is shown in Figure 5.7.

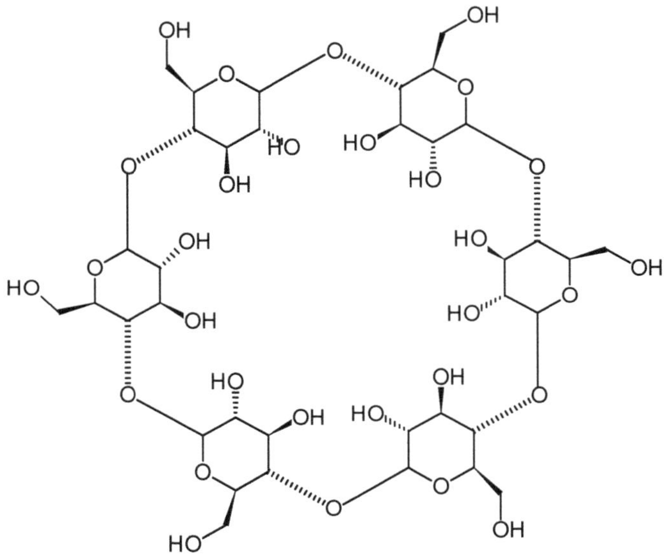

Figure 5.7 *β*-Cyclodextrin.

Unlike one-dimensional binders, the hyperbranched network structure of hyperbranched *β*-cyclodextrin exhibits multidimensional hydrogen-bonding interactions with the silicon particles and therefore offers robust contacts between both components. Even the silicon nanoparticles that had lost the original contacts with the binder during cycling can be recovered within the multidimensional binder network, thus creating a self-healing effect.

Thus, a hyperbranched *β*-cyclodextrin-based silicon electrode shows a markedly improved cycling performance in comparison to those of other conventional binder systems, especially when the electrode is combined with linear polymers at an appropriate ratio to form hybrid binders (21).

5.5.1.2 Guar Gum

Long-term cyclability of a composite Li-ion anode electrode composed of 82% Si/C lithium-ion active material along with 8% of a polymeric binder and 10% Super P conductive carbon black has been studied (22). Polymeric binders exhibiting different elastic/tensile moduli and tensile yield strengths were used.

Accordingly, electrochemically active Si/C composite synthesized by high energy mechanical milling (HEMM), exhibiting reversible specific capacities of around 780 $mA\,h\,g^{-1}$ and 600 mAh/g at charge/discharge rates of ca. 50 $mA\,h\,g^{-1}$ and 200 $mA\,h\,g^{-1}$, respectively, were selected as the Li-ion active anode. Poly(vinylidene fluoride) (PVDF) and purified guar gum with reported elastic moduli of around 1000 MPa and around 3200 MPa, respectively, were selected as the binders.

The results of characterization show that the composite electrode (Si/C + binder + conducting carbon) comprising the higher elastic modulus binder, i.e., purified guar gum, exhibits a better long-term cyclability compared to PVDF. 1H-NMR analysis of the polymer before and after cycling shows structural degradation/deformation of the low elastic modulus PVDF, whereas the high elastic modulus purified guar gum binder shows no permanent structural deformation or damage.

The results reveal that purified guar gum-based polymers exhibiting high elastic modulus are a promising class of binders with the desired mechanical integrity needed for enduring the colossal volume expansion stresses of Si/C-based composite anodes (22).

5.5.2 Nano Bioceramic Filler

A series of nanocomposite solid polymer electrolytes (NCSPE) consisting of poly(methyl methacrylate) (PMMA) as host polymer, lithium bisoxalatoborate, cf. Figure 5.8, as doping salt and a nano-hydroxy apatite as filler have been prepared by a membrane hot-press method (23).

To enhance the electrochemical properties and stiffness of polymer electrolyte film, a bioactive ceramic filler nano-hydroxy apatite was incorporated into the polymer matrix.

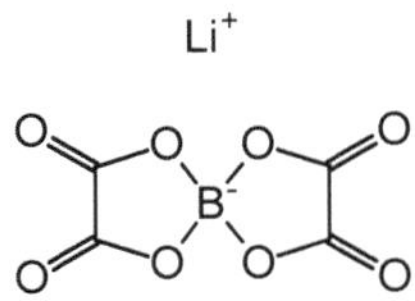

Figure 5.8 Lithium bisoxalatoborate.

The nanocomposite solid polymer electrolyte films with different weight contents were subjected to various electrochemical characterizations such as ionic conductivity, electric modulus and dielectric spectroscopy studies (23).

The complexation behavior and structural reorganization in polymer electrolytes are confirmed by means of Fourier transform infrared (FTIR) analysis. The electrical response and relaxation of dipole in polymer electrolytes were investigated by means of electric modulus and dielectric studies.

It has been found that the addition of a nano-hydroxy apatite compound significantly enhances the ionic conductivity and blocks the reorganizing tendency of the polymer matrix. The maximum ionic conductivity is found to be in the range of $10^{-4.8}$ $S\,cm^{-1}$ for a sample with 10% of the nanoceramic filler (23).

Similarly, plasticized nanocomposite solid polymer electrolytes consisting of PEO as polymer host, lithium bisoxalatoborate as salt with different weight ratios of succinonitrile and nano-hydroxy apatite was prepared by a membrane hot-press technique (24).

Here, also, the incorporation of different compositions of filler and plasticizer in the polymer matrix significantly enhanced the amorphous nature, resulting in increase in ionic conductivity of the plasticized nanocomposite solid polymer electrolyte. The maximum ionic conductivity was found to be in the order of $10^{-3.1}$ $S\,cm^{-1}$ (24).

5.5.3 *Polymer Binder-Free Anode*

A gold-coated silicon nanowire/graphene hybrid composite was fabricated as a polymer binder-free anode for rechargeable lithium-ion batteries (25). A large amount of silicon nanowires for the anode materials can be prepared by a metal-assisted chemical etching process.

Metal-assisted chemical etching is a direct electroless Si wafer etching process resulting in high crystalline quality and good conductivity (26–28).

The composite film on the current collector was obtained by vacuum filtration using an anodic aluminum oxide membrane and a hot-pressing method.

The results show that the gold-coated silicon composite has a stable reversible capacity of about 1520 $mA\,h\,g^{-1}$, which could be maintained for 20 cycles. The composite anode showed a much better cycling performance than a silicon nanowire/poly(vinylidene fluoride)-containing composite, and pure silicon nanowire anodes. The improved electrochemical properties of this composite anode material has mainly been attributed to the porous network structure of the composite (25).

5.5.4 *Overcharge Protection*

Functionalized separators have been fabricated that are capable of providing long-term overcharge protection for secondary lithium batteries (29).

Freestanding nonwoven fiber membranes consisting of an electroactive polymer and a supporting polymer were prepared by an inexpensive and scalable electrospinning technique. The polymers used are a regioregular poly(3-butylthiophene), poly(9,9-dioctylfluorene) end-capped with dimethylphenyl groups, PMMA, and PEO. To prepare the fibers and mats, polymer solutions were loaded into a syringe and electrospun at 20 kV onto aluminum foil substrates.

The membranes sustained large shunt current densities despite the presence of an inert polymer component that dilutes the electroactive polymer.

A bilayer fiber separator prepared by this method provided a reversible voltage-regulated current shunt for a $Li_{1.05}Mn_{1.95}O_4/Li$ cell for more than 1000 135% overcharge cycles at a 2/3 C rate, which is a very stable overcharge protection. This approach enables a better distribution of the electroactive polymer, which should reduce the cost of overcharge protection separators (29).

5.5.5 Electrode Protection

Actually, there has been a considerable interest in developing high energy density batteries with lithium-containing anodes (30). Lithium metal is particularly attractive as the anode of electrochemical cells because of its extremely light weight and high energy density.

The reactivity of lithium and the associated cycle life, dendrite formation, electrolyte compatibility, fabrication and safety problems can make problems for lithium cells.

A special electrode for a lithium electrochemical cell has been reported (30). The electrode has a base layer comprising an active electrode species, and a protective structure positioned to protect the electrode from an electrolyte when the electrode is arranged in an electrochemical cell. The protective structure contains a first side facing the active electrode species, and a second side is arranged to face the electrolyte. The protective structure has layers made from a polymer matrix with a plurality of cavities, and a ceramic material filling.

Examples of polymers that may offer good adhesion to inorganic materials and ceramics are poly(siloxane)s, which may provide flexibility and strength.

The fabrication of a protective structure including a composite of ceramic and polymer portions runs as follows (30):

Preparation 5–2: A shadow mask is first positioned on a substrate. Then, electron beam evaporation is used to deposit a 0.5 μm thick layer of an oxysulfide ceramic on the substrate. The shadow mask is then removed, leaving a pattern of ceramic islands separated by voids or trenches.

A spin coater is used to coat the top surfaces of the ceramic islands with a silicon oil. The silicon oil acts as a dewetting agent that prevents the polymer from adhering to the top surfaces of the ceramic islands. Then, a spin coater is used to fill the voids in the ceramic pattern with a 0.5 μm thick layer of a polymer, Oppanol B15, a poly(isobutene). The polymer is then dried. Finally, the polymer-ceramic structure is plasma treated to remove any silicon oil residue on the exposed ceramic surfaces.

The polymer-ceramic structure is then ready to be coated with lithium metal or with another protective layer, e.g., an additional ceramic-polymer structure. The protective structure can then be released from the substrate.

5.5.6 *Calix[4]quinone*

Calix[4]quinone (C4Q) has eight available carbonyl groups for binding lithium ions (31). Calix[4]quinone is shown in Figure 5.9. It has been exploited to prepare quasi-solid-state rechargeable lithium batteries with a poly(methyl acrylate)/poly(ethylene glycol)-based gel polymer electrolyte and a $LiClO_4$/dimethyl sulfoxide loading.

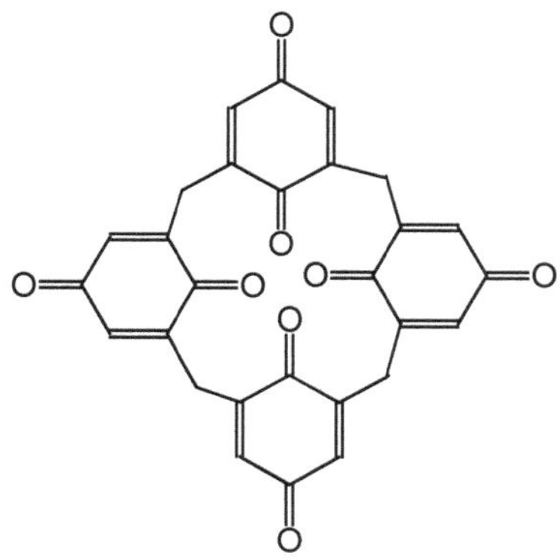

Figure 5.9 Calix[4]quinone.

It shows an initial discharge capacity of 422 $mA\,h\,g^{-1}$ and a capacity retention of 379 $mA\,h\,g^{-1}$ after 100 cycles (31).

5.5.7 *Copolymer of Methyl methacrylate and Ethylene oxide Electrolyte*

A polymer composition for a rechargeable lithium battery including a copolymer of methyl methacrylate (or acrylonitrile) and ethylene oxide has been described (32). The polymer composition may be used for a binder for a negative active material or a binder for a positive active material for a rechargeable lithium battery. In addition, the polymer composition may be used for an electrolyte for a rechargeable lithium battery.

A solid phase is preferable for the entire polymer composition in that a solid has a rigid property that may function as an electrolyte and a separating layer, or a binder, as well as having an appropriate ion conductivity.

A copolymer of methyl methacrylate and ethylene oxide can be prepared as follows (32):

Preparation 5–3: First, 10 *g* of methyl methacrylate and 10 *g* of ethylene oxide were added to 50 *g* of toluene, and then a radical polymerization initiator of dibenzoyl peroxide was added and reacted at 65°C for 9 *h* to provide a copolymer of methyl methacrylate and ethylene oxide. The copolymer of methyl methacrylate and ethylene oxide had a weight average molecular weight of 29,000 *Da*.

When the copolymer is a methyl methacrylate and ethylene oxide copolymer, the lithium salt may be added at about 5–25%. The physical phase of the polymer composition is changed depending upon the amount of the methyl methacrylate and the amount of lithium salt in the polymer composition. For example, when the methyl methacrylate is included in the polymer composition at about 31% or more, the physical phase of the polymer composition is changed depending upon the amount of lithium salt (32).

When the lithium salt is included at about 8% or less, a liquid polymer composition may be obtained. When the lithium salt is included at about 15% or more, a solid polymer composition may be obtained. As lithium salt, $LiClO_4$ can be used (32).

5.5.8 *Poly(vinylene carbonate) Electrolyte*

The process of the fabrication of poly(vinylidene fluoride-hexafluoropropylene)-based polymer electrolytes (33) is complicated and expensive owing to a large amount of fluorine substituents (34).

A novel kind of poly(vinylene carbonate)-based polymer electrolyte has been developed via a facile *in-situ* polymerization method, which possesses the merits of good interfacial compatibility with electrodes (34).

This polymer electrolyte shows a high ionic conductivity of $5.59 \times 10^{-4}\ S\ cm^{-1}$ and a wide electrochemical stability window exceeding 4.8 *V* vs. Li^+/Li at ambient temperature. Furthermore, the rigid cyclic carbonate backbone of poly(vinylene carbonate) results in superior mechanical properties.

$LiFe_{0.2}Mn_{0.8}PO_4$/graphite lithium-ion batteries that use this polymer electrolyte have a good rate capability and an excellent cyclability at room temperature.

This performance demonstrates that the poly(vinylene carbonate)-based electrolyte formed via *in-situ* polymerization is a potential alternative polymer electrolyte for high-performance rechargeable lithium-ion batteries (34).

5.5.9 *Graphene/Carbon Nanotube Foam Conjugated Polymers*

Graphene nanosheets/acid-treated multiwalled carbon nanotubes-supported 1,5-diaminoanthraquinone organic foams have been prepared by organic solvent displacement method followed by a solvothermal reaction (35). Then, an electrochemical polymerization was done to get three-dimensional porous carbon nanotube organic foam-supported poly(1,5-diaminoanthraquinone) nanocomposites. Here the ordered growth of homogeneous nanoparticles on the surface occurs. Such a structure facilitates the charge transportation and suppresses the dissolution of the poly(1,5-diaminoanthraquinone). 1,5-Diaminoanthraquinone is shown in Figure 5.10.

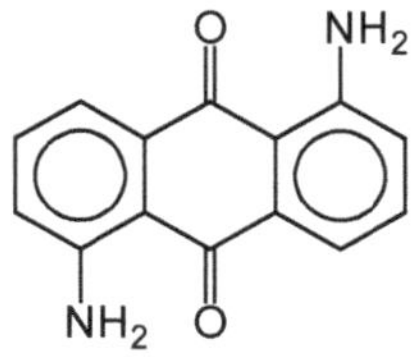

Figure 5.10 1,5-Diaminoanthraquinone.

Such a cathode for rechargeable lithium batteries delivers a high discharge capacity of 289 $mA\,h\,g^{-1}$ at 30 $mA\,g^{-1}$ and still retains 122 $mA\,h\,g^{-1}$ at extreme 10 $A\,g^{-1}$ for rapid charging and discharging. A superior cycling stability is achieved with only 14.8% capacity loss after 2000 cycles even at a high current density of 1 $A\,g^{-1}$ (35).

5.5.10 *Fibrous Nanocomposite Polymer Electrolyte*

A fibrous nanocomposite polymer electrolyte based on poly(vinylidene fluoride-*co*-hexafluoropropylene) was prepared through an electrospinning technology (36). The effects of SiO_2 nanoparticles and diethyl carbonate on the electrochemical properties of the fibrous nanocomposite polymer electrolyte have been investigated by linear sweep voltammetry, cyclic voltammogram and electrochemical impedance spectroscopy.

The electrolyte uptake and the ionic conductivity of the fibrous nanocomposite polymer electrolyte are enhanced due to the incorporation of SiO_2 nanoparticles. The addition of diethyl carbonate into the electrolyte promotes the electrochemical stability and also the ionic conductivity of the fibrous nanocomposite polymer electrolyte.

The fibrous nanocomposite polymer electrolyte has a high ionic conductivity up to $3.48 \times 10^{-3}\ S\,cm^{-1}$ at 25°C with an incorporation of 5% SiO_2. It exhibits good lithium stripping and depositing properties during cycling (36). The Li/$LiFePO_4$ cells that use this nanocomposite polymer electrolyte membrane as separator exhibit a good rate capability and cycling performance (36).

5.5.11 *Nanocomposite Fluoro Polymer Electrolyte*

A kind of nanocomposite polymer electrolyte based on poly(vinylidene fluoride-*co*-hexafluoropropylene) was prepared using a solution-casting technology (37).

Polymer solution-casting is a manufacturing process for making flexible plastic components (38,39). This manufacturing technology is unique in that the process does not require conventional extrusion or injection molding technologies. However, it readily incorporates components and features traditionally produced by these processes.

Here, a room-temperature ionic liquid, 1-ethyl-3-methyl imidazolium tetrafluoroborate, cf. Figure 5.11, was used as plasticizer to improve the thermal stability.

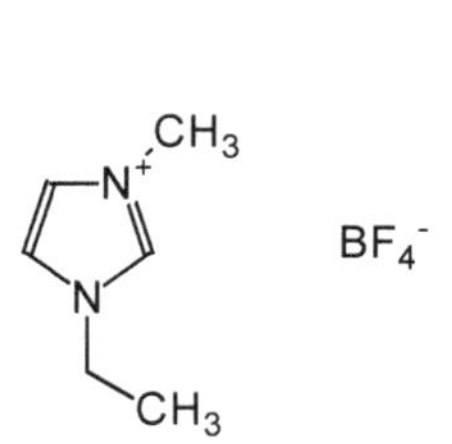

Figure 5.11 1-Ethyl-3-methyl imidazolium tetrafluoroborate.

The thus-obtained nanocomposite polymer electrolyte displayed a porous structure composed of many spherical polymer grains and its crystallinity decreased with the amount of SiO_2 nanoparticles (37).

The effect of the SiO_2 nanoparticles on the electrochemical properties was studied by impedance spectroscopy, linear sweep voltammetry and cyclic voltammetry. When the nanocomposite polymer electrolyte is filled with 2% SiO_2 nanoparticles, it has a room-temperature ionic conductivity of $4.7 \times 10^{-4}\ S\,cm^{-1}$. Furthermore, it exhibits a high decomposition temperature up to 289°C. Li/$LiFePO_4$ cells that use this nanocomposite polymer electrolyte as separator materials show a good rate capability and a satisfied cycling performance (37).

5.5.12 *Solid Polymer Electrolytes for Lithium Battery Applications*

Solid polymer electrolytes for lithium battery applications have been investigated (40). By studying diverse polymer chemistries, it has been discovered that the ion-solvation-site connectivity is an important feature of polymer electrolytes that is necessary for the conductance of high lithium-ion batteries (40).

5.5.12.1 *Solid Polymer Electrolyte Membranes*

Solid polymer electrolyte membranes for rechargeable battery with both high ionic conductivity and superior mechanical performance have been prepared (41). The composite polymer electrolyte contains lithium bis-trifluoromethanesulfonimide, succinonitrile, and PEO segmented poly(sulfone) copolymers with various PEO contents with a low molecular weight M_n of 1500 *Da*. This materials was synthesized by condensation polymerization.

The optimized composite polymer electrolyte membrane exhibits a remarkable amorphous state. This leads to its ionic conductivity of $1.6 \times 10^{-4}\ S\,cm^{-1}$ at room temperature. The tensile strength of the electrolyte membrane is still more than 4.3 *MPa* at 80°C. This indicates its excellent mechanical properties and a high thermal stability in a wide temperature range.

A Li symmetric cell and a Li/$LiFePO_4$ cell with the above electrolyte display a low voltage polarization and a good rechargeability (41).

5.5.12.2 *Poly(vinylidene fluoride)*

Solid polymer electrolytes consisting of PVDF and $LiCF_3SO_3$ plasticized with different amounts of ethylene carbonate as plasticizer were prepared by a solution-casting method. The addition of plasticizer significantly improves the ionic conductivity. The temperature dependence of ionic conductivity of the plasticized PVDF film follows the Vogel-Fulcher-Tamman equation (42) in empirical form, i.e., the migration of ions depends mainly on the segmental movements of the polymer chain in the amorphous region (43).

A composite gel polymer electrolyte based on poly(vinylidene fluoride-hexafluoropropylene) has been described (44). Here also a modified aluminum-doped lithium lanthanum titanate is used. A layer was fabricated through a solution-casting method followed by the activation in a liquid electrolyte.

The layer can protect the Li metal electrode in a Li O_2. The cell was effective in blocking the contamination of the Li electrode by oxygen gas or impurities diffused from the cathode side while suppressing the Li dendrites (44).

5.5.12.3 *Poly(vinyl alcohol)/Poly(acrylic acid) Blend*

A polymer blend of 25 mol% poly(acrylic acid) and 75 mol% poly-(vinyl alcohol) (PVA) was optimized based on its thermal, mechanical and structural properties (45). The ionic liquid electrolyte, i.e., 1-butyl-1-methylpyrrolidinium bis(trifluoromethanesulfonyl)imide with 0.2 *M* lithium bis(trifluoromethansulfonyl)imide, cf. Figure 5.12, was added to the polymer blend in different molar ratios.

A maximum ionic conductivity of 1 $mS\ cm^{-1}$ is observed at 90°C in the membrane with 70 mol% ionic liquid. Cyclic voltammetry of the polymer electrolytes shows peaks that correspond to lithium stripping and also deposition processes, indicating the occurrence of a highly reversible redox process.

The electrochemical stability window of these polymer electrolytes, as determined by linear sweep voltammetry, extends up to 5 *V*, suggesting that these electrolytes could be suitable for batteries that use high-voltage cathode materials.

A lithium transference number of 0.4 was determined for the polymer electrolytes by using chronoamperometry and impedance

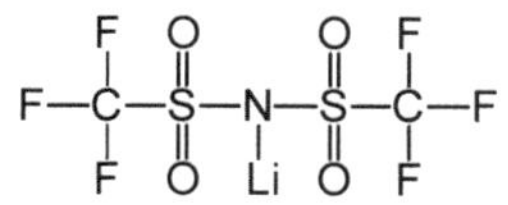

Lithium bis(trifluoromethanesulfonyl)imide

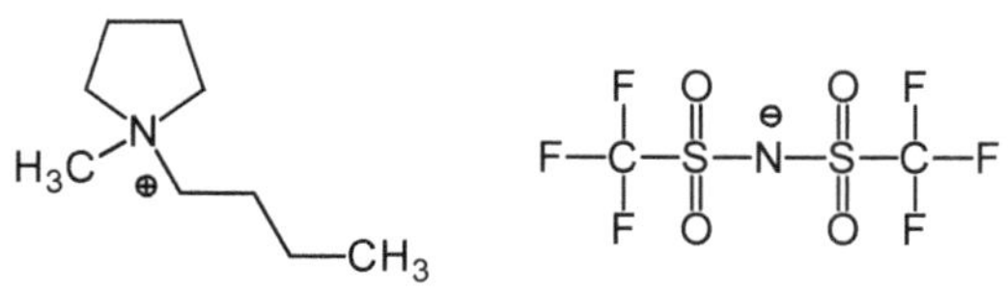

1-Butyl-1-methylpyrrolidinium bis(trifluoromethanesulfonyl)imide

Figure 5.12 Lithium bis(trifluoromethanesulfonyl)imide and 1-Butyl-1-methylpyrrolidinium bis(trifluoromethanesulfonyl)imide.

measurements. Galvanostatic charge-discharge studies of the polymer electrolytes in a lithium half-cell with $LiCoO_2$ as cathode shows a capacity of about 100 $mA\,h\,g^{-1}$ at a temperature of 60°C.

A coin-type half-cell with $LiFePO_4$ cathode and the polymer electrolyte containing 70 mol% ionic liquid shows a capacity of 172 $mA\,h\,g^{-1}$. The $LiFePO_4$ polymer composite cathode delivers a higher capacity of 215 $mA\,h\,g^{-1}$ at 60°C than the pristine $LiFePO_4$ cathode (45). Pristine is shown in Figure 5.13.

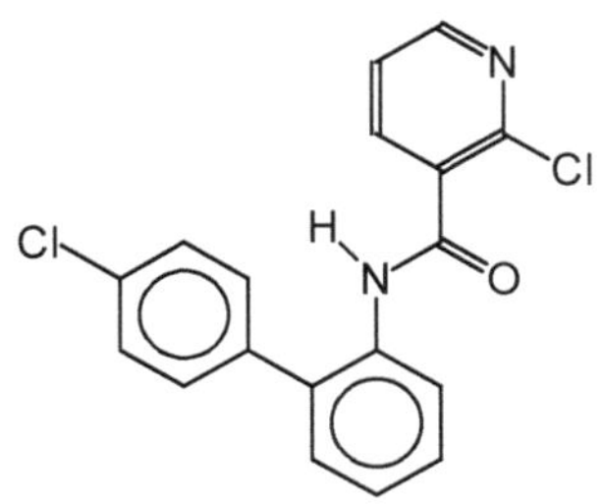

Figure 5.13 Pristine.

5.5.12.4 *Poly(vinyl alcohol)/Poly(acrylonitrile) Blend*

A polymer-ceramic phase separation porous membrane has been prepared from a PVA-poly(acrylonitrile) (PAN) water emulsion mixed with fumed nano-SiO_2 particles using the phase-inversion method (46). This porous membrane is then wetted by a nonaqueous Li-salt liquid electrolyte to form the polymer/colloid dual-phase electrolyte membrane.

In comparison to the liquid electrolyte in a conventional polyolefin separator, the electrolyte membrane obtained here has superior properties in high ionic conductivity of 1.9 $ms\,cm^{-1}$ at 30°C, a high Li^+ transference number of 0.41, high electrochemical stability, extended up to 5.0 V versus Li^+/Li on a stainless steel electrode, and also a good interfacial stability with the lithium metal.

A test cell with $Li/LiCoO_2$ with the above-described electrolyte membrane as separator also shows a high-rate capability and an excellent cycle performance (46).

5.5.13 *Porous Polymer Electrolytes*

Porous polymer electrolytes are attractive for their use in lithium-ion batteries because of the combined advantages of liquid and solid polymer electrolytes.

A porous polymer membrane doped with phytic acid, also known as inositol hexakisphosphate, has been prepared, which is used as a crosslinking agent in polymer electrolyte matrix (47). Phytic acid can also plasticize porous polymer electrolyte membranes, changing them into soft, tough flexible materials. A polymer membrane based on PEO and PMMA and $LiClO_4$ has been prepared by a simple evaporation method.

The effects of the ratio of the content of the polymers on the properties of the porous membrane, including morphology, porous structure, and mechanical property, have been studied (47). Phytic acid improves the porous structure and mechanical properties of polymer membrane. The maximum tensile strength and elongation of the porous polymer membranes are 20.71 MPa and 45.7% at 15% phytic acid, respectively. Porous polymer electrolytes with 15% content of phytic acid has a conductivity of 1.59×10^{-5} $S\,cm^{1}$ at

20°C, a good electrochemical window of greater than 5 *V*, and a low interfacial resistance.

These results demonstrate the compatibility of the mechanical properties and conductivity of the porous polymer electrolytes, thus indicating that porous polymer electrolytes have good application prospects for lithium-ion batteries (47).

5.5.13.1 *Semi-interpenetrated Network Solid Polymer Electrolytes*

Semi-interpenetrated network solid polymer electrolytes were fabricated by the UV-induced crosslinking of poly(ethylene glycol) diacrylate and divinylbenzene within a PEO matrix, comprising lithium bis(trifluoromethanesulfonyl)imide salt, at a molar ratio of ethylene oxide to Li of around 30:1 (48).

The influence of the content of divinylbenzene on the final solid polymer electrolyte properties was investigated in detail. The increase of divinylbenzene concentration results in self-standing polymer electrolytes. The incorporation of the divinylbenzene crosslinking agent was found to decrease the crystallinity of the PEO matrix from 34% to 23%, with a decrease in the melting temperature of the membrane from 50°C to 34°C (48).

In addition, the influence of the concentration of divinylbenzene on the ionic conductivity was determined for polymer electrolytes with 0%, 10%, 20%, and 45% divinylbenzene from room temperature to 80°C. The resulting semi-interpenetrated network solid polymer electrolytes showed a high electrochemical stability of 4.3 *V* as well as practical conductivity values exceeding 10^{-4} $S\,cm^{-1}$ at 70°C. The cycling performance of these semi-interpenetrated electrolytes have been shown with a Li metal polymer battery and an all-solid-state Li sulfur battery (48).

5.5.14 *Poly(anthraquinonyl sulfide) Cathode Material*

Poly(anthraquinonyl sulfide) has been synthesized and investigated as an organic cathode material for rechargeable lithium batteries (49). The synthetic route for poly(anthraquinonyl sulfide) is shown in Figure 5.14.

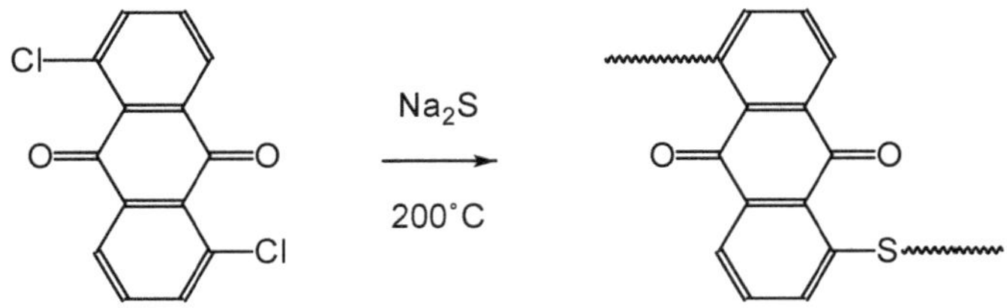

Figure 5.14 Synthesis of poly(anthraquinonyl sulfide) (49).

The theoretical capacity of polymers with quinone units is shown in Table 5.2. The above batteries show an excellent reversibility and cyclability.

The synthesis of self-assembled graphene/poly(anthraquinonyl sufide) composite aerogel has been reported (50). Poly(anthraquinonyl sufide) is shown in Figure 5.15.

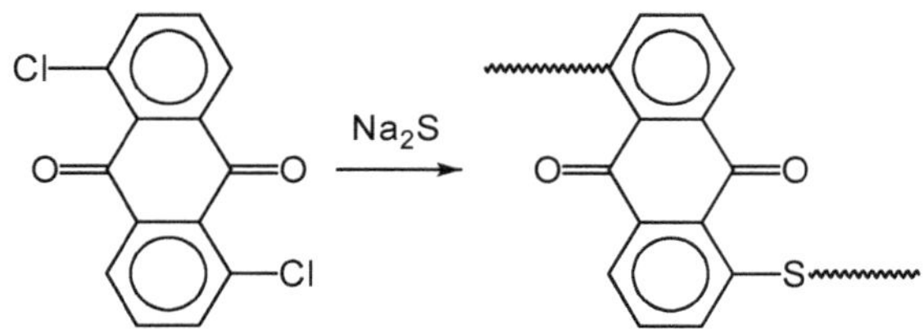

Figure 5.15 Poly(anthraquinonyl sufide).

An efficient integration of a three-dimensional graphene framework occurred here with electroactive poly(anthraquinonyl sufide) particles via a novel dispersion-assembly strategy, which can be used as a freestanding flexible cathode upon mechanical pressing.

The entire cathode can deliver the highest capacity of 156 $mA\,h\,g^{-1}$ at 0.1 C (1 C = 225 $mA\,h\,g^{-1}$) with an ultrahigh utilization of 94.9% of poly(anthraquinonyl sufide) and exhibits an excellent rate performance with 102 $mA\,h\,g^{-1}$ at 20 C in lithium batteries. Also, for Na batteries the performance is very good.

The excellent electrochemical performance could be ascribed to the fast redox kinetics and electron transportation within the composite aerogel, resulting from the interconnected conductive framework of graphene and the intimate interaction between graphene

Table 5.2 Properties of polymers with quinone units (49).

Polymer	Theoretical Capacity *mA h g*$^{-1}$
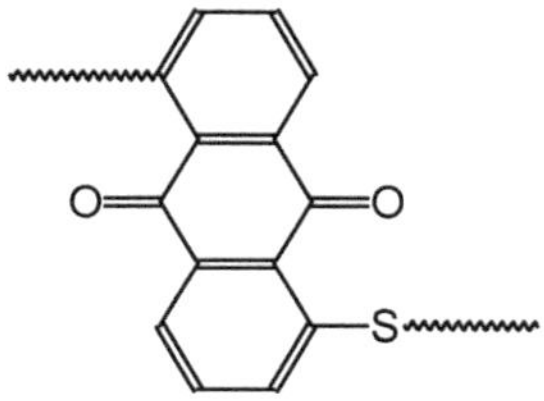	225
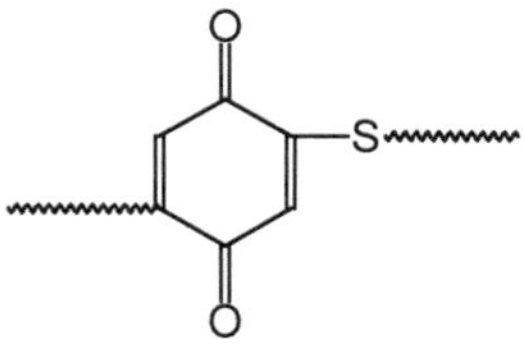	388
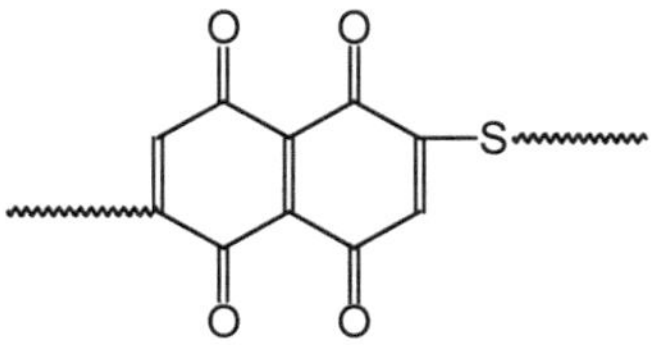	492
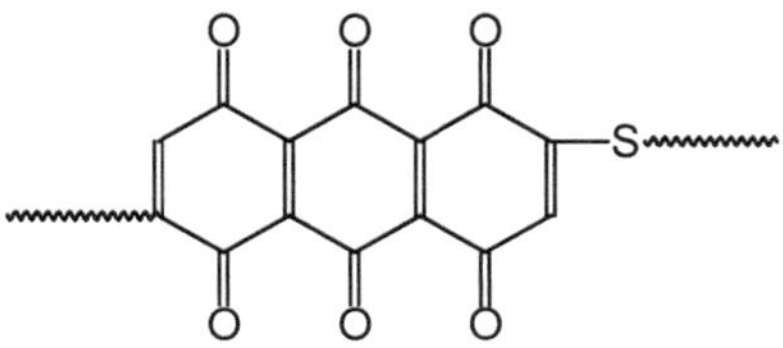	540

and poly(anthraquinonyl sufide) through an efficient wrapping structure (50).

5.5.15 *Poly(aniline) Cathode Material*

The aniline was polymerized onto functionalized multiwalled carbon nanotubes. In this way, a cathode material with core-shell structures for lithium batteries was obtained (51).

The structure and morphology of the samples were investigated by FTIR spectroscopy, scanning electron microscope, transmission electron microscope and X-ray diffraction. The electrochemical properties of the composite were characterized by the cyclic voltammetry, the charge/discharge property, coulombic efficiency, and AC impedance spectroscopy.

At a constant current density of 0.2 C, the first specific discharge capacity of the reduced and oxidized PANI/ multiwalled carbon nanotubes was 181.8 $mA\,h\,g^{-1}$ and 135.1 $mA\,h\,g^{-1}$ separately, and the capacity retention rates were corresponding to 76.75% and 86.04% for 100 cycles with a coulombic efficiency of 99%.

It was confirmed that the carbon nanotubes enhanced the conductivity and the electrochemical performance of PANI, and compared with the pure PANI, the reduced composite showed a good performance for the cathode of lithium batteries (51).

5.5.16 *Polymer Gel Electrolytes*

5.5.16.1 *Gel Polymer Electrolyte Precursor*

A gel polymer electrolyte precursor has been prepared from a bismaleimide monomer or bismaleimide oligomer. The bismaleimide oligomer is prepared by the reaction of barbituric acid and bismaleimide (52).

The bismaleimide oligomer is a multifunction bismaleimide oligomer with a hyperbranch architecture or multi-double-bond reactive functional groups. In the hyperbranch architecture, the bismaleimide serves as an architecture matrix. The radical barbituric acid is grafted to the bismaleimide's double bond to begin branching and ordering to form the hyperbranch architecture. The preparation of the bismaleimide oligomer is as follows (52):

Preparation 5–4: First, 19.9995 *g* 1,1-methylenedi-4,1-phenylene bismaleimide monomer particles or powders and 108.6008 *g* γ-butyrolactone were mixed in a 250 *ml* round-bottomed three-necked flask and heated to 130°C with stirring until the bismaleimide monomer was completely dissolved. Next, 7.1483 *g* barbituric acid powders was progressively added to the 130"C bismaleimide/γ-butyrolactone solution with 16 batches in a 15 *min* interval and stirred to perform the polymerization of the bismaleimide. After addition of the barbituric acid batches were completed, the polymerization continuously proceeded for 6 *h* to form bismaleimide oligomer. The mole concentration ratio of the bismaleimide and barbituric acid was 1:1.

1,1-Methylenedi-4,1-phenylene bismaleimide is shown in Figure 5.16.

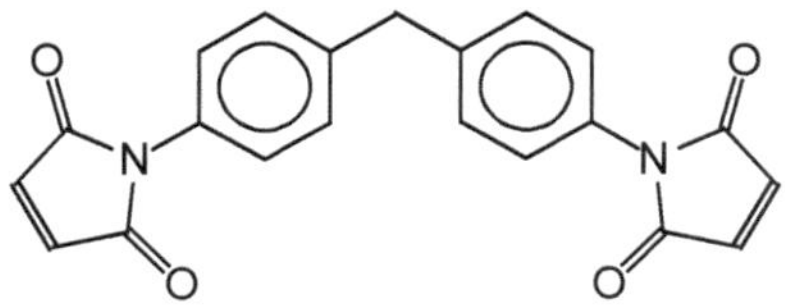

Figure 5.16 1,1-Methylenedi-4,1-phenylene bismaleimide.

The gel polymer electrolyte precursor is rapidly formed into a soft gel, thus improving the performance of an alkali metal rechargeable cell by, for example, high interface compatibility and high lithium-ion conduction between positive and negative electrodes (52).

The gel polymer electrolyte is prepared by heating polymerization/crosslinking of a gel polymer electrolyte precursor. The gel polymer electrolyte precursor is injected into an aluminum foil cell. After cell packaging, the gel polymer electrolyte precursor is heated by heating polymerization to form the gel polymer electrolyte, for example, crosslinked copolymers. The temperature of the heating polymerization ranges from 30–130°C. The gel polymer electrolyte can be tightly combined with electrode plates with a high fabrication compatibility.

Leakage of the lithium rechargeable cell utilizing the gel polymer electrolyte is avoided. The gel polymer electrolyte is rapidly crosslinked, leaving electrolyte exceeding 95%, with a high ionic conductivity (52).

5.5.16.2 *Semi-interpenetrating Polymer Network*

A semi-interpenetrating polymer network gel polymer electrolyte was developed. This is a membrane based on a crosslinked poly(ethylene glycol) diacrylate-*co*-poly(vinylene carbonate) and a PVDF hydrophobic fluorous linear polymer (53). This polymer could be synthesized by an UV-curing technology. The crosslinked poly-(ethylene glycol) diacrylate-*co*-poly(vinylene carbonate) can accommodate a large amount of liquid electrolyte inside the nonporous membrane due to its strong interaction with Li^+ and solvents, which avoids a leakage of the liquid electrolyte.

The ionic conductivity of the polymer network reaches 1.49×10^{-3} $S\,cm^{-1}$ at 25°C and the electrochemical stability window up to 4.2 V versus Li/Li^+. Also, an excellent interface stability to lithium metal electrode, superior thermal stability and good mechanical properties have been shown (53).

A symmetric Li/Li cell with the above electrolyte displays a lower voltage polarization and a longer valid cycle life than cells that are based on a conventional liquid electrolyte. Moreover, Li $Li/LiFePO_4$ cells using this electrolyte show a superior cycling stability and rate performance comparable to a cell based on a conventional liquid electrolyte (53).

5.5.16.3 *Lithium nonafluoro-1-butanesulfonate*

The preparation of a new category of gel polymer electrolytes has been reported (54, 55). This occurs by the immobilization of various compositions of a lithium nonafluoro-1-butanesulfonate salt and the less viscous 1-ethyl-3-methyl imidazolium nonafluoro-1-butanesulfonate ionic liquid in poly(vinylidene fluoride-*co*-hexafluoropropylene) matrix for their application in lithium-ion batteries.

The study showed that a composition with 80% 1-ethyl-3-methyl imidazolium nonafluoro-1-butanesulfonate-lithium nonafluoro-1-butanesulfonate and 20% poly(vinylidene fluoride-*co*-hexafluoropropylene) has the highest ionic conductivity of 10^{-2} $S\,cm^{-1}$.

The ionic liquid incorporated gel polymer electrolytes exhibit excellent properties and will facilitate their use as a potential separator for lithium-ion batteries (55).

Also, the ionic conductivity and the cation transport properties of polymer electrolytes can be improved by adding a bulky anion-based lithium bisnonafluoro-1-butanesulfonimidate salt (56).

5.5.16.4 *Poly(ethylene oxide) Gel Polymer Electrolyte*

The synthesis and characterization of a gel polymer electrolyte based on the polymer PEO, salt lithium bis(trifluoromethylsulfonyl)imide and various amounts of an added ionic liquid, i.e., 1-ethyl-3-methyl imidazolium bis(trifluoromethylsulfonyl)imide, has been reported (57).

Differential scanning calorimetry, thermogravimetric analysis, complex impedance spectroscopy, ionic transference number studies, linear sweep voltammetry, and cyclic voltammetry studies exhibited promising characteristics of the prepared gel polymer electrolytes for suitable application in lithium polymer batteries.

The gel polymer electrolytes show high thermal stability, i.e., no weight loss up to 310°C, a high ionic conductivity of 2.08×10^{-4} $S\,cm^{-1}$ at 30°C, a high lithium transference number of 0.39, and a high electrochemical stability window of ca. 4.6 V.

A low-cost simple thermal lamination technique was used to encapsulate the whole lithium polymer battery assembly by sandwiching the best performing gel polymer electrolyte between a $LiMn_2O_4$ cathode and a lithium metal anode. Galvanostatic charge/discharge cycles of the prepared cell exhibited a good electrochemical performance (57).

5.5.16.5 *Rhodanide-Based Gel Polymer Electrolytes*

Rhodanide anion-based ternary gel polymer electrolytes with high electrochemical and thermal stability have been developed (58).

They can be advantageously used with the temperature-responsive polymer poly(vinylidene fluoride-*co*-hexafluoropropylene) and a room-temperature ionic liquid, i.e., 1-ethyl-3-methylimiazolium rhodanide (thiocyanate). These polymer electrolytes were fabricated using a facile solution cast method by incorporating the ionic liquid and the lithium rhodanide into the polymeric-based membranes.

The membrane with 80% electrolyte mixtures showed a fine performance. The maximum ionic conductivity was found to be in the order of 2.8×10^{-4} $S\,cm^{-1}$ at 298 K. The inimitable properties should allow an effective use of the rhodanide-based electrolytes as active separators for the development of advanced lithium-ion batteries (58).

5.5.17 *Lithium-Oxygen Batteries*

A quasi-solid-state lithium-oxygen battery has been fabricated using a gel polymer electrolyte with an ionic liquid (59). The battery architecture incorporates a design feature that can be easily scaled up in size for use in large systems. A feasibility study demonstrated that the battery operates successfully for repeated discharge-charge cycles.

5.5.18 *Lithium-Sulfur Batteries*

Various polymer sulfur composites and their impact on the electrochemical performance have been reviewed (60). Also, the synthesis approaches toward these composites have been summarized.

Lithium-sulfur batteries are a particular type of rechargeable battery (61). Unlike most rechargeable batteries in which the ion actually moves into and out of a crystal lattice, the ion on lithium-sulfur batteries reacts with lithium in the anode and with sulfur in the cathode even in the absence of a precise crystal structure. In most lithium-sulfur batteries the anode is lithium metal. In operation lithium leaves the metal as lithium ions (Li^+) and enters the electrolyte when the battery is discharging. When the battery is recharged, lithium ions (Li^+) leave the electrolyte and plate out on the lithium metal anode as lithium metal. At the cathode, during the discharge process, particles of elemental sulfur react with the lithium ion in the electrolyte to form Li_2S. When the battery is recharged, lithium ions leave the cathode, allowing the reversion to elemental sulfur.

Sulfur is an attractive cathode candidate as compared to traditional lithium-ion battery cathodes because it offers an order of magnitude higher theoretical capacity of 1675 $mA\,h\,g^{-1}$ than the conventionally used cathodes and it operates at a safer voltage range of 1.5–2.5 *V*. In addition, sulfur is inexpensive and environmentally benign.

The major problem with a sulfur cathode is its poor cycle life. The discharge of sulfur cathodes involves the formation of intermediate poly(sulfide) ions, which dissolve easily in the electrolyte during the charge-discharge process and result in an irreversible loss of active material during cycling. The higher-order poly(sulfide)s produced during the initial stage of the discharge process are soluble in the electrolyte and move toward the lithium metal anode, where they are reduced to lower-order poly(sulfide)s (61).

This process results in irreversible capacity loss and causes the buildup of a thick irreversible Li_2S barrier on the electrodes during prolonged cycling, which is electrochemically inaccessible (61).

A polymer-coated, shaped sulfur-nanocomposite has been described that can be used as a cathode in lithium-sulfur rechargeable batteries. The preparation runs as follows (61):

Preparation 5–5: First, 4.963 *g* of sodium thiosulfate pentahydrate was dissolved in 160 *ml* decyltrimethylammonium bromide aqueous solution with magnetic stirring. Decyltrimethylammonium bromide consists of a hydrophilic head (trimethylammonium bromide) and a long hydrophobic tail (the C_{12} hydrocarbon chain). An amount of concentrated hydrochloric acid (4 *mL*) was then added dropwise. Decyltrimethylammonium bromide can form micelles with microsized/nanosized nonpolar environments in water, assisting the formation of individual sulfur particles from the reaction of sodium thiosulfate with dilute hydrochloric acid. The reaction proceeded at room temperature for 3 *h* and a yellow sulfur colloidal solution was obtained. The obtained sulfur colloidal solution contained microsized sulfur particles with a uniform bipyramidal shape. An appropriate amount of pyrrole was then added while the reaction mixture was cooled to 0–5°C in an ice bath, followed by the addition of ammonium peroxydisulfate. The pyrrole formed ultrafine poly(pyrrole) nanospheres of around 100 *nm* within the decyltrimethylammonium bromide micelles by the oxidation polymerization reaction under the surfactant concentration of 0.05 *M*. At the same time, the poly(pyrrole) nanospheres agglomerate to build a nanolayer on the surface of the sulfur particles due to their common hydrophobic features with the aid of the contracting effect of decyltrimethylammonium bromide micelles. The reaction proceeded at 0–5°C for 4 *h*, and the color of the reaction solution slowly turned black. The product was filtered, rinsed thoroughly with deionized water, and dried in an air oven at 50°C overnight to obtain a black powder. The obtained sulfur particles were coated with a poly(pyrrole) layer consisting of stacked poly(pyrrole) nanospheres.

Also, a rechargeable cathode has been described and a lithium-sulfur battery comprising this cathode (62). The cathode includes a solid, ionically conducting polymer material and electroactive sulfur. The battery also contains a lithium anode and an electrolyte.

The base polymer can be a poly(phenylene sulfide), a poly(ether ether ketone), or a liquid crystal polymer. The dopant is an electron acceptor such as 2,3-dichloro-5,6-dicyano-1,4-benzoquinone, sulfur trioxide or chloranil. Chloranil is also known as 2,3,5,6-tetrachlorocyclohexa-2,5-diene-1,4-dione. These compounds are shown in Figure 5.17.

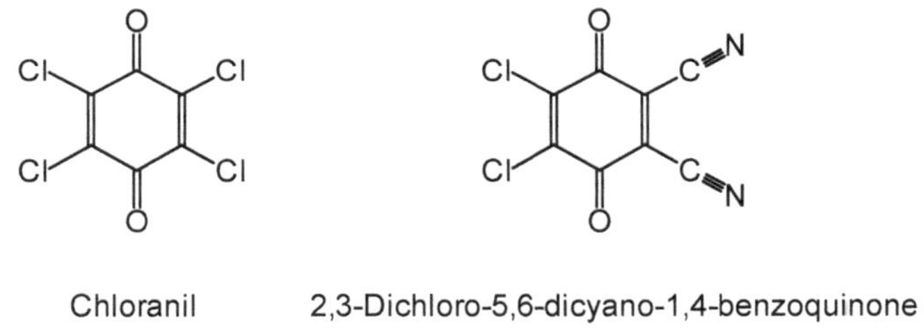

Figure 5.17 Electron acceptors.

The solid, ionically conductive polymer material can also be useful as a separator film, as it is electrically nonconductive, and ionically conductive (62).

5.5.18.1 *Sandwiched Gel Polymer Electrolyte*

A sandwiched gel polymer electrolyte has been prepared using a facile method as separator solely for rechargeable lithium-sulfur batteries (63). As a result of the strong physical shielding and chemical absorption of the gel polymer electrolyte, the separator can not only suppress the shuttle effect in an ether-based electrolyte, but also improves the usage of sulfur significantly, resulting in a high capacity.

The PVDF layers can absorb largely the ether-based electrolyte and then enhance Li^+ transfer. The PMMA layer can be utilized to trap the dissolved poly(sulfide)s.

Lithium-sulfur batteries with the sandwiched gel polymer electrolyte separator show an encouraging electrochemical performance. A high initial discharge capacity of 1711.8 $mA\,h\,g^{-1}$ is obtained, and the capacity is retained at 1145.3 $mA\,h\,g^{-1}$ after 50 cycles at 200 $mA\,g^{-1}$, which is higher than that of the cell with a conventional separator. These results indicate that the appropriate gel polymer electrolyte separator is more suitable in lithium-sulfur battery applications (63).

5.5.18.2 *Polymer-Coated Graphene Oxide Electrode*

Poly(diallyldimethylammonium chloride)-graphene oxide-sulfur composites were prepared by a chemical oxidation method (64). For the poly(diallyldimethylammonium chloride)-graphene oxide composites, the conducting polymers were coated on the surface of the graphene oxide sheets. Poly(diallyldimethylammonium chloride)-graphene oxide composites were expected to increase the electrical conductivity and to protect the restacking of the graphene sheets.

Then, sulfur particles were dispersed into the poly(diallyldimethylammonium chloride)-graphene oxide composites by mixing it in a CS_2 solvent. It has been expected that the poly(diallyldimethylammonium chloride)-graphene oxide-sulfur composites show the limited release of poly(sulfide)s due to the fact that they can provide a high surface area, because conducting polymer can be used as spacer between graphene sheets.

The poly(diallyldimethylammonium chloride)-graphene oxide-sulfur composites showed a high discharge capacity of 1102 $mA\,h\,g^{-1}$ at the first cycle and a good cycle retention of 60% after 100 cycles (64).

5.5.19 *Lithium-Ion Poly(sulfide) Batteries*

Aqueous electrolyte lithium-ion poly(sulfide) batteries are of great interest, due to the use of low-cost and abundant raw materials. A new practical battery chemistry coupling has been explored by using a well-known cathode material in Li-ion batteries, i.e., $LiMn_2O_4$ with a dissolved poly(sulfide) anode (65). This system has been improved by replacing the ceramic membrane with an ion-selective polymer membrane, thus allowing cost-effective and higher energy density options.

After tuning the osmotic movements inside the membrane, dissolved poly(sulfide) leakage from one-compartment to another could be successfully eliminated.

With the additional use of porous silica serving as an absorbent for sulfur-based gaseous products, a 1.5 V average voltage together with a stable cycling profile of more than 200 cycles at high current density regimes could be achieved (65).

5.5.20 *Lithium-Carbon Dioxide Batteries*

The utilization of carbon dioxide in lithium-carbon dioxide batteries has attracted extensive attention (66). However, the poor rechargeability and low applied current density are problematic.

A gel polymer electrolyte has been developed which is composed of a polymer matrix filled with a tetraglyme-based liquid electrolyte (66). Tetraglyme is also known as tetraethylenglycoldimethylether.

This electrolyte was used to fabricate a rechargeable $Li-CO_2$ battery with a carbon nanotube-based gas electrode. The discharge product of Li_2CO_3 formed in the gel polymer electrolyte-based $Li-CO_2$ battery exhibits a particle-shaped morphology with a poor crystallinity, which is different from the contiguous polymer-like and crystalline discharge product in conventional $Li-CO_2$ battery that uses a liquid electrolyte.

Thus, the gel polymer electrolyte-based battery shows a much improved electrochemical performance. The achieved cycle life (60 cycles) and rate capability (maximum applied current density of 500 $mA\ g^{-1}$) are much higher than most previously reported. This points out a new way for the development of high-performance $Li-CO_2$ batteries (66).

5.5.21 *Lithium Titanate Spinel*

The synthesis of a cubic mesostructured lithium titanate spinel $Li_4Ti_5O1_2$ with uniform pores of diameter of 15 nm and sub-10 nm grains has been reported (67). The material was prepared in powder form by sol-gel co-assembly through a soft-templating method using a poly(isobutylene)-block-poly(ethylene oxide) diblock copolymer structure-directing agent.

Electron microscopy demonstrated the mesoporous nature. Mesoporous $Li_4Ti_5O1_2$ obtained after heating to 600°C at 10°C/min is virtually single phase, with minor traces of Li_2CO_3 accumulated on the surface. Half-cells with a lithium metal anode display a superior cycling with a 5% capacity decay between the fifth and 300th cycles at C/2 (67).

5.5.22 *Selenized Poly(acrylonitrile) Electrodes*

The correlation between the structure of a selenized PAN composite material and the electrochemical properties for lithium batteries was studied (68).

Raman spectroscopy and X-ray photoelectron spectroscopy measurements demonstrate that a higher synthesis temperature results in a higher graphitization degree of the polymer skeleton and fewer Se–Se bonds. The selenized PAN electrodes present excellent rate capability and extra-long cycle life due to their fast electrochemical reaction kinetics and their high structural stability.

A reversible specific capacity of about 325 $mA\,h\,g^{-1}$ for the electrode composite synthesized at 500°C was obtained with a capacity decay of only 2.6% (based on the second cycle) after 1500 cycles. In addition, the correlation between their structure and the electrochemical performance was elucidated. The electrode composites obtained at higher temperature show a better cycling stability but a lower capacity (68).

5.5.23 *Flexible Rechargeable Thin-Film Batteries*

Flexible rechargeable thin-film lithium-ion batteries have been developed. These devices are based on all-solid-state materials. The flexible batteries were fabricated using low-temperature sequential physical vapor deposition techniques (69).

A thin-film battery architecture consisting of a $Ti/V_2O_5/LiPON/Li$ encapsulation multilayer was deposited on a flexible poly(imide) substrate. To the best of our knowledge, the obtained thin-film batteries are among the thinnest reported with an overall thickness of 50 μm, including substrate, active layers and encapsulation stack.

The fabricated thin-film batteries delivered a discharge capacity as high as 0.15 $mA\,h$ upon galvanostatic cycling at 30 $\mu A\,cm^{-2}$ within a voltage range of 3.8–1.5 V. The capacity decreased during cycling with an average fading rate of 0.25% over 100 cycles.

Electrochemical impedance spectroscopy measurements and modeling analysis revealed an increase of the internal resistance during cycling. In addition, it was shown that the internal resistance increase was induced by a progressive decrease of the contact area of electrolyte and electrodes. Thin-film batteries having the same architecture and cell design were fabricated onto two substrates: A flexible poly(imide) foil and a rigid silicon wafer. The electrochemical characterization showed a clear influence of the substrate type on discharge capacity of the thin-film lithium-ion batteries and variations of the internal resistance during cycling (69).

References

1. X.-G. Sun, Y. Fang, K. Yoshii, and S. Dai, Polymer gel membranes for aluminum deposition and rechargeable aluminum ion batteries, in *EC Meeting Abstracts*, number 3, pp. 213–213. The Electrochemical Society, 2015.
2. X.-G. Sun, Y. Fang, X. Jiang, K. Yoshii, T. Tsuda, and S. Dai, *Chemical Communications*, Vol. 52, p. 292, 2016.
3. C. Chen, X. Hong, A. Chen, T. Xu, L. Lu, S. Lin, and Y. Gao, *Electrochimica Acta*, Vol. 190, p. 240, 2016.
4. A. Guerfi, J. Trottier, I. Boyano, I.D. Meatza, J. Blazquez, S. Brewer, K. Ryder, A. Vijh, and K. Zaghib, *Journal of Power Sources*, Vol. 248, p. 1099, 2014.
5. Z. Liu, S. Zein El Abedin, and F. Endres, *Journal of Solid State Electrochemistry*, Vol. 18, p. 2683, October 2014.
6. J. Yang, T. Fujigaya, and N. Nakashima, A highly efficient and durable hybrid bifunctional catalyst of polymer-wrapped pristine multi-wall carbon nanotubes and nico2o4 for rechargeable zinc-air batteries, in *ECS Meeting Abstracts*, number 1, pp. 55–55. The Electrochemical Society, 2016.
7. J. Fu, D.U. Lee, F.M. Hassan, L. Yang, Z. Bai, M.G. Park, and Z. Chen, *Advanced Materials*, Vol. 27, p. 5623, 2015.
8. J. Fu, D.U. Lee, F.M. Hassan, L. Yang, Z. Bai, M.G. Park, and Z. Chen, *Advanced Materials*, Vol. 27, p. 5617, 2015.
9. A. Guerfi, J. Trottier, C. Gagnon, F. Barray, and K. Zaghib, *Journal of Power Sources*, Vol. 335, p. 131 , 2016.

10. V. Casasanta, Rechargeable organosodium polymer battery, US Patent 9 350 012, assigned to Empire Technology Development, LLC (Wilmington, DE), May 24, 2016.
11. H.J. Chang, X. Lu, J.F. Bonnett, N.L. Canfield, S. Son, Y.-C. Park, K. Jung, V.L. Sprenkle, and G. Li, *Journal of Power Sources*, Vol. 348, p. 150, 2017.
12. J. Bitenc, K. Pirnat, T. Bancic, M. Gaberšcek, B. Genorio, A. Randon-Vitanova, and R. Dominko, *ChemSusChem*, Vol. 8, p. 4128, 2015.
13. Q.D. Truong, M. Kempaiah Devaraju, D.N. Nguyen, Y. Gambe, K. Nayuki, Y. Sasaki, P.D. Tran, and I. Honma, *Nano Letters*, Vol. 16, p. 5829, 2016.
14. Y. Shao, N.N. Rajput, J. Hu, M. Hu, T. Liu, Z. Wei, M. Gu, X. Deng, S. Xu, K.S. Han, J. Wang, Z. Nie, G. Li, K.R. Zavadil, J. Xiao, C. Wang, W.A. Henderson, J.-G. Zhang, Y. Wang, K.T. Mueller, K. Persson, and J. Liu, *Nano Energy*, Vol. 12, p. 750, 2015.
15. H.N.M. Sarangika, M.A.K.L. Dissanayake, G.K.R. Senadeera, R.R.D.V. Rathnayake, and H.M.J.C. Pitawala, *Ionics*, October 2016.
16. J.-H. Baik, D.-G. Kim, J. Shim, J.H. Lee, Y.-S. Choi, and J.-C. Lee, *Polymer*, Vol. 99, p. 704, 2016.
17. B. Pan, J. Huang, Z. Feng, L. Zeng, M. He, L. Zhang, J.T. Vaughey, M.J. Bedzyk, P. Fenter, Z. Zhang, et al., *Advanced Energy Materials*, Vol. 6, 2016.
18. W. Xu, A. Read, P.K. Koech, D. Hu, C. Wang, J. Xiao, A.B. Padmaperuma, G.L. Graff, J. Liu, and J.-G. Zhang, *Journal of Materials Chemistry*, Vol. 22, p. 4032, 2012.
19. J.-M. Tarascon and M. Armand, *Nature*, Vol. 414, p. 359, November 2001.
20. C. Jarvis, D. Teagle, W. Fraser, S. Gilmore, A. Bracken, D. Betteridge, N. Ward, W. Zhang, and R. Frerker, Rechargeable lithium polymer electrolyte battery for oilfield use, US Patent Application 20 160 087 271, assigned to Schlumberger Technology Corp., March 24, 2016.
21. Y.K. Jeong, T.-w. Kwon, I. Lee, T.-S. Kim, A. Coskun, and J.W. Choi, *Nano Letters*, Vol. 14, p. 864, 2014.
22. R. Kuruba, M.K. Datta, K. Damodaran, P.H. Jampani, B. Gattu, P.P. Patel, P.M. Shanthi, S. Damle, and P.N. Kumta, *Journal of Power Sources*, Vol. 298, p. 331, 2015.
23. K. Karuppasamy, T. Linda, S. Thanikaikarasan, S. Balakumar, T. Mahalingam, P.J. Sebastian, and X. Sahaya Shajan, *Journal of New Materials for Electrochemical Systems*, Vol. 16, p. 116, 2013.
24. K. Karuppasamy, C. Vijil Vani, R. Antony, S. Balakumar, and X. Sahaya Shajan, *Polymer Bulletin*, Vol. 70, p. 2531, September 2013.

25. H.-J. Kim, S.E. Lee, J. Lee, J.-Y. Jung, E.-S. Lee, J.-H. Choi, J.-H. Jung, M. Oh, S. Hyun, and D.-G. Choi, *Physica E: Low-dimensional Systems and Nanostructures*, Vol. 61, p. 204, 2014.
26. J. Huang, S.Y. Chiam, H.H. Tan, S. Wang, and W.K. Chim, *Chemistry of Materials*, Vol. 22, p. 4111, 2010.
27. Z. Huang, N. Geyer, P. Werner, J. de Boor, and U. Gösele, *Advanced Materials*, Vol. 23, p. 285, 2011.
28. X. Li, *Current Opinion in Solid State and Materials Science*, Vol. 16, p. 71, 2012.
29. B. Wang, T.J. Richardson, and G. Chen, *Journal of the Electrochemical Society*, Vol. 161, p. A1039, 2014.
30. M.G. Laramie, Y.V. Mikhaylik, J.A. Phipps, and V.G. Viner, Ceramic/polymer matrix for electrode protection in electrochemical cells, including rechargeable lithium batteries, US Patent Application 20 150 086 837, assigned to Sion Power Corporation, Tucson (AZ), March 26, 2015.
31. W. Huang, Z. Zhu, L. Wang, S. Wang, H. Li, Z. Tao, J. Shi, L. Guan, and J. Chen, *Angewandte Chemie International Edition*, Vol. 52, p. 9162, 2013.
32. J.-W. Lee, Rechargeable battery with an electrode assembly having a polymer region, US Patent 9 209 481, assigned to Samsung SDI Co., Ltd. (Yongin-Si, KR), December 8, 2015.
33. A.S. Gozdz, C.N. Schmutz, and P.C. Warren, Hybrid lithium-ion battery polymer matrix compositions, US Patent 5 571 634, assigned to Bell Communications Research, Inc. (Morristown, NJ), November 5, 1996.
34. J. Chai, Z. Liu, J. Zhang, J. Sun, Z. Tian, Y. Ji, K. Tang, X. Zhou, and G. Cui, *ACS Applied Materials & Interfaces*, Vol. 9, p. 17897, 2017.
35. M. Sun, H. Li, J. Wang, and G. Wang, *Carbon*, Vol. 94, p. 864, 2015.
36. C.L. Yang, H.Y. Liu, Q.L. Xia, Z.H. Li, Q.Z. Xiao, and G.T. Lei, *Arabian Journal for Science and Engineering*, Vol. 39, p. 6711, September 2014.
37. Q.C. Xiao, H.Y. Liu, Q.L. Xia, Q.Z. Xiao, G.T. Lei, and Z.H. Li, *Arabian Journal for Science and Engineering*, Vol. 39, p. 6651, September 2014.
38. U. Siemann, Solvent cast technology – a versatile tool for thin film production in *Scattering Methods and the Properties of Polymer Materials*, number 130 in Progress in Colloid and Polymer Science Book Series, pp. 1–14. Springer Berlin Heidelberg, Berlin, Heidelberg, 2005.
39. Wikipedia, Polymer solution casting — wikipedia, the free encyclopedia, 2017. [Online; accessed 5-August-2017].
40. T.F. Miller, Z.-G. Wang, G.W. Coates, and N.P. Balsara, *Accounts of Chemical Research*, Vol. 50, p. 590, 2017.
41. Q. Lu, J. Fang, J. Yang, G. Yan, S. Liu, and J. Wang, *Journal of Membrane Science*, Vol. 425, p. 105, 2013.
42. A. Takeuchi, H. Kato, and A. Inoue, *Intermetallics*, Vol. 18, p. 406 , 2010.

43. N.S. Mohamed, S.A.H. Ali, and A.K. Arof, *Indonesian Journal of Physics*, Vol. 15, p. 55, 2016.
44. H.T.T. Le, D.T. Ngo, R.S. Kalubarme, G. Cao, C.-N. Park, and C.-J. Park, *ACS Applied Materials & Interfaces*, Vol. 8, p. 20710, 2016.
45. S. Thayumanasundaram, V.S. Rangasamy, J.W. Seo, and J.-P. Locquet, *Electrochimica Acta*, Vol. 240, p. 371, 2017.
46. Y. Huai, J. Deng, R. Li, Z. Deng, and J. Suo, *Journal of Solid State Electrochemistry*, Vol. 17, p. 209, January 2013.
47. B. Liang, Q. Jiang, S. Tang, S. Li, and X. Chen, *Journal of Power Sources*, Vol. 307, p. 320, 2016.
48. H.B. Youcef, O. Garcia-Calvo, N. Lago, S. Devaraj, and M. Armand, *Electrochimica Acta*, Vol. 220, p. 587, 2016.
49. Z. Song, H. Zhan, and Y. Zhou, *Chemical Communications*, pp. 448–450, 2009.
50. Y. Zhang, Y. Huang, G. Yang, F. Bu, K. Li, I. Shakir, and Y. Xu, *ACS Applied Materials & Interfaces*, Vol. 9, p. 15549, 2017.
51. P. Liu, J.-J. Han, L.-F. Jiang, Z.-Y. Li, and J.-N. Cheng, *Applied Surface Science*, Vol. 400, p. 446, 2017.
52. Y.-W. Lin, T.-H. Wang, J.-P. Pan, C.-R. Yang, and J.-M. Hsu, Gel polymer electrolyte precursor and rechargeable cell comprising the same, US Patent 8 304 117, assigned to Industrial Technology Research Institute (Hsinchu, TW), November 6, 2012.
53. Q. Lu, J. Yang, W. Lu, J. Wang, and Y. Nuli, *Electrochimica Acta*, Vol. 152, p. 489, 2015.
54. K. Karuppasamy, P.A. Reddy, G. Srinivas, A. Tewari, R. Sharma, X.S. Shajan, and D. Gupta, *Journal of Membrane Science*, Vol. 514, p. 350 , 2016.
55. K. Karuppasamy, P.A. Reddy, G. Srinivas, R. Sharma, A. Tewari, G.H. Kumar, and D. Gupta, *Journal of Solid State Electrochemistry*, Vol. 21, p. 1145, April 2017.
56. K. Karuppasamy, D. Kim, Y.H. Kang, K. Prasanna, and H.W. Rhee, *Journal of Industrial and Engineering Chemistry*, Vol. 52, p. 224, 2017.
57. L. Balo, Shalu, H. Gupta, V.K. Singh, and R.K. Singh, *Electrochimica Acta*, Vol. 230, p. 123, 2017.
58. K. Karuppasamy, K. Prasanna, D. Kim, Y.H. Kang, and H.W. Rhee, *RSC Advances*, Vol. 7, p. 19211, 2017.
59. K.-N. Jung, J.-I. Lee, J.-H. Jung, K.-H. Shin, and J.-W. Lee, *Chemical Communications*, Vol. 50, p. 5458, 2014.
60. H. Cheng and S. Wang, *Journal of Materials Chemistry A*, Vol. 2, p. 13783, 2014.
61. A. Manthiram and Y. Fu, Conductive polymer-coated, shaped sulfur-nanocomposite cathodes for rechargeable lithium-sulfur batteries and

methods of making the same, US Patent Application 20 150 349 323, assigned to Board of Regents, The University of Texas System, December 3, 2015.
62. M.A. Zimmerman, R. Leising, A.B. Gavrilov, K. Smith, and A. Teoli, High capactity polymer cathode and high energy dmensity rechargeable cell comprising the cathode, US Patent Application 20 150 280 218, assigned to Ionic Materials, Inc., October 1, 2015.
63. W. Yang, W. Yang, J. Feng, Z. Ma, and G. Shao, *Electrochimica Acta*, Vol. 210, p. 71, 2016.
64. H.-Y. Lee, Y. Jung, and S. Kim, *Journal of Nanoscience and Nanotechnology*, Vol. 16, p. 2692, 2016.
65. R. Demir-Cakan, M. Morcrette, and J.-M. Tarascon, *Journal of Materials Chemistry A*, Vol. 3, p. 2869, 2015.
66. C. Li, Z. Guo, B. Yang, Y. Liu, Y. Wang, and Y. Xia, *Angewandte Chemie International Edition*, Vol. 56, p. 9126, 2017.
67. J. Yue, C. Suchomski, T. Brezesinski, and B.M. Smarsly, *ChemNanoMat*, Vol. 1, p. 415, 2015.
68. J. Guo, Q. Wang, J. Jin, C. Chen, and Z. Wen, *Journal of The Electrochemical Society*, Vol. 163, p. A654, 2016.
69. S. Oukassi, C. Giroud-Garampon, S. Poncet, and R. Salot, *Journal of The Electrochemical Society*, Vol. 164, p. A1785, 2017.

Index

Acronyms

Chemicals

Boldface numbers refer to Figures

General Index

Also of Interest

Check out these other books by the author published by Scrivener Publishing

Fuel Cells, Solar Panels, and Storage Devices
Materials and Methods
By Johannes Karl Fink
Published 2018. ISBN 978-1-119-48010-5

Chemicals and Methods for Conservation and Restoration
Paintings, Textiles, Fossils, Wood, Stones, Metals, and Glass
By Johannes Karl Fink
Published 2017. ISBN 978-1-119-41824-5

Additives for High Performance Applications
Chemistry and Applications
By Johannes Karl Fink
Published 2017. ISBN 978-1-119-36361-3

Metallized and Magnetic Polymers
By Johannes Karl Fink
Published 2016. ISBN: 9781119242321

Marine, Waterborne, and Water-Resistant Polymers
Chemistry and Applications
By Johannes Karl Fink
Published 2015. ISBN 978-1-119-018486-7

The Chemistry of Printing Inks and Their Electronics and Medical Applications
By Johannes Karl Fink
Published 2015. ISBN 978-1-119-04130-6

The Chemistry of Bio-based Polymers
By Johannes Karl Fink
Published 2014. ISBN 978-1-118-83725-2

Polymeric Sensors and Actuators
By Johannes Karl Fink
Published 2012. ISBN 978-1-118-41408-8

Handbook of Engineering and Specialty Thermoplastics
Part 1: Polyolefins and Styrenics
By Johannes Karl Fink
Published 2010. ISBN 978-0-470-62483-5

Handbook of Engineering and Specialty Thermoplastics
Part 2: Water Soluble Polymers
By Johannes Karl Fink
Published 2011. ISBN 978-1-118-06275-3

A Concise Introduction to Additives for Thermoplastic Polymers
by Johannes Karl Fink.
Published 2010. ISBN 978-0-470-60955-2

Lightning Source UK Ltd.
Milton Keynes UK
UKHW01n1355231018
331048UK00003B/86/P

9 781119 480105